Psychotherapy for Pregnancy Loss

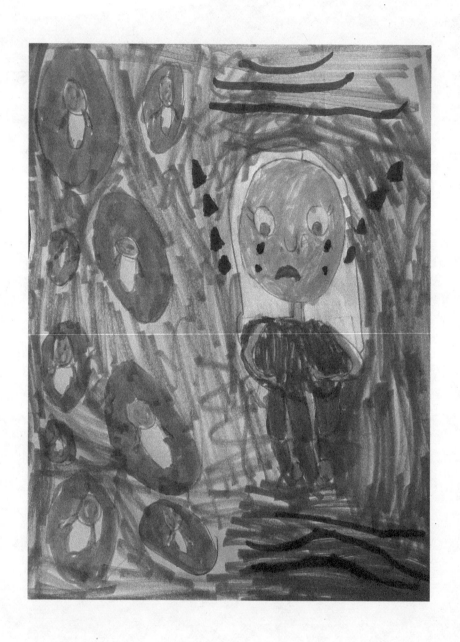

Psychotherapy
for Pregnancy Loss

*Applying Relationship Science
to Clinical Practice*

RAYNA D. MARKIN

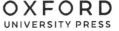

OXFORD
UNIVERSITY PRESS

Oxford University Press is a department of the University of Oxford. It furthers
the University's objective of excellence in research, scholarship, and education
by publishing worldwide. Oxford is a registered trade mark of Oxford University
Press in the UK and certain other countries.

Published in the United States of America by Oxford University Press
198 Madison Avenue, New York, NY 10016, United States of America.

Library of Congress Cataloging-in-Publication Data
Names: Markin, Rayna D., author.
Title: Psychotherapy for pregnancy loss : applying relationship science to clinical practice /
Rayna D. Markin
Description: New York, NY : Oxford University Press, [2024] |
Includes bibliographical references and index.
Identifiers: LCCN 2023032655 (print) | LCCN 2023032656 (ebook) |
ISBN 9780197693353 (pb) | ISBN 9780197693377 (epub) | ISBN 9780197693384 (ebook)
Subjects: LCSH: Grief therapy. | Miscarriage—Psychological aspects. |
Infertility—Psychological aspects. | Parental grief. | Loss (Psychology) | Psychotherapy.
Classification: LCC RC455.4.L67 M367 2024 (print) | LCC RC455.4.L67 (ebook) |
DDC 618.3/920651—dc23/eng/20230921
LC record available at https://lccn.loc.gov/2023032655
LC ebook record available at https://lccn.loc.gov/2023032656

DOI: 10.1093/oso/9780197693353.001.0001

Printed by Marquis Book Printing, Canada

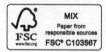

CONTENTS

ACKNOWLEDGMENTS

I would like to thank Drs. David Diamond, Martha Diamond, Janet Jaffe, and Irving Leon, pioneers in the field of reproductive trauma who paved the way for me to do this work that gives me such meaning and purpose. I thank Dr. David Diamond for his constant mentorship and support throughout the years and for his invaluable feedback on earlier versions of this book. Thank you, Sharon Covington, for your wisdom, guidance, and support in the area of infertility counseling; I have learned so much from you.

As a graduate student, I first read John Norcross's *Psychotherapy Relationships That Work* (Norcross, 2002) and it opened up a door for me that I did not even know was closed and inspired me to better understand how relationships can both harm and heal us in and outside of psychotherapy. Thank you, Drs. John Norcross, Michael Lambert, Bruce Wampold, and many others, in the field of relationship research, who made this possible. Thank you to my mentors throughout the years including, Charlie Gelso, Dennis Kivlighan, and Cheri Marmarosh.

A huge thank you to the very busy friends and colleagues who took time to read earlier versions of this book and offer their insights and feedback, including Drs. David Diamond, Catherine Eubanks, Kevin McCarthy, Janet Jaffe, and Sigal Zilcha-Mano. Thank you to all of my students throughout the years who have bravely listened to and learned from my clinical examples of immense reproductive trauma and loss with empathy and care. Thank you to my students, collaborators, and colleagues, especially Dr. Kevin McCarthy, for embarking on this journey with me. And, of course, a huge thank you to Sarah Harrington and the entire OUP team for giving me this opportunity and for your support of this project.

Thank you to all my patients throughout the years for teaching me about grief and loss, but also about a parent's enduring love. Thank you for trusting me with your stories, with your hopes and dreams that never got a chance to be realized, and with your memories of the babies that you never got a chance to meet.

Thank you to my family and teammates, Eric, Lily, Scarlett, and Justin, for your support, your love, and your understanding, especially when Mommy would disappear on weekends to write her book. Thank you for believing in me and for inspiring me.

Introduction

The guiding initiative behind this book was to take the most current research in the field on the therapy relationship and apply it to a specific clinical context, that of psychotherapy for pregnancy loss. This notion was born from over 60 years of research on the association between the therapy relationship and treatment outcome (Norcross & Lambert, 2019) and the author's clinical experiences conducting weekly outpatient psychotherapy with both individuals and couples struggling to come to terms with the loss of a pregnancy or unborn baby, during which a supportive and understanding relationship is often all one truly has to offer a grieving parent. Consistent with this, this book maps out an approach to psychotherapy for pregnancy loss wherein it is not the therapist's theoretical orientation or specific techniques per se that are believed to predict treatment outcome, but rather a focus on the relationship and the functions (e.g., affect regulation, self-esteem maintenance, empathy, support) it provides grieving parents.

Two overarching goals were kept in mind throughout the writing of this book. The first goal was to take what are often more general and abstract research findings on how the therapist–client relationship predicts the process and outcome of therapy and talk about them in more specific *how*, *what*, and *why* terms within a particular clinical context. The therapy relationship is broadly defined as "the feelings and attitudes that therapist and client have toward one another, and the manner in which these are expressed" (Gelso & Carter, 1985, p. 159). The therapy relationship can be thought of as a higher-order construct that consists of multiple relationship subcomponents to which therapists and clients both contribute (Gelso & Carter, 1985). While studies generally find that higher ratings of these various relationship components during the process of therapy predict better outcomes at termination (Norcross & Lambert, 2019), these findings, though important, leave practicing clinicians with many unanswered questions. For instance, *how* exactly do therapists (and clients) contribute to the cultivation and maintenance of various relationship components, and *what* does this process look like with certain clients? Moreover, *why* or *how* do these relationship components contribute to outcome (and which outcomes) within a particular therapeutic context, such as therapy for pregnancy loss?

Psychotherapy for Pregnancy Loss. Rayna D. Markin, Oxford University Press. © Oxford University Press 2024.
DOI: 10.1093/oso/9780197693353.003.0001

The pages ahead begin to address these important questions through providing detailed relational guidance to therapists on *how* to cultivate and maintain multiple facets or components of the therapist–client relationship that have been empirically linked to treatment outcome (hence the term *evidence-based relationships* [Norcross & Lambert, 2019]) within therapy for pregnancy loss. More specifically, the evidence-based therapy relationship components that are covered in this book include alliance in individual and couples therapy, empathy, emotional expression, countertransference, alliance ruptures, attachment, and, to a lesser extent, self-disclosure and immediacy, client feedback, and positive regard. Rather than taking a one-size-fits-all approach, the clinical guidance offered in this book on how to apply relationship research to psychotherapy for pregnancy loss considers the unique and complex psychological experience of such losses. Detailed clinical examples illustrate *what* the process of building and maintaining the relationship may look like during the course of treatment with this client population. Moreover, specific guidance is offered on *how* to utilize the therapy relationship to promote better treatment outcomes, in ways that are specifically tied to *why* the relationship is believed to help clients who have suffered a pregnancy loss "get better." In essence, while research strongly suggests that the relationship is related to outcome across theoretical orientations and treatment modalities (Norcross & Lambert, 2019), less is known about how the cultivation, maintenance, and utilization of the relationship may differ depending on client presenting problem and the psychological sequelae that typically follow particular presenting problems like pregnancy loss. In general, the nuances pertaining to *how* therapists can facilitate and utilize the relationship in treatment, *what* challenges lie in the way of building and maintaining it, and *why* it relates to outcome and what kinds of outcomes may differ depending on the specific clinical issue or presenting problem at hand in subtle yet meaningful ways.

The second overarching goal of this book was to begin to fill in what is an unfortunately large gap in the literature on psychotherapy for pregnancy loss, particularly therapy approaches that consider the complex psychological sequelae that typically follow such a loss. Existing interventions for pregnancy loss are generally brief and target immediate symptom relief following a loss (e.g., Kersting et al., 2013; Nakano et al., 2013). In general, studies on the efficacy of such relatively brief interventions for pregnancy loss, and for the related area of infertility, suffer from severe methodological flaws and yield inconclusive findings (see Diamond & Diamond, 2016; Verkuijlen et al., 2016, for reviews). Although perhaps effective for reducing distress in the short term (see Kersting & Wagner, 2012, for a review), such treatments may overlook other important therapeutic goals like the processing of trauma and loss and the restoration of self-esteem (Markin & McCarthy, 2020). During pregnancies after loss, for example, about 21 percent of women will meet post-traumatic stress disorder (PTSD) criteria (Turton et al., 2001), while often also struggling with acute feelings of shame and inadequacy (Jaffe & Diamond, 2011).

Following this, psychotherapy approaches that go beyond crisis intervention and immediate symptom relief and target underlying and unresolved feelings of trauma and loss, while helping to rebuild the client's damaged sense of self, are sorely needed for this client population (Markin & McCarthy, 2020). The author argues that relationally focused psychotherapies are better able to target these important, yet often overlooked, treatment goals, through providing a safe, supportive, and affect-regulating therapy relationship in which unresolved feelings of trauma and loss can be safely approached and processed, and in which the therapist's empathic support and attunement can help to restore the client's self-esteem.

DEFINITIONS

The following definitions are of common terms used throughout this book. Definitions of these terms often vary from study to study and from author to author, and thus it is important to clarify from the onset how these terms are used here.

Miscarriage is defined as the loss of a pregnancy up to 20 to 24 weeks gestation (Diamond & Diamond, 2016).

Stillbirth, fetal death, and *fetal demise* are terms that refer to losses that occur after 21 to 24 weeks gestation (Diamond & Diamond, 2016).

Perinatal loss is a more general term used to refer to losses during pregnancy and up to approximately 1 month after birth (Diamond & Diamond, 2016).

Pregnancy termination due to fetal anomaly (PTFA) is defined as terminating the pregnancy of a much-wanted but unhealthy fetus/baby, or one that has been diagnosed with a genetic anomaly, which in many cases may be lethal (Leon, 2017).

Pregnancy loss is a generic term used to refer to various types of losses, including those just listed above, all of which are believed to have much in common psychologically (Diamond & Diamond, 2016). It is often used as an umbrella term for the death of a conceptus, fetus, or neonate before the 21st day of life. This book focuses on pregnancy loss, which encompasses a wide range of types of losses that, while they all may differ in a number of important ways, still share core psychological components.

Reproductive loss refers to experiences of miscarriage, stillbirth, perinatal and infant death, and maternal death, and, more broadly, to the loss of "normal" reproductive experiences, such as those associated with infertility and assisted reproduction (Earle et al., 2008). Reproductive loss is often referred to in this book, as it so often encompasses pregnancy loss (for example, couples experiencing infertility often simultaneously experience recurrent pregnancy loss).

Reproductive trauma is a term introduced by Jaffe et al. (2005) and Jaffe and Diamond (2011) to refer to the traumatic nature of the losses just defined, along with infertility, premature or medically compromised births, and a variety of other adverse reproductive events that are believed to have similar psychological dynamics. Jaffe et al. (2005) argue that these adverse reproductive events are consistent with the more general definition of trauma as any event or feeling that (a) goes beyond the range of usual human experience and is overwhelming either physically, emotionally, or both; (b) typically involves a threat to a person's physical integrity or that of a loved one; and (c) may be the result of a single devastating event or a series of events that gradually build up and overwhelm a person. Similar to what clients may report after other kinds of traumatic events, following an adverse reproductive event like pregnancy loss, clients frequently report (a) re-experiencing the event in flashbacks (e.g., intrusive and disturbing images of a prior miscarriage when a woman gets her period after miscarriage); (b) experiencing a general hypersensitivity and irritability, which may alternate with a sense of numbness and withdrawal (e.g., during pregnancy after loss, a woman may be hypersensitive to signs of another possible loss, and, at the same time, distance herself from the fetus as a protective mechanism against the emotional pain of another loss); and (c) feeling anxious or depressed, or having difficulty concentrating (e.g., feeling hopeless that one will never realize one's dream of becoming a parent and anxious that despite all one's efforts to become pregnant "it" will never work). In essence, infertility and pregnancy loss are believed to be experienced as traumatic events because they attack both the physical and psychological sense of self, impacting relationships with others and with the self (Diamond & Diamond, 2016; Jaffe et al., 2005).

Reproductive story is a term introduced by Jaffe et al. (2005) to refer to an individual's partly conscious and partly unconscious narrative of how one's reproductive life will unfold. This set of expectations, plans, and fantasies makes up an individual's sense of parental identity. Disruptions in this aspect of identity, and the narrative underlying it, represent reproductive traumas that need to be grieved (Diamond & Diamond, 2016).

Dilation and curettage (D&C) refers to a procedure in which the cervix is dilated and a surgical tool is inserted to remove uterine contents. This procedure is often required after a pregnancy loss to remove fetal and uterine tissue that is not expelled naturally (Diamond & Diamond, 2016).

Dilation and evacuation (D&E) is a procedure that can be used after 12 weeks of pregnancy. The cervix is opened and the contents of the uterus are removed using instruments and a suction device (American College of Obstetricians and Gynecologists, 2022).

Assisted reproductive technology (ART) is a generic term referring to a wide range of medical interventions designed to achieve conception and pregnancy, including intrauterine insemination (IUI), in vitro fertilization (IVF), and other procedures. Many ART treatments involve invasive medical procedures and/or hormonal stimulation that significantly impacts mood and affect (Diamond & Diamond, 2016).

IVF is a sequence of medical interventions involving hormonal stimulation of ovaries, surgical removal of eggs, fertilization by sperm in the laboratory, and transfer of embryos to the mother's (or carrier's) uterus (Diamond & Diamond, 2016). IVF may involve the genetic testing of embryos.

Preimplantation genetic testing (PGT) is a technique used to identify chromosomal genetic abnormalities in embryos created through in vitro fertilization (IVF) *before* pregnancy. Preimplantation genetic testing is an umbrella term that refers to the assessment of embryos prior to implantation or pregnancy (Dayal et al., 2022).

Infertility is defined as not being able to get pregnant after 1 year (or longer) of unprotected sex (Practice Committee of the American Society for Reproductive Medicine, 2020).

Perinatal is the period of time during pregnancy and up to a year after birth.

A *fetus* is defined as an unborn baby more than 8 weeks after conception. In this book, the terms "fetus" and "unborn baby" are used interchangeably. When the author is referring to a baby after birth, this is so denoted. Some pregnancy loss clients prefer the term "fetus" or "it," while others prefer the terms "baby" or "unborn baby." This may have to do with the degree of attachment that the parent/client formed to the fetus/baby at the time of the loss, and, relatedly, the degree of personhood the parent assigned "it."

Perinatal bereavement is the experience of parents that begins immediately following the loss of an infant through death by miscarriage, stillbirth, neonatal loss, or elective termination for fetal anomalies. It is characterized by a complex emotional response, most commonly manifested as grief, but often expressed differently between parents/clients, depending on a number of factors including gender, culture, support, number of living children, personality, and attachment style (Fenstermacher & Hupcey, 2013).

Perinatal grief, or grief following the loss of a conceptus, fetus, or neonate, is a normal reaction to the loss of an attachment object (i.e., the fetus/baby). Research supports the presence of three subdomains of perinatal grief: (1) *active grief*, including feelings of sadness, missing the baby, and crying for the baby, (2) *difficulty coping*, which suggests difficulty in dealing with normal activities and with other people, and (3) *despair*, indicating withdrawal and depression and feelings of worthlessness and hopelessness (Toedter et al., 1988).

Bereaved (or grieving) parents is a term used in this book to denote parents mourning a pregnancy loss. Parenthood is believed to start long before the physical birth of a baby and even before conception, as parents fantasize about a future relationship to an imagined baby (Diamond & Diamond, 2016). Consistent with this, findings suggest that most mothers attach to the fetus and develop a subjective internal sense, or mental representation, of the fetus relatively early on in the pregnancy (Ammaniti, 1991; see Brandon et al., 2009, for a review). Thus, the term "parent" in this book does not necessarily denote that the person/client has living children.

INTENDED AUDIENCES

This book is for anyone who is passionate about understanding the psychological experience of pregnancy loss and how to help grieving parents to heal from the trauma and profound grief that often ensues. However, this book was written primarily for mental health practitioners conducting psychotherapy with clients specifically seeking treatment for perinatal grief and reproductive trauma, and for clients who experience a pregnancy loss during the course of psycho-therapy. Pregnancy loss is common and can occur unexpectedly, so even gener-alist practitioners need to be prepared to suddenly move in this direction during an ongoing treatment. Unfortunately, while there are numerous books written about the experience of infertility (which may include pregnancy loss) that are intended for fertility patients (e.g., Flemons, 2018; Jaffe et al., 2005), as well as sev-eral books written for infertility counselors conducting fertility counseling (which focuses on supporting and coaching intended parents through reproductive med-ical procedures and options) (e.g., Covington, 2015), there is a lack of resources for practicing clinicians conducting psychotherapy with clients who have suffered one or more pregnancy losses. This book aims to fill in this gap in the literature by offering evidence-based and practical relational guidance to psychotherapists working with both individuals and couples who have suffered a pregnancy loss, sometimes within the context of infertility.

This book is *not* intended for clinicians of any one theoretical orientation, but for clinicians of all theoretical orientations who have in common a focus on the therapist–client relationship (Markin, 2014). Consistent with this, the purpose of this book is not to offer an entirely distinct and new treatment approach, but rather to offer relational guidance, grounded in science, that can be integrated into a clinician's current way of practicing, regardless of theoretical orientation. After all, the therapy relationship is important to the process and outcome of treatment regardless of therapist theoretical orientation (Norcross & Lambert, 2019). More generally, relationally oriented clinicians may be able to extrapolate the relational guidance offered in these pages to therapies with other client populations and presenting problems, particularly other types of traumatic losses. In this sense, this book is intended for psychotherapists who want a better understanding of *how* to apply research on the therapist–client relationship to their clinical practice.

In addition, it is the author's hope that this book will be used in counseling and clinical training programs and related fields to train future psychotherapists to provide competent treatment to grieving parents. Overall, there is a startling lack of attention in clinical training programs on the psychosocial consequences of pregnancy loss and on how to treat bereaved parents who are struggling with the common effects of this kind of unique loss, such as chronic grief, post-traumatic stress symptoms, and a damaged sense of self (Diamond & Diamond, 2016). For the psychotherapy researcher, hopefully reading this book stimulates future studies on the process and outcome of therapy for pregnancy loss, and, in particular, the role of the therapist–client relationship. Next, although fertility counseling has different aims and purposes than psychotherapy per se, infertility counselors also provide relationships in which clients mourn the loss of their unborn babies, re-productive capacities, and hopes and dreams for the future. Fertility counselors can use the relational guidance and associated interventions offered in this book to support their clients through what is most often a stressful, even traumatic, fer-tility journey, which often includes recurrent pregnancy loss.

Lastly, the empathic support of medical professionals often plays a signif-icant role in how parents adjust after loss. Many studies have documented the importance of empathic support by medical health providers for the resolution of grief and improved self-worth following various kinds of perinatal losses (Geerinck-Vercammen & Kanhai, 2003; Gold, 2007; Lafarge et al., 2014; McCoyd, 2009). The relational guidance offered here, though primarily intended for therapists, may help medical providers to meet their patients' need for empathic support and validation during what is a vulnerable time in the immediate aftermath of a pregnancy loss.

TRAJECTORY OF THE BOOK

This book is composed of two introductory chapters, a conclusion chapter, and seven clinical chapters in between. Five of the seven clinical chapters focus on different relationship elements primarily provided by the psychotherapist, or what have been termed *evidence-based therapist contributions* to the therapeutic relationship (Norcross & Lambert, 2019), including alliance (Chapter 3), empathy (Chapter 4), emotional expression (Chapter 5), alliance rupture and repair (Chapter 6), and countertransference management (Chapter 7). Although these relationship components or elements are often treated as distinct in research and on a conceptual level, in practice, separating these various facets of the relationship into discrete parts is most likely akin to "reductionist fiction" (Elliot et al., 2018, p. 18). Instead, as Elliott et al. (2018) argue, it is probably more accurate to view each relationship element in context of the other relational elements, which are all part of a higher-order therapeutic relationship. Given this, the order of chapters in this book is not intended to imply that a certain relationship element should be focused on in psychotherapy before another, as all these elements are constantly occurring in tandem. Rather, the author begins with a chapter on alliance because of its pivotal and historical role in relationship research, followed by a chapter on empathy because of its clinical importance to pregnancy loss clients. For these clients, who frequently feel a lack of empathy from friends, family, medical professionals, and even society at large, empathy is often the anchor in psychotherapy without which the process tends to go afloat. A chapter on emotional expression follows that on empathy because of the close connection between the therapist's capacity to understand the client on a cognitive and affective level and to help the client to identify, express, and regulate important affects. Chapters on alliance rupture and repair episodes and countertransference management then proceed because of the conceptual link between rupture moments and unmanaged therapist countertransference.

The remaining two clinical chapters in this book focus on effective methods of adapting or tailoring the relationship and treatment to the individual client. Methods for adapting treatment to the individual client's transdiagnostic characteristics have been termed *evidence-based therapist responsiveness or adaptations* (Norcross & Wampold, 2019). While there are numerous client transdiagnostic characteristics to which therapists should or can adapt their treatment approach, this book focuses on how therapists should adapt their approach depending on client attachment style. The first chapter on attachment reviews attachment theory and research and how it relates to a client's experience of pregnancy loss (particularly recurrent pregnancy loss within the context of infertility) and to the process and outcome of therapy, and associated treatment implications. The second attachment chapter offers specific relational guidance on how the therapist should adapt to the client's attachment style in therapy for pregnancy loss based on attachment theory and research. More generally, an attachment perspective to the therapy process runs throughout all the clinical chapters and provides a way of understanding the experience of pregnancy loss, as well as how and why the therapy relationship is believed to be healing in this therapeutic context (see Chapter 2 for a full discussion).

ORGANIZATION OF CHAPTERS

All seven of the clinical chapters (Chapters 3 through 9) follow a similar outline: (a) brief introduction, (b) case vignette of a client seeking therapy for pregnancy loss that demonstrates the relationship component under discussion "in action," (c) summary of the most recent research (focusing on current meta-analyses in the field) on how a particular relationship component predicts the process and outcome of therapy, (d) clinical application of the research, including relational guidance on how to facilitate and maintain the relationship component, and how to utilize it to reach important goals or outcomes, in therapy for pregnancy loss, (e) therapist–client session dialogue demonstrating the suggested relational guidance and associated interventions (with the exception of the countertransference management chapter, which provides a detailed case vignette to demonstrate the relational guidance suggested), (f) common challenges to facilitating the relationship component in therapy for pregnancy loss, and (g) summary of clinical implications.

THE BACKGROUND: EVIDENCE-BASED RELATIONSHIPS AND RESPONSIVENESS

As Norcross and Lambert (2019) astutely observe, psychotherapy researchers and theoreticians alike have long been fascinated with two central questions pertaining to the therapist–client relationship: (1) what works in the psychotherapy relationship in general, and (2) what works in psychotherapy for specific clients. In 1999, a task force, established by the America Psychological Association (APA) Division of Psychotherapy, set out to answer these two all-important yet elusive questions based on current research at the time. Since then, that initial task force has resulted in three editions of the iconic book *Psychotherapy Relationships That Work* (Eds. Norcross, 2002; Norcross, 2011; Norcross & Lambert, 2019), multiple special journal issues based on the books, and hundreds of scholarly presentations and workshops (Norcross et al., 2018). Almost 20 years after the formation of the first task force, the third Interdivisional APA Task Force[1] on evidence-based relationships and responsiveness once again sought to identify what works in the therapy relationship and what works in therapy for particular clients based on updated meta-analyses that were later published in the third edition of *Psychotherapy Relationships That Work* (Norcross et al., 2018; Norcross & Lambert, 2019; Norcross & Wampold, 2019). Like its predecessors, this most recent edition published original meta-analyses on various relationship elements, including traditional features of the therapy relationship such as alliance, empathy, and positive regard, as well as what were termed "relational methods," such as alliance rupture and repair episodes, collecting client feedback, facilitating client emotional expression, and managing countertransference (Norcross & Lambert, 2019). In addition, a second volume, dedicated to therapist adaptations and responsiveness to individual client characteristics, such as client attachment style, was also included in the third edition (Norcross & Wampold, 2019).

The conclusions of the third Interdivisional Task Force are presented in Table 1.1, which summarizes the committee's findings regarding the degree to which current meta-analytic results provide evidence to suggest that a particular *relationship element* or *method of adaptation or responsiveness* predicts therapy outcome. The task force was careful to specify that these conclusions do not constitute practice or treatment standards; rather, they represent current scientific knowledge that should be understood and applied in the context of the clinical evidence available in each case (Norcross & Lambert, 2019). As seen in Table 1.1, the task force judged each relational element or method of adaptation as falling into one of four categories: (1) "demonstrably effective," (2) "probably effective," (3) "promising but insufficient research," or (4) "important but not yet investigated." These judgments were based upon the following criteria: (1) number of empirical studies included in the meta-analysis, (2) consistency of empirical results, (3) independence of supportive studies, (4) magnitude of association between the relationship element and outcome, (5) evidence for causal link between relationship element and outcome, and (6) the external validity of the research (Norcross & Lambert, 2019). Also denoted in Table 1.1 are those relationship elements or methods of adaptation that were specifically chosen for inclusion in this book. Facets of the relationship that were judged by the task force to have the most evidence for effectiveness or for predicting therapy outcome, as well as those deemed by the author and the clinical and theoretical literature to be the most relevant to psychotherapy for pregnancy loss, were ultimately chosen for inclusion in this book.

In most cases, an entire chapter (or two in the case of attachment style) is dedicated to each selected relationship component, apart from a few exceptions in

---

1. The Third Task Force was led by a 10-person steering committee, chaired by John Norcross. He and the author (Rayna D. Markin) were appointed as Division 29's representatives on the committee (Norcross et al., 2018; Norcross & Lambert, 2019).

Table 1.1. CONCLUSIONS OF THE THIRD INTERDIVISIONAL TASK FORCE

	Elements of the Relationship	Methods of Adapting
Demonstrably effective	Alliance in individual psychotherapy*	Culture (race/ethnicity)
	Alliance in child and adolescent psychotherapy	Religion/spirituality
	Alliances in couple and family therapy*	Patient preferences
	Collaboration	
	Goal consensus	
	Cohesion in group therapy	
	Empathy*	
	Positive regard and affirmation*	
	Collecting and delivering client feedback*	
Probably effective	Congruence/genuineness	Reactance level
	Real relationship	Stages of change Coping style
	Emotional expression*	
	Cultivating positive expectations	
	Promoting treatment credibility	
	Managing countertransference*	
	Repairing alliance ruptures*	
Promising but insufficient research	Self-disclosure and immediacy*	Attachment style*
Important but not yet investigated		Gender identity Sexual orientation

* Relationship component that is covered in this book.
Adapted from Norcross & Lambert (2019) and used with the permission of Oxford University Press and Dr. John Norcross.

which a relationship element is included more briefly in a related chapter. For example, self-disclosure and immediacy are included in the countertransference management chapter, positive regard in the empathy chapter, and collecting client feedback in the alliance chapter. The relationship elements not selected for inclusion in this book are not necessarily of any less importance or value. Rather, this initial book represents a reasonable starting place toward applying relationship research to psychotherapy for pregnancy loss. While the author chose to primarily focus on those relationship elements that constitute *evidence-based therapist contributions*, future work should apply research on therapist responsiveness to client transdiagnostic characteristics to therapy for pregnancy loss. In particular, examining how therapists should adapt to client culture in therapy for pregnancy loss is an important area of future study.

META-ANALYSIS: WHAT, WHY, AND HOW?

While a comprehensive understanding of meta-analysis is not needed for this book, because the chapters ahead focus heavily on the clinical application of research findings derived from recent meta-analyses in the field, it is important to first have a basic understanding of what meta-analysis is and how to interpret the results. Following this, this section answers three important questions: (1) what is a meta-analysis, (2) why conduct one, and (3) how do I interpret the results? To answer the first of these three questions, meta-analysis is a quantitative study design used to ascertain estimates of the magnitude and direction (positive or negative) of an association in the form of effect sizes by systematically assessing the results of previous studies. A meta-analysis is performed to assess the utility or relative effectiveness of an intervention. For instance, meta-analysis can help answer the question: To what extent and in which direction is some relationship element, such as client-perceived empathy, during the process of therapy, associated with therapy outcome? Importantly, a meta-analysis, ideally, is used to obtain a single summary estimate of an observed effect that is more precise than any individual study contributing to the pooled analysis. Continuing with the earlier example, a meta-analysis on the association between empathy and outcome yields a more precise estimate of the extent to which empathy and outcome are related than any of the individual studies that went into the meta-analysis. Because results typically vary from study to study, the results of a meta-analysis can improve precision of estimates of effect, settle controversies arising from apparently conflicting studies, and generate new hypotheses (Haidich, 2010; Norcross & Lambert, 2019).

The meta-analyses referred to in subsequent chapters of this book all examined the association between some relationship element during the process of therapy and therapy outcome. The goal of these meta-analyses was to estimate the magnitude of the association (and the direction) between a particular relationship element and outcome in the form of effect sizes, using a weighted r and/or its equivalent d or g. The Pearson r correlation is a parameter of effect size that summarizes the strength of the relationship between two continuous variables (McLeod, 2019). To aid in interpretation, in many cases, r values are converted into Cohen's d values. These meta-analyses included studies that were correlational in nature; that is, client ratings of some relationship element during the process of therapy and their association to outcome at termination (Norcross & Lambert, 2019). As exceptions, a few meta-analyses referred to in subsequent chapters compared groups; for example, one meta-analysis looked at the relationship between client feedback and outcome in a group of clients at risk for deterioration and all clients (Lambert et al., 2019). These meta-analyses report Cohen's d and Hedge's g, which are standardized differences between two group means divided by the (pooled) standard deviation. The resulting effect size is in standardized deviation units.

Regardless, the larger the magnitude of r or d, the higher the probability of client success in psychotherapy based on the relationship variable under examination

(Norcross & Lambert, 2019). By convention (Cohen, 1988), an r of .10 in the behavioral sciences is considered a small effect, .20 a medium effect, and .50 a large effect. By contrast, a d of .30 is considered a small effect, .50 a medium effect, and .80 a large effect. Across the meta-analyses conducted on various relationship components and therapy outcome in *Psychotherapy Relationships That Work* (Eds. Norcross & Lambert, 2019; Norcross & Wampold, 2019), researchers tended to find beneficial and helpful, yet small to medium-sized, effects. This is perhaps to be expected given the large number of factors contributing to client success and the complexity of psychotherapy (Norcross & Lambert, 2019). Table 1.2 presents a summary of meta-analytic associations between those relationship components that were chosen for inclusion in this book and psychotherapy outcome, as originally reported in Norcross and Lambert (2019) and Norcross and Wampold (2019), along with the third Interdivisional Task Force's conclusions regarding evidentiary strength (Norcross et al., 2018; Norcross & Lambert, 2019).

PUTTING THE TASK FORCE'S CONCLUSIONS AND RECOMMENDATIONS INTO ACTION

Based on its evaluation of the various relationship–outcome meta-analyses, the task force made a number of conclusions and recommendations in the areas of practice, training, and research (for a complete list of the task force's conclusions and recommendations see Norcross & Lambert, 2019). Perhaps one of the most important conclusions was that "the psychotherapy relationship makes substantial and consistent contributions to patient outcome independent of the specific type of psychological treatment" and "accounts for client improvement (or lack of improvement) as much as, and probably more, than the particular treatment method" (Norcross & Lambert, 2019, p. 631). Based on their conclusions, the task force went on to recommend that practitioners "make the creation and cultivation of the therapy relationship a primary aim of treatment," particularly for those relationship elements found to be demonstrably or probably effective (Norcross & Lambert, 2019, p. 633). Despite this "call to action," there still exists little guidance on how exactly to apply relationship research to the clinical context, especially when taking into consideration a specific client population like those affected by pregnancy loss. Accordingly, this book provides specific relational guidance on how to cultivate and maintain evidence-based relationships, and, moreover, on how to use the relationship to promote successful outcomes within the context of therapy for pregnancy loss. The task force also recommended that "practitioners assess relational behaviors (e.g., alliance, empathy, cohesion) vis-a-vis cut-off scores on popular clinical measures in ways that lead to more positive outcomes" (Norcross et al., 2018, p. 9). Accordingly, the appendix of this book provides a summary table of easy-to-administer and easy-to-score measures of the various relationship components focused on in this book that can be used in clinical practice. A reference is provided for each measure for practicing clinicians to refer to for further information.

Table 1.2. SUMMARY OF META-ANALYTIC ASSOCIATIONS BETWEEN RELATIONSHIP COMPONENTS AND PSYCHOTHERAPY OUTCOMES

Relationship Element	# of Studies (k)	# of Patients (N)	Effect Size (r)	Effect Size (d or g)	Consensus on Evidentiary Strength
Alliance in individual psychotherapy	306	30,000+	.28	.57	Demonstrably effective
Alliances in couple and family therapy	40	4,113	.30	.62	Demonstrably effective
Empathy	82	6, 138	.28	.58	Demonstrably effective
Positive regard and affirmation	64	3,528		.28	Demonstrably effective
Self-disclosure and immediacy	21	≈140	NA	NA	Promising but insufficient research
Emotional expression	42	925	.40	.85	Probably effective
Managing countertransference	9	392 therapists	.39	.84	Probably effective
Repairing alliance ruptures	11	1,318	.30	.62	Probably effective
Collecting and delivering client feedback	24	10,921		.14–.49[a]	Demonstrably effective
Attachment	32	3,158		.35[b]	Promising but insufficient research to judge

NA, not applicable; the chapter employed qualitative meta-analysis, which does not produce effect sizes.

[a] The effect sizes depended upon the comparison group and the feedback method; feedback proved more effective with clients at risk for deterioration and less effective for all clients.

[b] Represents correlation between pretreatment security attachment and psychotherapy outcome; more secure attachment/less insecurity predicted better treatment outcomes.

Adapted from Norcross & Lambert (2019) and used with the permission of Oxford University Press and Dr. John Norcross.

Next, Chapter 2 provides a deeper look into the psychological experience and consequences of pregnancy loss, and provides a conceptual rationale for why, given the unique psychosocial consequences of pregnancy loss, the relationship may be particularly important to therapy for this client population.

2

Understanding and Treating Pregnancy Loss

Rates, Risk Factors, Symptomatology, and Implications for the Therapeutic Relationship and Treatment

There is something very distinct about the pain a parent feels upon the loss of a pregnancy or unborn baby that is hard to put into verbal language, but as the clinician you can feel it the second a grieving mother walks into your office, shakingly sits down across from you in her chair, and looks at you as if she is drowning and you are the only lifeboat around. Maybe it's that you instinctively sense her fragility, or how the trauma of loss has shattered her to her very core. Maybe it's because you feel the desperate sting in her longing for the baby that died, or maybe you simply intuit that the woman standing before you is a raw shell-like version of the woman she used to be. Regardless of the exact reason, something feels both unfamiliar and raw the second a grieving mother or her partner steps into the therapy room. Because of this, psychotherapy for pregnancy loss grief requires clinicians to possess an in-depth understanding of the psychology of pregnancy loss and how to treat its effects. As such, in this chapter, common symptomatology associated with pregnancy loss is discussed. Complicated versus noncomplicated pregnancy loss grief reactions are examined and understood within an attachment framework. Prior interventions to treat symptoms associated with pregnancy loss are reviewed. It is argued that, unlike these prior interventions, future therapy approaches should focus on the relationship as a vehicle for processing feelings of trauma and loss and associated symptoms of depression and anxiety, as well as restoring self-esteem, after pregnancy loss.

RATES AND RISK FACTORS

Perinatal loss occurs in about 25 percent of all pregnancies and includes miscarriage rates of approximately 15 to 25 percent (Hutti et al., 2016; MacDorman et al.,

Psychotherapy for Pregnancy Loss. Rayna D. Markin, Oxford University Press. © Oxford University Press 2024.
DOI: 10.1093/oso/9780197693353.003.0002

2015; Sapra et al., 2016). Furthermore, in the United States, the rate of stillbirths is approximately 6.05/1,000 live births (MacDorman et al., 2015). A 2012 systematic review looked at the overall chance of pregnancy loss during the first and second trimesters of pregnancy and found it to be between 11 and 22 percent in weeks 5 through 20, although risk of loss decreased as gestational age increased. Further, the chance of pregnancy loss was found to vary from person to person depending on a variety of factors, including age and overall health (Ammon Avalos et al., 2012). Several other studies have found maternal age to be a significant predictor of miscarriage and stillbirth, which is important given recent trends for women to postpone childbearing (Ammon Avalos et al., 2012; Magnus et al., 2019; Nybo Andersen et al., 2000). These losses have been found to occur across all cultural and socioeconomic groups, although rates of miscarriage appear higher among Black women for pregnancies achieved spontaneously or through IVF, as compared to Caucasian women (Harb et al., 2014). Thus, pregnancy loss poses a major public health problem for women and their families (Hutti et al., 2016; Johnson et al., 2015; Macdorman et al., 2015; Sapra et al., 2016).

SYMPTOMATOLOGY ASSOCIATED WITH PREGNANCY LOSS

Although pregnancy loss is a relatively common event, clinical experience and research suggest that many women and their partners suffer long-lasting and devastating psychosocial consequences after loss, although reactions can greatly vary. Women may experience a wide range of normal or typical responses to pregnancy loss, including feelings of profound grief (Hutti et al., 2013). Yet, not every woman who experiences such a loss will feel intense grief (Hutti, 1992), and some may feel little or no grief, particularly if the process of prenatal attachment has yet to begin (Hutti, 1992; Hutti et al., 1998, 2013). Importantly, even if the loss is not experienced as a grief-inducing event, it may still be experienced as a traumatic, painful, and disruptive event in a woman's life (Adolfsson, 2011). Overall, studies suggest that 15 to 25 percent of affected women have enduring adjustment problems and may seek professional help to support them in the aftermath of loss (Hughes et al., 2002; Klier et al., 2000). Some have estimated that up to 30 percent of pregnancy losses are followed by significant emotional distress (Zeanah et al., 1995). Further, studies suggest that approximately 10 percent of the time women after loss experience diagnosable disorders, including acute stress disorder, PTSD, anxiety disorders, depressive disorders, or substance use disorders (Janssen et al., 1996; Sham et al., 2010). In fact, several studies have found a risk of substance misuse following pregnancy loss (Dingle et al., 2008; Grauerholz et al., 2021), perhaps as a way of coping with feelings of loss, depression, and/or comorbid PTSD. Substance misuse can lead to increasing feelings of shame for women following pregnancy loss, increasing their sense of isolation and discouraging them from seeking help. Despite all this, clinicians are often unfamiliar with the psychological dynamics or psychosocial consequences of pregnancy loss and may genuinely not know how to identify, understand, and treat the symptoms with which pregnancy loss clients often present to treatment (Diamond & Diamond, 2016). To begin to address this limitation, research on common symptomatology associated with pregnancy loss is discussed below.

Depression

While much of the research has focused on depression following pregnancy loss, as elaborated upon later, it is important to note from the onset that trauma and anxiety symptoms may be more prominent and lasting after such losses (Diamond & Diamond, 2016). One reason why studies have typically focused on depressive symptoms as a consequence of pregnancy loss may be that depression is, unfortunately, often confused with grief. The line between depression and complicated grief in particular is not always clear or consistent across studies. Even noncomplicated grief and depression can look similar on the surface; however, depression typically involves more significant and lasting impairment in functioning and is associated with decreases in self-esteem and increases in self-criticism, or negative feelings about the self (Diamond & Diamond, 2016). Further, while grief is an adaptive emotion that activates a process through which the bereaved can mourn and move on, depression is generally maladaptive and keeps the bereaved stuck in feelings of hopelessness and despair.

Despite what is often a blurry line between grief and depression, a large number of empirical and systematic reviews on mood disorders following pregnancy loss have been conducted (Brouquet, 1999; Frost & Condon, 1996; Klier et al., 2002; Lee & Slade, 1996; Slade, 1994; Stirtzinger & Robinson, 1989). Some of the studies included in these reviews assess depressive disorders that meet the full Diagnostic and Statistical Manual of Mental Disorders (DSM) criteria, while others assess subclinical levels of depressive symptomatology that do not necessarily meet the full criteria set forth in the DSM, but rather look at depressive symptoms as existing on a continuum. There is now fairly consistent agreement that subclinical levels of depression and even clinical-level depressive disorders follow pregnancy loss in a substantial percentage of cases (Diamond & Diamond, 2016). In studies where appropriate comparison groups are used, major depressive disorder or depressive disorder not otherwise specified appear to occur at higher rates among women following pregnancy loss as compared to general population controls (Beutel et al., 1995; Neugebauer et al., 1992), non-loss pregnant women (Neugebauer et al., 1992; Thapar & Thapar, 1992), and post–live birth mothers (Clarke & Williams, 1979).

In a recent meta-analysis of 29 studies from 17 different countries, Herbert et al. (2022) found that women who experienced perinatal loss ($n = 31,072$) were more likely to experience depression than women in a control group who did not experience loss ($n = 1,261,517$), regardless of whether depression was assessed as a categorical (presence or absence of depression) or dimensional variable (mean depression scores). When depression was assessed as a categorical variable, moderator analysis revealed that type of loss did not significantly impact the strength of the association between loss and depression, although recurrent loss had the largest effect on depression, followed by neonatal death, stillbirth, fetal terminations due to genetic anomalies, and grouped loss, which included studies that grouped different types of losses together. When depression was assessed as a continuous variable, type of loss did significantly moderate the relation between loss and depressive symptoms, with terminations due to fetal anomalies producing the largest effect, or the strongest relation between loss and depressive symptoms, followed by stillbirth, recurrent loss, and grouped loss (Herbert et al., 2022). One way of understanding these differing moderator results is that significant findings are just more likely when variables are assessed continuously rather than categorically. At the same time, assessing depression as a continuous variable allows researchers to capture individuals who are clearly affected by the loss, but do not fit within the narrower categorical definition of a depressive disorder. It is also important to consider the possibility that certain types of losses emerge as better predictors of depressive symptoms not because of the type of loss per se but because certain types of losses are more likely to be experienced as traumatic, and future studies should take this possibility into account. Lastly, rather than examining which type of loss is "worse" and has the strongest association with symptoms, future studies may want to consider using qualitative methodologies to better understand the subjective experiences of different types of losses, rather than trying to compare one against the other.

In contrast to Herbert et al. (2022), in a study that compared 137 miscarrying women to a comparison group of randomly selected pregnant women on rates of depressive disorder (according to International Classification of Diseases [ICD-10] criteria) and complicated grief, the relative risk of developing a depressive disorder after miscarriage was not significantly higher compared to pregnant women, after taking into account age and period of amenorrhea. However, almost half the women developed complicated grief after miscarriage, and of these a significant proportion also showed features of a depressive disorder, even though they did not meet the full ICD criteria (Kulathilaka et al., 2016). These findings point to the importance of assessing depression and complicated grief in the same study and looking at subclinical levels of depressive symptomatology.

The duration of depressive symptoms following pregnancy loss varies from study to study, and, unfortunately, the fact that depressive symptoms are not always differentiated from grief in the research makes it difficult to draw definitive conclusions. While some studies have suggested that depressive symptoms decrease substantially by 4 weeks post-miscarriage (e.g., Friedman & Garth, 1989), others have found that grief and sadness can persist for up to 14 years post-loss (e.g., Dyson & While 1998; see Wright, 2011, for a review). Further, feelings of depression often fluctuate and are nonlinear over time (Robinson et al., 1994). Because studies have yielded conflicting findings regarding the duration of depressive symptoms after loss, more research is needed on risk factors that predict chronic levels of post-loss depression. Initial research in this area suggests that the personal significance that a miscarriage has to a woman may mediate the relationship between certain demographic variables and depression (Swanson, 2000). For example, in one study, women who miscarried and remained involuntarily childless were found to have the highest risk for depression and poor life satisfaction compared to other groups of women, perhaps because the miscarriage, in the context of involuntary childlessness, represented a loss of opportunity for adult identity development and advancement (Schwerdtfeger & Shreffler, 2009). A deeper understanding of what the pregnancy and the loss means to a woman may help clinicians and researchers better predict her risk for severe and/ or long-term depressive symptoms and plan treatment accordingly (Diamond & Diamond, 2016).

PTSD

Many cases of pregnancy loss can be classified as traumatic events, for feelings of fear, helplessness, and horror are commonly reported (Engelhard et al., 2001; Walker & Davidson, 2001). Pregnancy loss can be both a psychologically and physically traumatic event for women, who are often surprised by the intensity of physical pain experienced (particularly with ectopic pregnancies, in which the embryo attaches outside of the uterus), and the amount of blood and other scary bodily sensations involved. Physical symptoms of pregnancy loss sometimes unfold gradually, over the course of hours or days, and are often accompanied by feelings of confusion and a loss of control. Women may feel scared and overwhelmed, and, in some cases, even fear that they are dying. Some may struggle with the horror of witnessing a dead fetus or infant. Feelings of distress are typically compounded when the woman undergoes certain surgical procedures that are often required in conjunction with miscarriage. These experiences can lead to classic post-traumatic–like symptoms such as shame and guilt, as well as a dissociative state in which women are simultaneously devastated and numb, merely going through the motions as if these events are occurring to someone else (Diamond & Diamond, 2016). Other classic post-traumatic–like symptoms and experiences commonly reported after pregnancy loss include re-experiencing, avoidance, and hyperarousal symptoms (Dyregrov, 1990; Engelhard, 2004; Lee & Slade, 1996; Walker & Davidson, 2001).

From this, Diamond and colleagues (Jaffe & Diamond, 2005) use the term *reproductive trauma* to describe the subjective experience of pregnancy loss, which, like other traumas, is often shocking and devastating and violates one's basic sense of safety. Framing pregnancy loss as a reproductive trauma helps clinicians understand that bereaved parents are forced to work through their grief while they are also processing their trauma; thus, treatment needs to address feelings of trauma and loss (Leon, 2015). In fact, studies find that PTSD correlates highly with grief, especially complicated grief, depression, and anxiety following pregnancy loss (Bennett et al., 2008; Dyregrov et al., 2003), though it is an independent construct (Bennett et al., 2008).

While the exact percentage of women who experience pregnancy loss as a traumatic event and may subsequently develop PTSD or another trauma-related disorder varies between studies, most studies find relatively high, even shocking, rates of trauma among affected women. In one study, 57 percent of women characterized their prenatal loss as a potentially traumatic event, with more than a third nominating the loss as their worst or second-worst traumatic exposure (Hamama et al., 2010). In another study of pregnant women who previously experienced stillbirth, 94 percent of the women characterized it as something so uncommon and horrible that it would be very distressing to almost anyone (Turton et al., 2001). It is unknown exactly how many of these women will go on to meet the DSM criteria for a trauma-related disorder, but several studies suggest that acute and post-traumatic stress disorders are common. For instance, Bowles et al. (2006) found that 28 percent of women met criteria for acute stress disorder soon after miscarriage, and 39 percent met criteria for PTSD at 1 month post-loss. Moreover, in their study, women who developed acute stress disorder were significantly more likely to exhibit subsequent PTSD. Similarly, Engelhard et al. (2003) found that 25 percent of the women in their sample met criteria for PTSD at 1 month post-loss, while much higher percentages met partial criteria for PTSD and were clearly feeling the effects of trauma. In a study that looked at rates of probable full, partial, and no PTSD for women following stillbirth, 60, 28, and 12 percent met the diagnostic criteria, respectively (Chung & Reed, 2017), suggesting that it is critical to look at the effects of trauma for women who fall outside the full DSM criteria. Specific to pregnancies after loss, about 21 percent of women pregnant after a miscarriage or stillbirth have been found to meet PTSD criteria (Fernández Ordóñez et al., 2018; Lamb, 2002; Turton et al., 2001).

Several systematic reviews and meta-analyses have looked at the relation between pregnancy loss and PTSD and other trauma-related disorders. In one systematic review that included 46 articles based on 31 different studies of PTSD in parents bereaved by losses occurring prior to, during, or up to 1 year after birth, the PTSD prevalence in mothers was found to differ widely across studies, with estimated rates at 0.6 to 39 percent. This review did not include studies on pregnancy terminations due to fetal anomalies and only included studies with more strict PTSD DSM requirements, which fails to capture women experiencing the effects of trauma but who fall outside the criteria set forth in the DSM. This review also looked at rates of PTSD in bereaved fathers, which has been less extensively studied, and found that PTSD levels were generally much lower than in mothers, with reported prevalence rates at 0 to 15.6 percent across studies. Lastly, PTSD symptoms were not found to differ much depending on whether the death occurred prior to, during, or following birth, nor was gestational age consistently associated with PTSD severity (Christiansen, 2017). Contrary to this review, a recent meta-analysis of 29 studies across 17 countries failed to find a significant relationship between perinatal loss and post-traumatic stress outcomes; however, this may have been due to the inclusion of relatively few heterogeneous studies (Herbert et al., 2022). These inconsistent findings in the literature point to the need for more research on when and for whom pregnancy loss is most likely to be experienced as traumatic and lead to post-traumatic stress outcomes. It has been argued that recent changes to the criteria for PTSD in the DSM-5 are responsible for a substantial reduction in prevalence rates of PTSD following perinatal loss, as compared to rates based on DSM-IV criteria (Kilpatrick et al., 2013). Consequently, future studies should examine the effects of trauma on women who fall outside the DSM-V diagnostic criteria. Future research should also include fathers and more non-Caucasian mothers, who are typically underrepresented in bereavement research. Black women in the United States are twice as likely as White women to suffer stillbirth or neonatal loss, and both Black and Hispanic mothers are more likely to suffer from PTSD than White mothers (Gold et al., 2015; Youngblut et al., 2013).

Lastly, specific traumatic aspects of pregnancy loss have been investigated in quantitative and qualitative studies to help us ultimately understand what aspects of the loss experience are most likely to predict post-traumatic stress reactions. Defrain et al. (1996) noted that both mothers and fathers reported flashbacks, nightmares, and feelings of going crazy. Suicidal thoughts were reported by 11.4 percent of the 172 mothers in their study and actual attempts by 1.8 percent. None of the 21 fathers in the study reported suicidal thoughts or attempts, although this may be due to small sample size. The authors emphasized the sense of losing control during the experience as a major contributor to the traumatic effects of pregnancy loss. In addition to perceived lack of control during the event, Engelhard et al. (2003) found that what they called peritraumatic dissociation, which involves dramatic changes in cognition and perception at the time of the trauma, was associated with both acute and chronic PTSD symptoms following pregnancy loss. They also reported that a sense of coherence, which is a trait like what others have called ego strength or reflective functioning (Fonagy et al., 1998), seems to provide some resilience against the traumatic effects of pregnancy loss, partly because women high in this trait were better able to mobilize social support (Engelhard et al., 2003). More generally, studies have found that perceived threat and intense acute emotional responses, such as peritraumatic dissociation, fear, helplessness, horror, anger, and numbing, have all been found to increase the risk of PTSD following pregnancy loss (Bennett et al., 2008; Engelhard, 2004; Engelhard et al., 2003a, 2003b; Séjourné et al., 2010). In essence, it has been suggested that extreme reactions to trauma at the time of the loss that are either overly responsive or hyperaroused, or, on the contrary, nonresponsive or dissociative may hinder future adaptation (Engelhard, 2004).

Anxiety Disorders

The anxiety symptoms frequently observed among women following pregnancy loss can be understood as a natural reaction to a traumatic event. Anxiety, or hyperarousal, has long been associated with trauma and trauma-related disorders, and, in fact, anxiety disorders and trauma-related disorders show high comorbidity

(Ginzburg et al., 2010). In their review, Diamond and Diamond (2016) unfortunately concluded that while a number of studies have looked at anxiety disorders and pregnancy loss specifically, problems with methodological quality preclude the ability to make any definitive conclusions regarding how many women meet the criteria for an anxiety disorder as a consequence of pregnancy loss. It is particularly important for future research to account for anxiety disorders that existed before pregnancy loss.

In one controlled study, Geller et al. (2001) examined the incidence of and relative risk for anxiety disorders (obsessive-compulsive disorder [OCD], panic disorder, and phobic disorders), as defined by the DSM-III, within 6 months following miscarriage. Using a cohort design, they tested whether women who miscarried were at increased risk for a first or recurrent episode of an anxiety disorder in the 6 months following loss. The miscarriage cohort consisted of 229 women attending a medical center for miscarriage, whereas the comparison group was a cohort of 230 women drawn from the community. Among miscarrying women, 3.5 percent experienced a recurrent episode of OCD, compared with 0.4 percent of community women. In fact, miscarrying women were eight times more likely to experience a recurrent episode of OCD as compared to the community cohort. A significant increase in OCD among miscarrying women was maintained even after comorbid cases of anxiety and depression were removed from the analysis. On the other hand, while the relative risk for non-comorbid panic disorder was substantial, it was not statistically significant, perhaps due to issues with statistical power. Similarly, there was no strong evidence for increased risk for phobic disorders or agoraphobia, combined or considered separately. In conclusion, in least in this cohort study, miscarriage emerged as a substantial risk factor for an initial and in particular a recurrent episode of OCD. It could be that the lack of control experienced by many women following miscarriage exacerbates pre-existing obsessive-compulsive tendencies. In general, the traumatic nature of miscarriage tends to engender obsessive and intrusive thoughts and images (flashbacks, nightmares) related to the events around the loss, as a person attempts to process the shock and horror of the event (Brier, 2004).

Separately, in a prospective study of 2,140 first-trimester women, women who went on to miscarry reported higher levels of somatic symptoms and anxiety up to 6 months after the loss as compared to non-miscarrying women. However, these two groups did not differ on anxiety 1 year after the loss (Janssen et al., 1996). In their review of the research on anxiety and pregnancy loss, Geller et al. (2004) concluded that anxiety symptoms seem to be consistently elevated until 4 months post-loss, while a subsequent review that looked at a smaller number of studies with greater methodological rigor concluded that anxiety symptoms seem to be elevated until approximately 6 months post-loss and are frequently accompanied by symptoms of OCD and PTSD (Brier, 2004). Lastly, in their meta-analysis, Herbert et al. (2022) found a small to moderate significant effect of perinatal loss on anxiety, when anxiety was assessed as a categorial (presence/absence) and continuous variable. When anxiety was assessed as a categorical variable, neonatal death showed the largest effect of loss on increased rates of anxiety, followed by fetal terminations due to genetic anomalies, stillbirths, and miscarriages, with the late-term loss group showing a larger effect than the early-term loss group. Similarly, moderator analysis also identified a significant effect of type of perinatal loss on continuous anxiety outcomes. A large effect was identified for fetal terminations due to genetic anomalies and a moderate effect for stillbirths, with a larger effect for late loss than early loss. These moderator findings refer to women in the aggregate and may not generalize to an individual woman's or parent's experience of loss in a clinical situation. A client's level of distress after loss is likely influenced by the unique meaning that the pregnancy and pregnancy loss held to that particular client.

Other studies have looked at anxiety specifically in the context of pregnancies after loss (see Diamond & Diamond, 2016, for a review). This research suggests that pregnancies after loss are most often characterized by *pregnancy-specific anxiety*, or the fear of yet another loss (Côte-Arsenault & Mahlangu, 1999). Evidence suggests that pregnancy-related anxiety is more strongly associated with maternal and child outcomes than general anxiety and depression and constitutes a distinct and multifaceted concept (Bayrampour et al., 2016). For instance, a recent meta-analysis of 19 studies representing 5,114 women with previous perinatal loss, 30,272 controls, 106 male partners with previous perinatal loss, and 91 control men, found a significant and large effect of previous perinatal loss on anxiety during subsequent pregnancies (Hunter et al., 2017). One reason anxiety during pregnancies after loss has garnered empirical and clinical attention is the concern that high levels of pregnancy-related anxiety interfere with prenatal attachment. Supporting this, Gaudet et al. (2010) found that pregnant women with prior perinatal loss reported significantly higher scores of grief, depression, and anxiety as compared to a control group, which predicted lower prenatal attachment. Thus, treating anxiety, and associated feelings of grief and loss, may benefit the mother and her future baby (Markin, 2018).

NORMAL VERSUS COMPLICATED PERINATAL GRIEF: DIAGNOSTIC FEATURES, RISK FACTORS, AND SOCIOCULTURAL CONSIDERATIONS

While symptoms of depression and anxiety are often most visible when clients who have suffered a pregnancy loss first enter treatment, these more overt symptoms typically represent an outward manifestation of underlying feelings of grief and loss that need to be processed and worked through. There is now substantial evidence that feelings of pregnancy loss grief can be intense and long-lasting (see Diamond & Diamond, 2016, for a review). For instance, in a study that looked specifically at bereaved parents after pregnancy loss, Lin and Lasker (1996) found that grief scores were initially relatively high and declined most steeply over the first year. In a 2-year follow-up, their evaluation of the grief process showed an interesting result: While 41 percent of participants showed a normal decline of grief scores, the remaining 59 percent showed different patterns of pervasive presence or delayed resolution of grief, suggesting that perinatal grief is often nonlinear and events such as subsequent pregnancies and anniversaries may evoke or re-evoke strong feelings of loss. Further, despite popular belief that a subsequent healthy pregnancy somehow eradicates a woman's grief over a prior loss, a large-scale and longitudinal study found no evidence that a subsequent healthy pregnancy resolves feelings of grief and related affective symptoms such as depression and anxiety that are associated with previous prenatal loss. Rather, previous prenatal loss appeared to be a persistent predictor of depressive and anxiety symptoms well after what would conventionally be defined as the postnatal period (Blackmore et al., 2011).

In terms of the quality of pregnancy loss grief, in their reviews, Covington (2006) and Brier (2008) describe the typical grief reaction as likely to include initial shock and confusion, a sense of unreality, interferences with sleep and appetite, loss of energy, somatic complaints, preoccupation with thoughts about the baby, and powerful experiences of sadness, anger, shame, and guilt. As with other forms of grief, bereaved parents are often preoccupied with thoughts about the lost person/baby and experience a painful sense of yearning for the deceased (Diamond & Diamond, 2016). Concerning the quality of perinatal grief for men, Obst et al. (2020) reviewed 46 articles that examined grief reactions of fathers. They concluded that men's grief experiences are highly varied and that current grief measures may not capture all of the complexities of grief for men. In particular, from qualitative studies identified in their review, these researchers concluded that in comparison to women, men often face different challenges when mourning a pregnancy loss, including expectations to support female partners and a lack of social recognition for their grief and subsequent needs (Obst et al., 2020).

Complicated Grief

While many women experience normal grief reactions in response to perinatal loss, about 25 to 30 percent may have significant, prolonged, highly intense, complicated grief reactions, which may negatively affect their psychological well-being (Heazell et al., 2016; Kersting et al., 2012). These highly intense grief reactions may be associated with high levels of anxiety (Heazell et al., 2016; Gausia et al., 2011; Woods-Giscombé et al., 2010), depression (Heazell et al., 2016; Gausia et al., 2011; Sutan et al., 2010), and post-traumatic stress (Armstrong et al., 2009; Heazell et al., 2016). Because of the potentially harmful consequences of severe or complicated grief, researchers have attempted to distinguish what characteristics constitute "normal" versus "pathological" or complicated grief in general and in cases of pregnancy loss specifically.

With other types of losses, complicated grief has been defined as the persistence of early symptoms to the point where they are chronic and maladaptive and cause significant functional impairment (Lobb et al., 2010). There are often persistent traumatic reactions with complicated grief like disbelief, anger, shock, and detachment. However, unlike with other types of losses, pregnancy loss is typically experienced as a traumatic loss, and thus the persistence of trauma-like symptoms may be a natural reaction to a stressful event rather than a sign of complicated grief (Diamond & Diamond, 2016). Other researchers have sought to distinguish normal versus complicated grief in the context of pregnancy loss by identifying the typical duration of perinatal grief. In practice, however, this approach may be problematic in that rigid categorical distinctions pertaining to what amount of time is "normal" versus "not normal" to grieve the loss of a pregnancy may not be particularly meaningful, as such losses are highly individualized and psychologically complex (Diamond & Diamond, 2016).

Not surprisingly, findings from various studies have yet to converge on a standard amount of time in which it is normal or typical for parents to grieve the loss of a pregnancy. Janssen et al. (1996), for example, found that parents often mourn for a year or more. In fact, as many as 20 percent of bereaved parents in their sample had not accepted the loss 2 years later. Other researchers, in one small qualitative study of mothers' experiences after stillbirth, found that sadness and grief may persist for 14 years post-loss (Dyson & While, 1998). Brier (2008), based on a review of multiple studies, concluded that, although intense reactions were very common in the early weeks following pregnancy loss, these usually declined substantially by 6 to 7 months post-loss, but substantial individual variation existed. It is important to recognize that intense and/or long-lasting grief is not necessarily pathological grief, but rather a reflection of a parent's healthy capacity to create deep and enduring attachment bonds to an unborn child. Because Western society often dismisses or minimizes perinatal grief instead of seeing it as the flip side of a healthy attachment, women and their partners typically lack the social support and societal validation needed to effectively grieve. This may result in unresolved or complicated grief reactions that are the result of a society that invalidates feelings of pregnancy loss grief and not of a parent's internal conflicts or deficits, as often assumed (Markin & Zilcha-Mano, 2018).

Risk Factors of Severe Grief

While what exactly constitutes complicated pregnancy loss grief is still being debated, identifying risk factors of more pervasive and severe grief reactions can help clinicians and researchers better target those grieving parents most in need. Risk factors for complicated grief after other types of losses (not necessarily pregnancy loss) include prior losses and traumas, pre-existing emotional disorders, attachment and separation problems in childhood, traumatic or violent circumstances of death, and lack of social support after loss (Lobb et al., 2010). The primary risk factor for complicated grief among those mourning a pregnancy loss specifically has been found to be poor psychological functioning prior to the loss, with lack of social support, other life stressors in pregnancy, poor physical health, and a history of other reproductive losses as additional risk factors (Covington, 2006). Brier's (2008) review similarly cited lack of social support and poor pre-loss psychological functioning as risk factors for significant anxiety and depression after pregnancy loss. In this review, several qualitative studies were found indicating that a strongly desired pregnancy, history of abortions or other losses, and lack of warning signs of the impending loss all predict complicated pregnancy loss grief. Lastly, in their review, Kersting and Wagner (2012) found that predictors of complicated grief after prenatal loss include lack of social support, pre-existing relationship difficulties, absence of surviving children, ambivalent attitudes toward the pregnancy, and perception of the pregnancy as real. The risk of complicated grief was found to be especially high after terminations due to fetal abnormalities.

There are several reasons why fetal terminations due to genetic abnormalities may pose a particular risk for complicated grief, as well as for numerous other psychological symptoms (Herbert et al., 2022). Parents typically approach ultrasound appointments as a rite of passage with a sense of hope and optimism and are often shocked and horrified when, instead, they learn of a fetal genetic anomaly (Leon, 2017). When the abnormality is lethal to the fetus, parents are often trapped between two horrific choices:(1) sign on the dotted line to terminate a much-wanted child, or (2) continue the pregnancy knowing the baby will likely die in utero and the mother will have to give birth to a stillborn baby. While there are no known studies comparing the psychological consequences of terminating versus continuing pregnancies in cases of a fetal lethal genetic anomaly, anecdotal evidence suggests that both options are horrific to grieving parents and that the "right" choice is likely highly individualized. When parents do elect to terminate, they often face social stigma, contributing to a lack of understanding and support, as well as feelings of shame, all of which can interfere with the grieving process (Leon, 2017). These parents are seen by some as having had an abortion (which, to these parents, typically feels like an incorrect label since they are terminating a wanted pregnancy and abortion is defined as the termination of an unwanted pregnancy), and by others as having had a miscarriage (which these parents often report "wishing" they had, so that they did not have to make "that" awful decision). In essence, the decision to terminate a much-wanted child, even if it is the "right" decision for that particular parent or couple, never feels like a "good" decision, or like a decision at all for that matter, to many parents (Leon, 2017).

From this, couples typically confront the decision to continue or terminate these pregnancies with a sense of confusion, ambivalence, and sometimes horror at being placed in this position in the first place (Lafarge et al., 2014; McCoyd, 2009b; Sandelowski & Barroso, 2005). One interesting longitudinal study of a nationally representative cohort ($n = 3,935$) examined psychological outcomes following termination of wanted versus unwanted pregnancies. They found that women who terminated wanted pregnancies experienced a 43 percent higher risk of affective problems compared to women terminating unwanted pregnancies, particularly risk of depression and suicidality, but risk of alcohol misuse was high for both the unwanted and wanted pregnancy groups (Sullins, 2019). Together, these studies clearly suggest that clinicians should pay careful attention to the psychological effects of terminating a wanted pregnancy due to the diagnosis of a genetic anomaly, as these bereaved parents are at particular risk. Clinicians should be aware that in States with restricted abortion access, women may not have the choice to terminate a wanted pregnancy due to a lethal genetic anaomly, potentially increasing the rate of stillbirth, which has been shown to predict maternal PTSD and complicated grief (Chung & Reed, 2017; Herbert et al., 2022). For instance, a recent report found that in 2019, fetal or infant death rates in the first week of life occurred at a 15% higher rate, on average, in states with abortion restrictions than in states with wider abortion access (Eugene Declercq et al., 2022).

In conclusion, complicated grief following pregnancy loss is important to study because it has been connected to the risk of serious depression, suicide, cardiac disease, and other health consequences (Covington, 2006; Prigerson et al., 1997). Further, while estimates of complicated grief among those who have experienced a pregnancy loss do not appear to significantly differ than for those who have experienced other types of losses (Brier, 2008; Janssen et al., 1996), it is important to keep in mind that given the sheer number of women who experience some type of pregnancy loss, even relatively low percentages translate into many affected women. Of the estimated 6 to 7 million pregnancy losses that occur each year in the United States, 10 to 20 percent are thought to lead to complicated grief reactions (Saraiya et al., 1999). This represents a large number of women, about 600,000 to 1.4 million, who are suffering complicated pregnancy loss grief reactions and may need clinical attention (Diamond & Diamond, 2016). Moving forward, defining complicated pregnancy loss grief should consider the unique aspects of perinatal grief.

REFLECTIONS ON THE UNIQUE ASPECTS
OF PERINATAL GRIEF

The grief a parent feels following the loss of a pregnancy is distinct from other kinds of grief experienced after other types of losses (Covington, 2005; Diamond & Diamond, 2016; Leon, 2015). For one, when a pregnancy or unborn baby is lost, the woman/mother typically feels as if a most precious and vulnerable part of herself has died, complicating the grieving process. In contrast, other kinds of losses are typically experienced as if the bereaved has lost a separate other in the world. It is important to understand that at the same time these women are grieving the loss of a baby, who is quite literally experienced as a part of the self, they are also grieving the loss of other important aspects of self and identity. For instance, a woman's gender identity and sense of self as a "real woman" may feel threatened (Diamond & Diamond, 2017; Leon, 2015). Reproduction is frequently seen as a skill and pregnancy loss as "proof" of the woman's profound personal failure and brokenness, resulting in the loss of self-esteem (Diamond & Diamond, 2017). Further, bereaved parents often feel as if their identity as a parent has been "stolen," as they watch peers have healthy babies and enter a new stage of adult identity development that they feel powerless to obtain (Diamond & Diamond, 2017). These bereaved parents are forced to go through a process of repairing the self at the same time they are grieving the loss of their baby (Leon, 2015).

Diamond and Diamond (2017) argue that grieving parents must first regain a sense of themselves as "whole and intact" before they can grieve "that which was lost" as separate from the self (p. 374).

Second, grieving parents are often forced to mourn at the same time they are struggling to make sense of and process the trauma associated with the loss (Diamond & Diamond, 2016; Leon, 2015). Pregnancy loss is often experienced as a traumatic event because it violates one's sense of trust in one's own body to function as it is "supposed to." The death of a baby defies a person's sense of fairness, of right and wrong, and of the world as a basically safe, just, and predictable place in which babies are not supposed to die and modern medicine is supposed to prevent these kinds of harrowing loses from occurring (Markin, 2017). The physical horror of losing a pregnancy and of associated medical procedures and events often leaves women feeling violated, ashamed, and out of control. As a result, feelings of powerlessness, devastation, and shock paint over a woman's experience of loss in a color unseen with other kinds of losses. For example, one woman was given a medication by her doctor to inject vaginally at home for "miscarriage management," which is used when bleeding has not begun but a pregnancy has been deemed as not viable. While she felt this was the right medical decision, the trauma of feeling like her baby's "executioner" interfered with her ability to mourn, for she did not know how to grieve someone who she would do anything to protect yet felt she had murdered.

Third, no one really knows how to process the loss of a life that has yet to be lived. As opposed to other types of losses, grieving parents lack memories with the deceased that they can hold on to and reflect upon, and that others also share (Diamond & Diamond, 2016). Family and friends, accustomed to *retrospective grief*, wherein the mourner has actual past memories of the deceased that are shared by others, may unintentionally dismiss or invalidate a grieving parent's *prospective grief*, wherein fantasies, hopes, and an imagined future must be mourned (Covington, 2005), telling the parent to move on and focus on having another child (Leon, 2015). Therapists may similarly struggle with how to help their clients grieve the loss of an imagined future and relationship with a baby that never came to be (Leon, 2015; Markin, 2016).

All these aspects and more make perinatal grief unique. However, perhaps the one aspect of perinatal grief that stands out above all the others as entirely different and devastating is that it is both deafeningly loud and shockingly silent. It is loud in that it never stops talking and parents do not have the option of simply not listening. The voice of grief is with them all the time, in every facet of their life and being, and though that voice will change over time, it will always be there, whether it be in the foreground or the background. The loss of a pregnancy or unborn baby is not just one event that grieving parents need to "get over" but a part of their ongoing life story (Diamond & Diamond, 2017). At the same time, perinatal grief can be deafeningly silent in that no matter how devastating and pervasive, the loss is rarely spoken about, and the grief is seldom acknowledged (Markin & Zilcha-Mano, 2018). In many cases, as the therapist, you will be the first person to whom the client has told her story of loss from beginning to end. Consistent with this, perinatal grief has been likened to *disenfranchised grief* (Doka, 1989), meaning it is not publicly recognized or supported. The lack of understanding and support that grieving parents typically report after pregnancy loss is not any one person's fault, but a function of, in least in part, the cultural taboo against the public recognition and expression of perinatal grief (Markin & Zilcha-Mano, 2018). Supporting this, pregnancy loss is the only kind of loss that lacks culturally sanctioned mourning rituals that provide grieving parents with a sense of validation, support, and socially prescribed ways to mourn (Markin & Zilcha-Mano, 2018). As a result, grieving parents often feel as if they must grieve in silence and isolation (Lang et al., 2011).

HOW ATTACHMENT THEORY HELPS TO UNDERSTAND THE PSYCHOLOGICAL EXPERIENCE OF PREGNANCY LOSS GRIEF: IMPLICATIONS FOR TREATMENT

Throughout this book, attachment theory is used as a guide for how to understand and treat pregnancy loss grief. More broadly, attachment theory has had a tremendous impact on how we understand grief, and, consequently, how, as clinicians, we treat it. Historically, in the grief literature, the dominant thinking was that one must completely detach from a deceased loved one to successfully grieve (Rothaupt & Becker, 2007). Any continued attachment to the deceased was considered pathological or complicated grieving (Covington, 2006; Jaffe & Diamond, 2011; Rothaupt & Becker, 2007). Bowlby's (1969) attachment theory provided a radically different and new model of grief that, contrary to prior models, encouraged continued bonds to deceased loved ones. In an attachment grief model, the bereaved maintains emotional ties to the deceased and forms a new relationship with that person based on memories (Diamond & Diamond, 2016). This is accomplished through the bereaved constructing an internal representation of the deceased that one can always subjectively "carry," while learning to live without the actual loved one. Culturally supported methods and rituals such as funerals, memorial services, storytelling, writing letters to the deceased, visiting grave sites, and talking to the deceased all aid in this process (Diamond & Diamond, 2016).

Bowlby's continued bonds theory is particularly useful for clients grieving the loss of a pregnancy because it considers the role of attachment in the reproductive process (Diamond & Diamond, 2016). Robinson et al. (1999) believed that the intensity of a mother's grief reaction after pregnancy loss is related to the depth of attachment she formed with the fetus and the meaning she assigned the pregnancy at the time of the loss. In fact, research has found that when predicting grief intensity following pregnancy loss, it is crucial to look at the degree of attachment the mother formed to the fetus, not just the gestational age at which the loss occurred (Greenfield & Walther, 1991; Robinson, et al., 1999; Serrano & Lima, 2006). Diamond and Diamond (2016) go even further and argue that attachment to one's child begins long before it is conceived, as individuals dream about becoming a parent and what their parenting or reproductive journey will look like. In a healthy pregnancy, by the time the baby is born, parents have a sense of knowing their child and have expectations about how the baby will fit into family life (Robinson et al., 1999). In fact, Beutel et al. (1995) found that most women in their study formed representations of their babies in the first trimester of pregnancy. In essence, perinatal grief can be seen as an understandable reaction to loss of an attachment object, or as the flip side of an enduring attachment bond that was solidified during pregnancy, yet started long before conception in a parent's fantasies of an imagined future baby.

Implications for Treatment

It is essential for therapists to validate and encourage grieving parents' healthy need for continued bonds to the deceased baby. The therapist simply validating a parent's attachment to the deceased baby as real and a parent's grief as legitimate can be extremely therapeutic and healing. Contrary to messages that these parents may receive from others to "move on," the therapist should encourage bereaved parents to find healthy ways of continuing their bond to the deceased baby and of internalizing and transforming their relationship. For example, one woman who was pregnant after stillbirth, over the course of her subsequent pregnancy, internalized the deceased baby as a protective and loving sibling of the baby she currently carried, who was watching over and rooting for her and the current unborn baby all the way to "the finish line" of a healthy delivery. This allowed the mother to continue her relationship to the deceased baby, while also attaching to the subsequent baby, without feeling as if she was simply replacing one baby with another. Memorial services, funerals, memory boxes, writing letters to the deceased baby, and talking to the deceased baby are all ways of helping grieving parents to transform and continue their bond.

PSYCHOLOGICAL TREATMENT OF PREGNANCY LOSS: A SYMPTOMATIC VERSUS RELATIONAL FOCUS

Research on Psychosocial Interventions for Pregnancy Loss in Healthcare Settings

A recent meta-analysis from the field of nursing looked at 15 randomized controlled studies of psychosocial interventions for pregnancy loss with mothers and fathers, and found a significant effect on symptoms of depression, anxiety, and grief (Shaohua & Shorey, 2021). Because type of intervention varied greatly between included studies, results from this meta-analysis do not suggest that any one type of intervention is effective, but rather that psychosocial interventions in general may be helpful in this context. Further, as appropriate for medical settings, psychosocial interventions for pregnancy loss within the field of nursing typically take place in the immediate aftermath of the loss and are relatively brief, supportive and/or psychoeducational, and crisis-oriented or symptom-focused. These types of interventions are surely sufficient for some bereaved parents, particularly those who have not yet attached to the fetus at the time of loss, have strong social support, and/or experience uncomplicated bereavement reactions. Such interventions may also be a necessary, yet not sufficient, first-wave treatment for other bereaved parents with more intense or complicated grief reactions. Supporting this, immediate follow-up interventions have been shown to significantly reduce the risk of negative and prolonged psychological outcomes for bereaved mothers, though not all immediate follow-up interventions are helpful to all bereaved mothers, and some may even be harmful without proper support (Koopmans et al., 2013). In particular, grieving parents who experience pregnancy loss as a traumatic event may benefit from subsequent psychotherapy intervention. Supporting this, psychological debriefing offered soon after miscarriage does not appear to have an effect on intrusion and avoidance symptoms, though it may be perceived as helpful (Lee et al., 1996). Additionally, bereaved parents who experience recurrent pregnancy loss, loss in the context of other reproductive traumas such as infertility, and/or an elevation of grief during subsequent life events such as anniversaries may require longer-term or follow-up care.

While more research is needed on what kinds of interventions are helpful to whom immediately after loss in healthcare settings, one thing is clear: It is critical for bereaved parents to feel understood and validated by their medical providers and to perceive them as caring and compassionate following a loss (Geller et al., 2010; Swanson et al., 2009). Unfortunately, studies have revealed that adequate care after pregnancy loss is often missing in healthcare settings from the patient's perspective. Routine treatment for mothers who experience pregnancy loss often fails to consider the psychological problems and emotional reactions that these mothers experience after loss, and even less so for fathers (Geller et al., 2010). While recent advances have been made in attending to parents' emotional reactions after late-term losses or stillbirths, less attention has been given to losses that occur before 20 weeks gestation. Many of these women report feeling dissatisfied with the follow-up care they receive from healthcare professionals, which tends not to focus on their emotional well-being (Geller et al., 2010). While prior authors have argued that more training for healthcare professionals is needed on empathic responding in the aftermath of loss (Geller et al., 2010; Sereshti et al., 2016), it is also perhaps true that given the sheer number of women impacted by pregnancy loss, and the complex psychosocial effects of pregnancy loss on grieving parents, it is unrealistic to expect medical professionals to treat all the psychological and emotional needs of all bereaved parents. Unfortunately, the field of psychotherapy, with some important exceptions (e.g., Jaffe & Diamond, 2005; Leon, 2015), has been largely silent in this area, leaving the burden of emotional care to healthcare professionals who have contact with this patient population for only a brief amount of time in medical settings. There is thus great need for more clinical attention in this area.

Prior Research on Psychotherapy for Pregnancy Loss: A Brief and Symptomatic Focus

Very few studies of bona fide psychotherapy treatments for pregnancy loss exist, and those that do tend to suffer from the same methodological flaws that are often found in studies of psychosocial interventions for pregnancy loss within the field of nursing, including small sample sizes, sampling bias, patient attrition, and lack of baseline scores or appropriate comparison groups (see Diamond & Diamond, 2016, for a review). Like psychosocial interventions in medical settings, existing psychotherapy studies tend to exclusively examine relatively brief symptom-focused or crisis-oriented interventions that take place in the immediate aftermath of the loss (Kersting et al., 2013; Nakano et al., 2013), which, as already discussed, may not meet the needs of all bereaved parents. Ironically, very few studies have focused on therapy for perinatal grief itself, with most assessing symptoms of depression and anxiety instead.

Neugebauer et al. (2007), for example, found that subclinical levels of depressive symptoms declined among miscarrying women who received one to six sessions of manualized, telephone, interpersonal counseling, although the sample was small and no follow-up was administered.

In addition to perinatal grief often being overlooked in intervention research for pregnancy loss, very few studies include PTSD as an outcome measure when evaluating the effectiveness of psychotherapy treatments after perinatal loss (Christiansen, 2017). This is despite the fact that previous studies have found that a substantial number of women experience pregnancy loss as a traumatic event and may develop a trauma-related disorder (e.g., Chung & Reed, 2017). As rare exceptions, two studies evaluated the effectiveness of a 5-week online cognitive-behavioral therapy (CBT) intervention on symptoms of post-traumatic stress and prolonged grief, relative to a waitlist control group, for women who suffered a pregnancy loss. Significant improvement in all symptoms of PTSD and prolonged grief at the final session and long-term follow-up were found, though problems with significant attrition at follow-up make it difficult to interpret these results (Kersting et al., 2011, 2013). Another study similarly found that four sessions of psychological grief counseling, which relied heavily on CBT techniques such as identifying dysfunctional beliefs and cognitive restructuring, reduced PTSD severity for mothers who experienced a stillbirth, yet the control group also showed a significant decrease in PTSD severity (Navidian et al., 2017). In a review of the literature, Christiansen (2017) concluded that existing brief interventions for pregnancy loss PTSD do not appear effective in the long term, and that this may be due to parents most in need prematurely dropping out of studies, or because longer-term treatments are needed to meaningfully address the trauma of pregnancy loss.

While psychotherapy studies that focus on mitigating symptoms are important, more can be done to address the deeper psychological wounds left behind by pregnancy loss (Diamond & Diamond, 2016). The author argues that researchers and clinicians should build upon existing research by focusing on both short-term supportive treatments for clients with uncomplicated grief and more intensive long-term or follow-up treatments for clients who are likely to experience more severe, nonlinear, or complicated grief reactions, such as those who have experienced recurrent pregnancy loss, stillbirth, termination due to fetal anomaly, and/or infertility (Herbert et al., 2022). Whether treatment is short or long, it is argued here that the therapist–client relationship plays an important role in healing the deeper-level wounds often inflicted upon grieving parents by the traumatic loss of a pregnancy.

How Psychotherapy Can Help from a Relational Perspective

Psychotherapy can help bereaved parents through offering them a relationship in which to grieve, wherein they no longer feel alone in their feelings of sadness and loss but feel supported and understood (Leon, 2015; Markin & Zilcha-Mano, 2018). Through the client sharing her fantasy of the baby that died, she is no longer the only one who can keep the dead baby's memory alive. Through the therapist hearing her grief and knowing her sadness, her loss is no longer silent or invisible. Similarly, as the therapist recognizes the partner's "right" to grieve and despair over feeling powerless to protect one's partner and save their baby, that partner's pain is legitimized and given a space to heal. The empathy, normalization, and validation that the therapy relationship provides helps bereaved parents to process feelings of trauma and loss and restore healthy self-esteem (Leon, 2015, 2017). Studies have shown the clinical benefit of multiple sessions that focus on empathic caring for couples in ameliorating depression and grief after miscarriage (Swanson et al., 2009). Essentially, while of course specific techniques matter, the basic premise of this book is that, especially in this therapeutic context, the relationship matters more. Grief needs to speak, but it also needs an understanding and supportive other to listen.

WHY IS THE RELATIONSHIP IMPORTANT IN PSYCHOTHERAPY FOR PREGNANCY LOSS?

The therapy relationship may play an especially important role in promoting positive outcomes in psychotherapy for pregnancy loss, making it an ideal therapeutic context in which to explore the clinical application of relationship research (see Chapter 1 in this book). It is important to understand why the relationship is believed to be so vital to the process and outcome of psychotherapy for pregnancy loss because the *why* is directly related to *how* the relationship can be utilized to help affected clients heal from the trauma of loss. Specifically, as introduced below and expanded upon throughout this book, the relationship is proposed to be critical to therapy for pregnancy loss because (a) it provides clients the support and understanding sometimes missing in society yet necessary to grieve, (b) it helps clients restore healthy self-esteem and identity, (c) it is within a secure attachment relationship with the therapist that clients feel safe to approach and process feelings of trauma and loss, and (d) a trusting and affect-regulating therapy relationship can serve as a vehicle for revisiting and revising early adverse attachment experiences that are currently making it difficult for clients to process separation and loss.

Providing Clients with Support and Understanding

While the loss of a loved one is emotionally painful, even unbearable and devastating, there is nothing pathological or problematic about grief itself. Grief is an adaptive emotion that allows the bereaved to mourn the loss of a loved one, and, in the case of pregnancy loss, one's hopes and dreams for the future. However, mourning is an inherently interpersonal process in which the loss itself, and any associated feelings and experiences, needs to be seen, heard, validated, and emotionally contained by others (Markin & Zilcha-Mano, 2018). This is supported by the fact that although the specific response to death varies between cultures, every culture defines its own traditions and rituals for grieving in ways that foster connections among the living (Covington, 2006; Littlewood, 1996; Markin & Zilcha-Mano, 2018). Unfortunately, because pregnancy loss is not seen as a legitimate loss in Western society, grieving parents often lack the support needed to adaptively grieve (Markin & Zilcha-Mano, 2018). Instead, grieving parents often feel as if their support persons minimize, dismiss, and invalidate their grief (Covington, 2005; Lang et al., 2011; Layne, 2003; Leon, 2015). The invalidation that grieving parents often report in close relationships can be understood as a reflection of a larger society that treats pregnancy loss, especially miscarriage, as a "nonevent," and actively inhibits the public expression of perinatal grief (Frost & Condon, 1996; Markin & Zilcha-Mano, 2018). Psychotherapy can offer these clients what they are sometimes missing in other close relationships and in society at large: an empathic, emotionally containing, and validating relationship in which to mourn (Markin & Zilcha-Mano, 2018). The therapist's empathic support and sharing of sadness helps clients to feel less alone and facilitates the processing of trauma and loss (Leon, 2010, 2015).

Restoring Clients' Self-Esteem and Identity

Pregnancy loss is often experienced as an attack on one's self-worth, personal agency, and gender identity that evokes strong feelings of shame and inadequacy (Diamond & Diamond, 2017; Leon, 1996). The therapist's empathic attunement, validation, and affirmation support the client's capacity to repair and maintain healthy self-esteem and to stabilize what is most often a damaged sense of self and identity that has been shattered by the loss of a pregnancy and perhaps other reproductive traumas (Leon, 2010; Markin & McCarthy, 2020). As the client feels understood by the therapist, she typically begins to rebuild a more positive and realistic sense of self, for what is understood by another can then feel understandable to the self and not all that different or "bad" (Leon, 2010). Further, processing traumatic experiences within a trusting and empathically attuned therapy relationship helps clients to see the traumatic event as something bad that happened to them and not because of them, which helps to repair self-esteem (Courtois & Sack, 2014).

A Secure Attachment Relationship

Pregnancy loss and related adverse reproductive events are often experienced as traumatic events that engender overwhelming and chaotic feelings within grieving parents (Jaffe & Diamond, 2011). According to attachment theory, in such times of trauma and loss, we need sensitive and responsive attachment figures to turn to for support and comfort in order to process the trauma and cope with feelings of sadness and loss (Bowlby, 1969). In psychotherapy for pregnancy loss, the therapist acting as a sensitive secure attachment figure facilitates the client's experience of the therapist as a safe base, from which overwhelming feelings of trauma and loss can be safely approached and processed (Leon, 2015). In general, the client's experience of safety and trust within the therapy relationship has been argued to be important to therapy outcomes with adults who have experienced other forms of trauma, particularly interpersonal or attachment trauma (Courtois & Brown, 2019; Ellis et al., 2018).

Revisiting and Reworking Early Adverse Attachment Experiences

The intense distress that individuals experience following pregnancy loss can trigger the attachment system and the individual's need for support and comfort from close others. This can evoke prior experiences of not feeling supported, understood, and/or comforted by early attachment figures during other times of trauma and loss (Markin, 2018). With these past attachment experiences evoked and/or magnified after pregnancy loss, clients with a more insecure or negative attachment history tend to have more difficulty trusting the therapist and feeling supported and understood (Leon, 2015). Put another way, past adverse attachment experiences of feeling unsupported, misunderstood, or alone in one's intense distress, particularly related to separation and loss, are likely to be evoked after a pregnancy loss and replayed or "revisited" within the therapy relationship. While this presents unique challenges to treatment, it also provides an opportunity to revise negative or insecure attachment internal working models, as the client comes to experience a safe, trusting, attuned, and responsive therapy relationship in which feelings of trauma and loss can be safely approached and processed, unlike in early attachment relationships.

THERAPY GOALS AND OUTCOMES

From an attachment-relational perspective, the ultimate goal of therapy for pregnancy loss is to utilize the therapy relationship as a mechanism through which clients (a) process feelings of trauma and loss, (b) restore healthy self-esteem, and (c) develop more secure attachment internal working models of self and other, as they come to experience the therapist as responsive, supportive, and understanding, and themselves as worthy of and effective at eliciting the care and concern of others (see Diamond & Diamond, 2016; Leon, 2015). When psychotherapy for pregnancy loss is framed in terms of these specific goals, then the relative effectiveness of treatment can be assessed via changes in scores on validated measures of perinatal grief, post-traumatic stress symptoms, self-esteem, and attachment style (see Markin & McCarthy, 2018, for an example). The success of this kind of therapy, however, is not solely determined by the absence of something negative, but also by the presence of something positive, such as the client's experience of post-traumatic growth (Markin, 2017).

In addition to the more immediate goals of processing trauma and loss and rebuilding self-esteem, therapy for pregnancy loss must sometimes also address clients' previous psychological disorders that have been exacerbated by the pregnancy loss (Diamond & Diamond, 2016). In fact, a history of psychiatric illness has been found to be a risk factor predisposing women who miscarry to psychological morbidity (see Lok & Neugebauer, 2007). Of note, in one large-scale longitudinal study of 998 women, a history of medically diagnosed depression or anxiety before miscarriage was a significant predictor of downward trajectories in mental health over time after miscarriage (Rowlands & Lee, 2010). From this, it is important for clinicians to assess previous psychological disorders and to understand that these may be exacerbated by the loss of a pregnancy and in need of clinical attention.

Clinically, it has been observed that pregnancy loss can resurrect prior traumatic experiences in the client's life, leading to increased post-traumatic-stress–like symptoms (Diamond & Diamond, 2016; Leon, 2015; Markin, 2018). Supporting this, Watson (2005) found that in clients with a history of abuse, feelings of shame and self-blame associated with miscarriage re-evoked similar feelings from past traumas. Similarly, a prior history of promiscuity, sexually transmitted disease, or substance abuse can also increase feelings of guilt, shame, or blame associated with pregnancy loss (Hart, 2002). Particularly for clients with a history of sexual abuse, the physical experience of pregnancy loss and of associated medical interventions can reawaken earlier trauma(s) and the feeling of being out of control and violated. Unfortunately, clients often do not volunteer this information easily and a strong therapy relationship can help them feel safe to disclose past traumas (Diamond & Diamond, 2016).

Pregnancy loss can also reawaken prior experiences of loss, particularly those experienced as traumatic losses and/or those that are unresolved. Because the loss of a pregnancy is a nebulous one in the sense that many times there is no physical baby to mourn or actual memories of the deceased, it is naturally vulnerable to merging with other unresolved losses from a client's past, often leading to layered and complicated grief reactions (Leon, 2015). For example, for one client, the experience of a sudden and devastating stillbirth resurrected past unresolved feelings of trauma and loss from suddenly losing her brother and father at a young age in a motor vehicle accident. Clinicians should assess for past experiences of trauma and loss and understand that, for some clients, to process the loss of a pregnancy, they must first process past experiences of trauma and loss, temporarily shifting the focus of therapy (Leon, 2015). However, clinicians should be careful not to unintentionally invalidate the client's grief over the loss of a pregnancy by suggesting the client is "really" sad about other past losses.

Recommendations

It is the paradox of this kind of work that while clinicians must be attuned to the trauma and deep psychological wounds that pregnancy loss inflicts, they must also recognize that most clients who have suffered a pregnancy loss do not seek therapy for personality change. Rather, they come to treatment because they are traumatized, grief-stricken, and full of feelings of shame and inadequacy (Diamond & Diamond, 2016; Leon, 1996). Especially when there are multiple losses and/or the losses occur within the context of infertility, clients enter treatment in a state of trauma and crisis. They often exhibit symptoms of PTSD, depression, and grief, including emotional lability, cognitive confusion, flashbacks, and difficulty concentrating, all of which can leave them feeling as if they are "going crazy" (Diamond & Diamond, 2016). In this state, it is imperative for the therapist from the beginning of treatment to focus less on technique or a structured assessment and more on the relationship, normalizing and validating the client's experience as an expectable and inevitable reaction to traumatic loss and developing a safe environment in which the client feels supported and not judged (Diamond & Diamond, 2016).

CONCLUSION

Because pregnancy loss profoundly impacts so many women and their partners and has the potential for severe and varied psychosocial consequences, the lack of clinical and empirical guidelines for practicing clinicians working with clients who have experienced such losses is both surprising and concerning. The longstanding lack of recognition by some medical professionals and nonspecialist mental health researchers of the profound psychological impact of adverse reproductive events in general has real-world implications (Diamond & Diamond, 2016). As Diamond and Diamond (2016) argue, while it has been noted that reproductive events like pregnancy loss and infertility, and even childbirth, may account for the higher general incidence of depression and certain other emotional disorders that women experience compared to men, researchers tend to assume the link is primarily a biological one (Serrano & Warnock, 2007). This is perhaps why more clinical guidelines and therapeutic approaches do not exist for individuals who have experienced different kinds of reproductive traumas. To fill in this gap in the literature, this book offers practical clinical guidance that is based on pan-theoretical therapy relationship research and principles to help affected parents.

3

The Alliance in Individual
and Couples Therapy
for Pregnancy Loss

Like most other therapies, fundamental to psychotherapy for pregnancy loss is a shared sense between the therapist and client that they are working together to ease the client's pain. Such mutual collaboration is predicated upon grieving parents experiencing the therapist as someone who is capable of understanding their pain, including feelings of grief and loss, horror and powerlessness, isolation and loneliness, desperation and longing, a sense of brokenness and inadequacy, and anger in an unjust and unfair world. When "the client" is a couple, therapists have the task of establishing themselves as someone who is capable of understanding and subsequently easing the suffering of both partners, individually and as a unit. From this, the treatment goals of both individual and couples therapy flow from first understanding the client's pain and include the processing of reproductive trauma and loss and the restoration of healthy self-esteem. While these treatment goals are relatively consistent across clients, the process by which therapists and clients work together to reach them will vary depending on the unique characteristics of the treatment, client, and therapist, as well as the relationship that they forge. As argued below, in individual and couples therapy for pregnancy loss, a therapist–client bond that is characterized by understanding and mutual collaboration is believed to lead to certain positive therapeutic outcomes directly, as well as indirectly through facilitating the success of certain therapeutic tasks, which then lead to successful outcomes (Leon, 2015).

This chapter begins with a brief empirical review of the alliance in individual and couples therapy. Evidence-based relationship principles derived from research on the alliance in individual and couples therapy is then applied to the treatment of clients who have suffered a pregnancy loss. Based on theory and research, the author describes how characteristics of the treatment, client, therapist,

Psychotherapy for Pregnancy Loss. Rayna D. Markin, Oxford University Press. © Oxford University Press 2024.
DOI: 10.1093/oso/9780197693353.003.0003

and relationship may facilitate or hinder the alliance in this therapeutic context. Specific therapeutic goals and tasks are discussed within an empathic, safe, and collaborative alliance. Therapist–client vignettes are given to demonstrate the application of these concepts. These vignettes are derived from a combination of real clinical examples so that no one person can be identified. Finally, common challenges to establishing and maintaining the alliance in psychotherapy for pregnancy loss and clinical implications are discussed.

CASE VIGNETTE: THE ALLIANCE IN COUPLES THERAPY

Scott and Stephanie were a married couple in their mid-thirties who attended therapy after suffering multiple pregnancy losses and unsuccessful IVF cycles. Their most recent loss was a late-term miscarriage, occurring after Stephanie had been on bed rest for several weeks. Scott worked as a construction worker. He presented as quiet and introverted and expressed a great deal of fear over saying the "wrong thing" in therapy and angering Stephanie. For example, he stated that he was "not good" at talking about feelings and never knew the "right" thing to say to support Stephanie when she was upset, which led to conflict in their relationship. He appeared eager to please Stephanie and caring of her. In fact, Scott stated that he came to therapy to learn how to better support her. Stephanie, on the other hand, was outgoing, vivacious, funny, but emotionally volatile at times and quick to anger, often yelling at and blaming Scott. Although the exact reason for their difficulties maintaining a viable pregnancy was unknown, Stephanie blamed Scott, stating that he wanted to wait to have children and would not listen to her when she tried to warn him that waiting to have children would almost certainly lead to problems conceiving. As a result, Scott reported feeling incredibly guilty and as if the couple's fertility problems and losses were all his fault. He felt a high degree of pressure to perform sexually and feared disappointing Stephanie if he could not "get" her pregnant. As a result, Scott developed symptoms of erectile dysfunction, which only reinforced his feelings of guilt and shame and Stephanie's feelings of anger and disappointment. A central area of conflict in their relationship revolved around how to communicate about grief and loss, for they both had very different ways of coping with grief. Stephanie reported that every time she would try to talk about her feelings, especially as related to their last late-term loss, Scott would withdraw and go outside to the backyard to work on his "latest project," which was building a greenhouse. In response, Stephanie would become enraged and feel emotionally abandoned. She would sometimes follow Scott outside in a rage, which only led him to withdraw even more, and her to subsequently amplify her efforts to elicit a response from him. Scott, on the other hand, reported feeling overwhelmed by Stephanie, afraid of saying the wrong thing, and always guilty for not "doing the right thing," leading him to withdraw.

It was clear to the therapist that this couple lacked a sense of safety with one another and that each partner felt very alone. The first thing the therapist focused on was making interventions to increase shared purpose, reflecting out loud that they both wanted to feel closer and safer with one another. She then validated their common struggle: "You both have different ways of coping with grief, and that causes conflict between you two, but you are both struggling to grieve and neither of you wants to do it alone." An important moment in the therapy occurred when Scott eventually felt safe enough to disclose his reasons for building and retreating to the backyard greenhouse. The therapist asked, "Why a greenhouse? Why not build something else?" He responded that he was building it for Stephanie because she loved gardening, and Scott wanted to feel like he could help her create something and watch it grow. Scott stated he honestly doesn't know what to say or do when Stephanie gets upset and feels helpless. "What I can do," he stated, "is build her something to make her feel better." It became clear that this greenhouse was Scott's way of trying to ease Stephanie's pain and support his own damaged self-esteem through feeling as if he could do something to help her bring something to life. This gave Stephanie a different perspective on why Scott retreats to the greenhouse. She was now able to see his withdrawal not as an abandonment or rejection of her, but as an act of love. The therapist asked Stephanie, "If the anger toward Scott wasn't there, what feelings do you think would come up for you?" Stephanie replied thoughtfully, "I guess I would just feel angry with myself and my body and very sad and empty." This more direct communication of her feelings helped Scott understand Stephanie's anger not as a reflection of his personal inadequacies, but as a symptom of the enormous sense of pain she felt underneath.

When Stephanie broke down crying in session (in contrast to the rage Scott was accustomed to seeing), Scott helplessly said that he didn't know what to do to fix this or what to say. The therapist encouraged Scott to "lean in" to Stephanie's feelings, rather than withdraw as typical. In response, Scott gave Stephanie a big bear hug and the two sat there in the therapy room holding each other for several minutes. This also opened the door for Scott to disclose his own feelings of grief and loss, after being reassured that this would not burden Stephanie, but rather help her feel less alone. While initially the couple's within-couple alliance was badly shattered by the trauma of reproductive loss, the therapeutic alliance, or an empathic and trusting bond with each partner and the couple as a whole, served as a bridge in this treatment to build back trust, safety, and a sense of togetherness in the couple's relationship. Scott and Stephanie eventually agreed to finish the greenhouse together. Scott became more skilled at simply listening to Stephanie, as they worked alongside one another building the greenhouse, which met Stephanie's need for support and comfort and his need to feel helpful and efficacious. When the greenhouse was complete, they decided to plant a special tree for each baby they had lost and felt a moment of release when they cried together as they watched them grow.

ALLIANCE: AN EVIDENCE-BASED RELATIONSHIP PRINCIPLE

Alliance Defined

The alliance, sometimes referred to as the *therapeutic, working,* or *helping* alliance, has captured the attention and fascination of researchers and practitioners alike, across psychotherapy orientations and treatment modalities (Flückiger et al., 2018; Friedlander et al., 2019). While meaningful differences exist between how authors define the term, the alliance, at its core, captures the collaborative aspects of the therapist–client relationship (Hatcher & Barends, 2006). In psychotherapy for pregnancy loss, the client's collaboration with the therapist, feeling a sense of ownership and agency in the treatment, is essential to a high-quality therapy relationship and process (Leon, 2015). These clients typically enter treatment feeling out of control of their own body, future, and *reproductive story,* or the conscious and unconscious narrative of how one's path to parenthood is supposed to unfold (Jaffe, 2014). They sometimes have undergone invasive medical procedures during which they experienced a lack of agency. Contrary to these experiences, these clients need a therapy relationship and process defined by mutual collaboration in order to feel safe and empowered.

While all definitions emphasize the collaborative aspects of the alliance, how exactly the concept is operationalized has evolved over time (for a review of alliance definitions see Flückiger et al., 2019). As reported in Flückiger et al. (2019), the idea of the alliance originated with Freud (1913), who came to believe that there existed a reality-based (non-transferential) collaboration between the therapist and client as they work together to conquer the client's pain (Freud, 1927). The term *therapeutic alliance* was later used by Zetzel (1956) to refer to the client's ability to use the healthy part of her or his ego to join with the analyst to accomplish the therapeutic tasks. Luborsky (1976) expanded upon Zetzel's definition and offered a phased conceptualization of alliance that could be applied to therapies outside of psychoanalysis. The first phase involved the client's belief that the therapist could help him or her through offering a warm, supportive, and caring relationship, while the second phase involved the client's investment and faith in the therapeutic process itself and a sense of joint ownership over the therapeutic process. Finally, Bordin (1975, 1979, 1994) proposed a pan-theoretical version of the alliance that he called the *working alliance,* which was built on three components: (a) agreement on therapeutic goals, (b) consensus on the tasks that make up therapy, and (c) a client–therapist bond. In this chapter, Bordin's (1975) tripartite definition of the alliance is used because of the ease with which it is applied to various types of therapies and treatment modalities. On a more phenomenological level, this chapter emphasizes the aspects of the alliance in which the therapist joins or aligns with the client's subjective experience, and the client joins with the therapist as co-owners of the therapeutic process. This way, both participants can collaboratively work together toward the tasks and goals of therapy.

In couples therapy, the complexity of how to best define and conceptualize the alliance grows exponentially, as there are multiple alliances that interact with one another in "covert as well as overt ways" (Friedlander et al., 2019, p. 117). Each partner forms a personal alliance with the therapist but also observes the unfolding alliance between the therapist and one's partner. The couple, or system as-a-whole, also forms an alliance with the therapist (Friedlander et al., 2019). A *split alliance* refers to an imbalance among these multiple alliances, wherein person X's alliance is stronger than person Y's alliance, which can be determinantal to therapy (Escudero & Friedlander, 2017; Friedlander et al., 2006; Pinsof & Catherall, 1986). Split alliances can prevent the alliance and treatment from getting off the ground or precipitate alliance ruptures (Escudero et al., 2012). In this sense, ruptures can be viewed as opportunities to heal split alliances and, once repaired, for all participants to get on the same page of the therapeutic process. In couples therapy for pregnancy loss, a split alliance sometimes occurs early in the therapy when a male partner presents to treatment with the stated goal of better supporting his female partner and is less personally invested in treatment. The focus of treatment is then often placed on the woman, partly as a result of the male partner's stated lack of personal investment and partly because the loss involved her body (Leon, 2015). In lesbian couples, the focus of treatment is often placed on the woman who carried the child, while her partner often feels like she does not "deserve" to have feelings about the loss because she did not have to go through the horrific physical experience of loss and associated medical procedures that her partner did (Markin, 2023). Yet, for couples therapy to be successful, both partners must feel an investment and sense of ownership in the therapeutic process. To circumvent this kind of split alliance, Friedlander et al. (2019) suggest that the therapist defines the treatment goals and tasks in such a way that both partners "sign on" or "join in." This requires the therapist to align with and empathically connect to both partners to understand their sense of distress and associated therapy goals (Friedlander et al., 2019). For example, as seen in the case of Scott and Stephanie, men and women often have different ways of coping with perinatal grief that can cause conflict in relationships (Leon, 2015). Despite these differences, the therapist can emphasize that each partner is grieving and is in emotional pain and, moreover, feels alone in their own distress, yet wants comfort and connection from the other. Accordingly, Stephanie and Scott's therapist said, "You both have different ways of coping with grief and that causes conflict between you two, but you are both struggling to grieve and neither of you wants to do it alone." The treatment goals can then be defined in terms of helping each partner to respect the other's way of coping with grief so that they can approach the pain of loss together, rather than feeling so alone in their distress (Leon, 2015; also see Markin, 2023).

Alliance and Outcome

Like other therapy relationship principles, research has yet to examine the association between alliance and therapy outcome with pregnancy loss clients specifically. However, there is an impressive body of literature on how alliance relates to psychotherapy outcome with other client populations from which to draw. Research consistently finds a moderate but robust relation between alliance and outcome across a broad array of treatments in individual therapy (Horvath & Bedi, 2002; Horvath et al., 2011; Horvath & Symonds, 1991; Martin et al., 2000) and couples therapy (Friedlander et al., 2011, 2019). In the individual therapy literature, most recently, Flückiger et al. (2019) conducted a meta-analysis based on 295 independent alliance–outcome relations. They found an alliance–outcome association of r = .278, suggesting that the alliance accounts for about 8 percent of variability in outcome. This relation did not change depending on the therapist's theoretical orientation. Their results are consistent with past meta-analyses (Del Re et al., 2012; Flückiger et al., 2012; Horvath & Bedi, 2002; Horvath et al., 2011).

In the couples therapy literature, Friedlander et al. (2019), in their meta-analysis across 39 independent samples, found a significant correlation between alliance and outcome (r = .297), suggesting that stronger alliances are associated with better outcomes. Furthermore, in their meta-analysis, based on seven independent samples, the correlation between split alliance and outcome was also significant (r = −.316), indicating that more split/unbalanced alliances contribute to worse treatment outcomes (Friedlander et al., 2019). Interestingly, in their meta-analysis, while significant correlations indicated that alliance predicted outcome across theoretical orientations, the strongest alliance–outcome correlation was found for CBT treatments, as compared to attachment/emotion-focused therapy (EFT) or integrative therapies, and the lowest correlation was found for structural/functional and multisystem models. These results suggest that the alliance is important to the outcome of couples therapy regardless of theoretical orientation but is even more important, or contributes even more to outcome, in certain types of treatments. Lastly, Friedlander et al. (2019) found that with couples the highest correlations emerged for systemic alliances, as compared to each individual's alliance with the therapist, highlighting the importance of the therapist's alliance with the couple-as-a-whole. This represents an important mental shift for many clinicians accustomed to working with individuals.

CHARACTERISTICS THAT FACILITATE THE ALLIANCE

Given that there is substantial evidence supporting an alliance–outcome association in individual and couples therapy, it is important to identify treatment, therapist, client, and relationship factors that have been shown to facilitate a strong alliance, and to explore these factors within the context of therapy for pregnancy loss. While not an exhaustive list, characteristics that have been shown in prior studies to predict alliance quality and are theoretically most relevant to therapy for pregnancy loss are discussed below.

Treatment Characteristics: Feedback

Results from a recent meta-analysis suggest that ongoing feedback, or feedback-assisted psychotherapy, outperforms treatment as usual (Lambert et al., 2019). While the specific mechanism that explains why feedback predicts better outcomes is unknown, feedback presumably works through supplying therapists with new information, correcting overly optimistic or pessimistic views of therapeutic progress, and increasing therapist–client collaboration (Lambert et al., 2019). One study found that the working alliance mediated the effect of routine outcome monitoring (a systematic feedback process) on posttreatment impairment (Brattland et al., 2019), suggesting that feedback "works" through facilitating therapist–client collaboration and joint investment in treatment.

In psychotherapy for pregnancy loss, Leon (2015) suggests dedicating the first few sessions toward (a) gathering the client's history, (b) hearing the client's story of loss and reproductive trauma, and (c) establishing rapport. Giving and receiving feedback during these early sessions is believed to be imperative to establishing rapport and a collaborative therapist–client relationship (Leon, 2015). Collecting and then empathically responding to client feedback, particularly concerning the client's experience of feeling understood and supported by the therapist, is believed to be important throughout therapy (Leon, 2015). From the first session to the last, it is recommended that the therapist elicit feedback from the client regarding areas in which the therapist may not fully understand the client's subjective experience of loss, making clients the expert on their reproductive story. It is also important to elicit client feedback regarding the tasks and goals of therapy so that clients feel as if the work of therapy is centered around their personal needs rather than the therapist's theoretical orientation or what the therapist thinks the client needs. Pregnancy loss clients, especially those who experience recurrent loss and/or infertility, often come to therapy accustomed to feeling like passive recipients of their medical care and decisions (Covington, 2005; Diamond, 2011). For example, one client who was unknowingly experiencing an ectopic pregnancy called her doctor's office multiple times crying that she was in severe pain. She was dismissed as having the "typical pains" of miscarriage and told to "wait it out," which led to a potentially life-threatening situation. Contrary to such experiences, the therapist eliciting and responding to client feedback about the therapy process helps the client feel a sense of agency, control, and validation.

Therapist Characteristics

Some research suggests that the ability to form an alliance is a therapist characteristic that predicts outcome (Ackerman & Hilsenroth, 2001, 2003; Del Re et al., 2012). In other words, some therapists tend to be more skilled at forming alliances with clients than others, regardless of the client or treatment (Del Re et al., 2012). For instance, therapists who have an interpersonal style that is colder and more detached tend to form worse alliances with clients (Hersoug et al., 2009). In the context of pregnancy loss, there are likely multiple therapist characteristics that facilitate or hinder the alliance. First, therapists who possess less anxiety, or are better able to manage their anxiety around death and dying, and specifically around the loss of a baby, are perhaps better able to collaborate and affectively join with the client on the difficult task of processing reproductive trauma and loss.

Second, therapists that are adept at pointing out client strengths, at a time when many women (and men) feel woefully inadequate and like a failure, may tend to form better alliances with these clients (Leon, 2015). Third, therapist flexibility, or the therapist's willingness to put "ideological purity" aside for the sake of "therapeutic efficacy," may facilitate therapist–client collaboration and ultimately treatment outcome (Leon, 2015, p. 228). For example, how structured and directive the therapist should be depends less on therapist theoretical orientation and more on the level of client crisis, which is usually higher when the loss is recent and calls for more therapist direction (Leon, 2015). In the author's experience, many alliances never have the chance to get off the ground after clients prematurely drop out of therapy because their level of distress over a recent loss was not adequately acknowledged or responded to by the therapist (Diamond & Diamond, 2017). This is consistent with research that has examined therapist flexibility or responsiveness as an interpersonal skill that promotes an empathic alliance and successful therapy outcome (Hatcher, 2015).

Client Characteristics

While most research suggests that therapists make the largest contribution to the alliance, certainly the client also contributes to the development of the alliance, as it is a *mutual* collaboration (Flückiger et al., 2019). Consistent with this, in their meta-analysis Flückiger et al. (2019) found that client characteristics, such as diagnosis, moderated the alliance–outcome association. Pregnancy loss clients, like all other clients, vary in terms of diagnostic presentation and history. For example, a client with borderline personality disorder who suffers a pregnancy loss may experience the loss as an abandonment or rejection, reinforcing her pre-existing conflict over separation-individuation. In turn, this may exacerbate this client's tendency to form problematic therapeutic alliances (see Flückiger et al., 2019) in which she craves closeness with the therapist yet fears rejection or engulfment (McWilliams, 1994).

Relatedly, the alliance–outcome association has been found to be not as strong for clients with more problem severity (Flückiger et al., 2019). Problem severity, in the context of pregnancy loss, can be defined in terms of the intensity of perinatal grief and/or severity of general psychiatric symptoms. Perinatal grief intensity is related to the degree to which a parent perceives the lost baby as a real person versus a "fetus/it," and to the quality of attachment to the fetus/unborn baby at the time of the loss (Robinson et al., 1999). In the author's clinical experience, "severe" perinatal grief does not negatively impact the alliance; in fact, these clients are often more invested in the treatment. On the contrary, clients with relatively severe psychiatric symptoms that predated but have been exacerbated by the loss are more likely to have difficulties forming an alliance, perhaps because clients with more psychiatric symptoms have been found to display more interpersonal problems in general (Siegel et al., 2015).

Attachment style has been conceptualized as one important client characteristic that impacts the quality of the alliance in psychotherapy for pregnancy loss (Leon,

2015; see Chapters 8 and 9 in this book). Supporting this, a recent meta-analysis showed that attachment avoidance and anxiety had a moderate yet significant negative association with working alliance ratings (Bernecker et al., 2014). Clients with an insecure attachment style are likely to have a difficult time collaborating on the primary goal and associated tasks of treatment having to do with the processing of trauma and loss. This is likely because of their difficulty using the therapist as a secure base from which to approach and process overwhelming and often chaotic affects associated with the loss and other adverse reproductive events (Leon, 2015). Furthermore, their negative internal working models of self and/or other may interfere with the formation of a trusting bond and with internalizing therapist empathy. Without a secure, trusting, and affect-regulating therapist–client bond in place, tasks related to the processing of trauma and loss may only further traumatize the client (Leon, 2015). Consistent with this, Mallinckrodt and Jeong (2015), in their meta-analysis, found that the client's pre-therapy attachment style significantly predicted the parallel type of attachment style to the therapist, which in turn generally predicted the quality of the working alliance. This supports the idea that the client's pre-therapy attachment style impacts the quality of the therapeutic relationship and, in particular, the client's capacity to form a trusting and collaborative bond with the therapist. Because a strong alliance is so fundamental to the client being able to use the therapist as a safe base from which to approach painful and overwhelming feelings of grief and loss, clients with an insecure attachment style may first need to develop more positive internal working models of self and other before the therapy can focus on the processing of reproductive trauma and loss.

Client Characteristics in Couples Therapy

With heterosexual couples, evidence suggests that men's and women's self-reported perceptions of alliance quality predict outcome differently (e.g., Glebova et al., 2011; Halford et al., 2016; Knobloch-Fedders et al., 2007). In their review, Friedlander et al. (2019) found that, overall, a male partner's ratings of the alliance early in treatment tended to be more strongly associated with outcome than their female partners. Less frequently, women's alliance scores from later in treatment emerged as the stronger predictor of outcome. These authors suggest that, perhaps, when couples invest in long-term therapy, the woman's alliance may be more critical, but in short-term therapies, where men are typically the more reluctant partner, the man's alliance may be more predictive of outcome (Anker et al., 2010).

In therapy for pregnancy loss with heterosexual couples, the woman is typically the one seeking treatment, and, while her male partner is usually willing to come and support her, he is usually less personally invested in treatment at the onset (Leon, 2015). From this perspective, the therapist forming an early alliance with the male partner seems especially important to securing his investment in and commitment to the therapeutic process. Importantly, in couples therapy, clients' feelings of safety in the therapeutic context seem important to connecting with the therapist, engaging in the treatment, disclosing more, and being more emotionally vulnerable in session (Escudero & Friedlander, 2017; Friedlander et al., 2006, 2010). To promote safety in couples therapy for pregnancy loss, it is important from the very first session to validate each partner's experience of loss and way of coping with grief, and to frame communication problems not as any one person's fault but rather as the result of different ways of coping with loss (Leon, 2015).

Relationship Characteristics: Empathy

Although empathy is sometimes conceptualized as a therapist skill or ability (Rogers, 1980), Elliott et al. (2019) found, in their meta-analysis, that who clients are and the kinds of problems they experience also contribute to empathy. Thus, it is probably more accurate to think of it as a relational, mutually constructed, construct (Elliott et al., 2019). Importantly, empathy is believed to be fundamental to psychotherapy for pregnancy loss (Leon, 2015). Empathy helps to heal the narcissistic wounds left behind by the loss of a pregnancy and to rebuild the client's self-esteem. Additionally, feeling understood by the therapist helps the client to process feelings of reproductive trauma and loss (Leon, 2015; see Chapter 4 in this book). Because empathic attunement is believed to be critical for pregnancy loss clients, empathy may be especially important to facilitating the alliance with this clinical population. Several studies on non-pregnancy loss clients support an empathy–alliance association. Nienhuis et al. (2018), for example, found that ratings of the alliance were significantly related to clients' perceptions of therapist empathy and genuineness. Furthermore, McClintock et al. (2018) found that early experiences of empathy strengthened the alliance, which in turn facilitated improvements in depressive symptoms and psychological well-being. Just as empathic attunement likely facilitates a good therapeutic alliance, lack of client-perceived therapist empathy may contribute to misunderstanding events, or ruptures in the alliance. Of course some empathic "misses" in the therapy relationship and subsequent alliance ruptures are inevitable and potentially healing (Leon, 2015). The therapist remaining open to repairing the rupture, and to understanding the client's experience of it, promotes a sense of collaboration and empowers the client through validating her experience (Leon, 2015). Empathy is therefore important not only to building a strong alliance, but also to maintaining and even strengthening it in the face of empathic failures and ruptures.

CLINICAL APPLICATION: THE ALLIANCE IN THERAPY FOR PREGNANCY LOSS

Based on Bordin's (1975) tripartite conceptualization of the alliance, special considerations regarding the therapist–client *bond*, and therapist–client agreement on the *goals* and *tasks* of treatment, in individual and couples therapy for pregnancy loss, are explored below and demonstrated in hypothetical client vignettes.

THERAPIST–CLIENT BOND

Bereaved parents often arrive to therapy shattered by the trauma of loss; thirsty for help, support, and understanding; and motivated to collaborate with the therapist. Because they are often in desperate need of comfort and understanding, a collaborative therapeutic bond may be quick to build yet easy to break, particularly when the client does not experience the therapist as empathic, nor the context as safe. In therapy for pregnancy loss, the bond dimension of the alliance, encompassing a trusting, empathic, and collaborative relationship, is believed to directly facilitate certain positive outcomes, like the increasing of client self-esteem, as the therapist understands, normalizes, and validates the client's experience. The bond dimension may also indirectly contribute to other outcomes, like the processing of trauma and grief, for the client no longer feels alone in her sense of sadness and loss and thus feels safer to approach these feelings (Leon, 2015).

AGREEMENT ON GOALS AND TASKS OF THERAPY FOR PREGNANCY LOSS

Agreement on the tasks and goals of therapy is an essential component of the alliance (Bordin, 1975). Leon (2015) suggests that the primary goals of therapy for pregnancy loss involve (a) processing trauma, (b) grieving, and (c) repairing the self (or self-esteem). While Leon (2015) also conceptualized "defining that which was lost" as a treatment goal, here, the author views this as a therapeutic task that works toward the goal of processing grief.

Processing Trauma

Processing the trauma of loss is an important goal of treatment that needs to be agreed upon and negotiated from the first session of therapy. Often just framing the loss as a traumatic event helps clients better understand their reaction and validates their experience. Processing the trauma or horror of loss most often involves the client telling the story, sometimes over and over, each time with a little bit more coherence and integration (Leon, 2015). As clients retell their story of loss, they relive the events as if they are happening in the moment, except this time within an empathic and affect-regulating relationship with the therapist, enabling traumatic affects to be safely approached and processed (Leon, 2015). The tasks intended to process trauma involve the client talking about personal experiences and feelings surrounding the loss, and the therapist and client collaboratively working together to better understand and organize these often chaotic and overwhelming experiences. In couples therapy, each partner serves as a witness to the other's experience of trauma and loss and the therapist serves as an emotional container within which the couple can process their individual and joint experience of trauma. Processing trauma can give these clients the sense of control they have been pining for. While many factors related to reproduction lie outside one's control, through talking about and processing feelings of trauma and loss, clients can come to feel in control of their internal subjective experience.

Facilitating Grieving

Grieving should be an agreed-upon goal from the start of treatment. By establishing grieving as a goal, the therapist validates the client's grief as legitimate and her loss as real. While grieving the loss of a pregnancy involves many of the same processes as grieving other types of losses, such as working through shock, disbelief, sadness, and anger, it is also unique in that pregnancy loss is a traumatic loss, is accompanied by intense feelings of shame and inadequacy, is not a socially acknowledged loss, and involves retrospective instead of prospective mourning (Leon, 2015). Tasks for facilitating the process of pregnancy loss grief involve (a) establishing the imagined identity of the deceased baby, as the baby existed in the parent's mind, (b) constructing memories of interactions (for example, ultrasounds, quickening, or, in the event of a stillbirth, holding or seeing the deceased baby), (c) establishing rituals or traditions that help the parent to grieve, and (d) defining how parents can continue their bond with the baby, such as writing letters to the deceased baby or creating a memorial site (Leon, 2015). For example, after a late-term miscarriage, Leah created a memory box that included ultrasound pictures, a picture of her deceased grandmother whom she envisioned was with her baby in heaven, a small Bible, and a Jizo statue, which in Japanese culture represents the soul of the deceased infant or fetus and is also the deity who takes care of children on the other-world journey. Yet, through the process of grieving, often the most important task does not involve "doing" anything, but the therapist being with the client emotionally and joining with the client's sadness (Leon, 2015). For instance, while creating and revisiting the memory box was healing for Leah, being able to share the memory box and what the items within it meant to her with her therapist helped Leah to feel as if something had been "lifted" and ready to move on.

Defining the Loss: A Task to Facilitate Grieving

Before bereaved parents can mourn and move forward, first the client or couple needs to define that which was lost (Leon, 2015). Defining the loss should be a collaborative process in which clients share their experience of loss, the therapist attempts to crystalize and expand upon their understanding of what and/or who was lost, and then the clients correct, edit, or add to the therapist's understanding. During this process, it is important for the therapist to keep in mind that pregnancy loss typically involves multiples losses. How the client or couple defines what or who was lost will vary depending upon the degree to which the parent(s) was invested in the pregnancy, attached to the fetus, and viewed the fetus as an "it" versus a "baby." When the fetus is conceptualized as a baby, bereaved parents have of course lost a baby, but also what the baby represented or symbolized to them

(Leon, 2015). For example, when Mary found out she was pregnant with a girl, she fantasized about having the kind of close relationship with her daughter that she was so deprived of with her own absent mother as a child, thereby working through early childhood trauma. Similarly, Jessica became pregnant immediately after the sudden and traumatic death of her father. The timing of the pregnancy, in combination with finding out the baby was a boy, led Jessica to feel the baby represented a special connection to her deceased father, a connection that was lost all over again when she miscarried. Moreover, the loss of a pregnancy is often layered on top of other associated losses, such as the loss of a parent's hopes and dreams for the future, innocence that a pregnancy will automatically equal a healthy baby, sense of control, femininity or womanhood, identity as a parent, and trust that one's body will function the way it is "supposed to" (Leon, 2015). In couples therapy, each partner may have a different individual experience of what was lost but share a common joint sense of loss. Bill's greatest sense of loss after miscarriage was that his dying father would not live to meet his first grandchild, while his partner Sally, who was an accomplished marathon runner, deeply felt a loss of identity as someone who is in control of one's body, healthy, and physically strong and capable. As a couple, they both mourned their hopes and dreams of becoming a parent to this baby and moving to the next stage of life and adult identity development.

Repairing the Self

Pregnancy loss can be experienced as a huge narcissistic injury and attack on one's self-esteem, self-worth, and gender identity (Leon, 2015). The therapist validating and normalizing the client's experience of loss is an important first step to ultimately restoring self-esteem. Further, as Leon (2015) describes, the therapist and client must work together to define those parts of self and identity that have been injured by the loss of a pregnancy. It is when valued parts of our very self are injured or threatened that our self-esteem suffers. For instance, after experiencing repeated miscarriages of pregnancies achieved through IVF and other invasive medical procedures, Alexa and her doctors concluded that considering a gestational carrier would be the best next step. Alexa was devastated and felt a complete loss of femininity and like she was no longer a real woman. Interestingly, while Alexa was not generally confident in her body and had a history of an eating disorder, she always assumed that being pregnant and going through labor and delivery would be something she would be "really good" at. The inability to maintain a viable pregnancy attacked her sense of self and gender identity as a woman who was capable and "good at" reproduction and represented the loss of a valued part of self.

Often, identifying, clarifying, and understanding these assaults to self-esteem and identity are enough to heal the narcissistic wounds brought about by pregnancy loss (Leon, 2015). For instance, Kylee grew up in a home with two parents who had high standards and expectations for their children. As a result, Kylee's self-esteem was always fragile at best because it was dependent upon her parents' approval, which she constantly felt was lacking. Suffering multiple pregnancy losses was deeply injurious to Kylee's already low self-esteem because these losses were experienced as yet another way she failed to live up to the expectations of her parents, husband, and society. This understanding led Kylee to want to work toward developing a sense of self-esteem based on internal characteristics, rather than external achievements and approval of others, in the therapy. At the same time, the therapist normalizing the fact that pregnancy loss is often experienced as an attack on self-esteem to most affected women helped Kylee to experience these losses as something bad that happened to her and not because of her. This shift helped Kylee to grieve her losses, rather than blaming herself for them. As seen here, it is often critical to the processing of different kinds of traumatic events for the client to move from a stance of blaming oneself to grieving for the self (Courtois, 2020).

Goals and Tasks in Couples Therapy

The therapist should actively pursue, from the very start of treatment, the investment of both individuals within the couple to avoid "split alliances." With heterosexual couples, because the focus of treatment is often placed on the woman, fathers are often the forgotten mourners (Leon, 2015). As one bereaved father once said after he and his wife experienced multiple losses and fertility setbacks, "Just because it didn't happen to me, doesn't mean it didn't affect me." Both partners are in pain and need to be invested in the treatment to feel as if they are in this together and for the therapy to be successful. Thus, it is important for the therapist from the beginning of treatment to align with both partners and pay careful attention to validating the male partner's experience of loss and way of coping with grief, which is often overlooked. Similarly, in same-sex couples, the therapist should validate that both partners are grieving, regardless of who physically carried and/or was genetically tied to the baby they lost. In essence, the therapist's empathic understanding and validation of each partner's experience of loss helps both partners to feel personally invested in the treatment and avoids harmful split alliances. The therapist emphasizing that each partner has valid feelings of grief that need to be acknowledged and worked through in the therapy sets the stage for the overarching therapeutic goal—for the partners to support and understand one another's different way of coping with grief and emotional needs.

Typically, men and women have different ways of coping with loss, which can cause conflict in relationships and mask the degree to which the man is suffering (Leon, 2015; Peterson, 2015). Because men are socialized to express anger over sadness, the male client's suffering may be less overt and is thus often overlooked, and the woman may feel as if she is the only one grieving (Leon, 2015). Men are often coming up against their own feelings of helplessness and powerlessness to save or protect their partner and baby (Leon, 2015). Perhaps because of this, men tend to use more problem-solving and active coping strategies to deal with grief and loss, while women typically want a place to share their sadness and receive emotional validation and support. Sometimes it is helpful for the woman to reframe her male partner's problem-solving strategies as a caring (albeit misattuned) attempt to rescue her from further pain and suffering and as a reflection of his own feelings of helplessness. At the same time, the man may need assurance from the therapist that merely listening will help soothe his partner's sadness, for she will no longer feel alone in her distress, and will not make her feel even worse (Leon, 2015). Although we lack research on ways of coping with grief following a pregnancy loss in same-sex couples, clinical experience suggests that partners in any couple become polarized, to varying degrees, in stressful situations, with one partner "holding" the emotional distress and sadness and the other engaging in more problem-solving behaviors, but more research is needed. These different ways of coping with grief can lead to partners feeling as if their needs are not being met and as if they are adversaries, when, in the therapy, both partners need to work together to feel as if they are not alone in their grief and for the treatment to be successful. The therapist making interventions to increase "shared purpose" and "validate common struggles" (for example, "You both have different ways of grieving, but you are both struggling to grieve") and framing the overall goal of treatment in terms of this shared purpose (for example, "What you both want is for your way of grieving to be validated and respected") helps each partner to respect and understand the other's way of coping with loss and how to best offer support and comfort (see Friedlander et al., 2019; Markin, 2023).

THERAPIST–CLIENT VIGNETTE

Below, specific considerations related to the bond, goal, and task dimensions of the alliance in therapy for pregnancy loss are demonstrated within a hypothetical vignette, with a client named Rose who is pregnant following a fetal death at 28 weeks gestation. In general, pregnancies after loss are characterized by perinatal grief and post-traumatic stress symptoms, depression and anxiety, fear of yet another potential loss, and prenatal attachment problems (see Chapter 2 in this book for a review). Women pregnant after loss typically struggle with how to grieve the loss of a prior baby, while attaching to the subsequent one, all while fearing yet another potential loss (O'Leary, 2004). It is a common clinical mistake to assume that the client's grief is somehow resolved upon a subsequent healthy pregnancy (Markin, 2016). Though common, such a clinical mistake or empathic failure can damage the alliance or prevent it from even getting off the ground. The first part of the vignette below is from an individual therapy session with Rose, while the second part is from a couple's session with Rose and her partner, Roger. While traditionally it was considered a boundary violation to see the couple in treatment when one of the partners is the individual client, in therapy for pregnancy loss, the partner of the individual client is often included since the loss impacts both partners (Leon, 2015).

Individual Session

ROSE: My mother threw a surprise baby shower for me this past week.

THERAPIST: How was that for you?

ROSE: Awful! I was so angry at her the entire time. I was so uncomfortable with all the attention, and everyone commenting on my belly, and saying congratulations. I ended up hiding in the bathroom most of the time. Afterwards, my mom and I got in a huge fight. She yelled, "You don't appreciate anything I do for you." Then, I yelled even louder, "I told you, I didn't want a baby shower!"

THERAPIST: It sounds like you were angry with your mother, but maybe you also felt hurt.

ROSE: Yes. I feel like nothing is for certain. I could lose this pregnancy any day. There are so many things that could go wrong, and I'm struggling to get through every day. So, I think it did hurt my feelings that she was celebrating.

THERAPIST: It feels like she misses how hard this has been for you, and just how much pain the fear of yet another loss is causing you.

ROSE: Exactly! I don't understand how she can celebrate when her daughter is in pain and her grandchild is dead.

THERAPIST: Maybe it feels like you are the only one grieving?

ROSE: Absolutely. Everyone keeps telling me to focus on this pregnancy. Yes, of course I'm grateful for this pregnancy, but every time I have an ultrasound, or go for an OB visit, or even when someone says congratulations on your pregnancy, all I can see is Jordyn [*sobbing*], and I can't get that horrific image of holding him so lifeless out of my head, and I just want to throw up or run away.

THERAPIST: I want to come back to that, that's so incredibly powerful and important, but I just want to check in with you about something first. When you first told me that you were pregnant again, I think I also said "congratulations." I wonder if you maybe had a feeling toward me about that at the time, given everything you've been through? [*Therapist attempts to address possible rupture in the alliance so that the therapeutic bond is strong enough for the client to safely process the trauma and loss of her stillborn baby named Jordyn.*]

ROSE: Well, like I said, I just don't feel pregnant. I mean, I feel like half-pregnant. So, when people say "congratulations," I don't want to hear that because what if I lose this pregnancy too? I feel like other people don't understand that's a real possibility.

THERAPIST: It sounds like with friends and family, and, sometimes, maybe with me in here, you are left feeling like other people just don't understand how unsafe and vulnerable you feel in this pregnancy and how badly you need to protect yourself.

ROSE: Right, but I feel like other people just think I'm being crazy and overdramatic and like I should just appreciate being pregnant now, but I'm *not* being crazy. I used to think pregnancy equals a healthy baby, but that's just not true for me, so when people say "congratulations" it feels like they don't recognize that. *[Client is articulating what was lost, including the loss of a cherished baby and the loss of innocence that a pregnancy equals a healthy baby.]*

THERAPIST: So, when I said "congratulations," I imagine you must have felt invalidated and misunderstood, is that right? *[Therapist invites client feedback and uses empathy to help repair the rupture and build their bond.]*

ROSE: Yes—I mean, I know you didn't mean it that way, but that's how I felt.

THERAPIST: That makes sense to me. I think I really do understand why you felt that way, and I'm glad you are telling me this now. *[Pause]* I agree, my comment was "off" and not at all where you were emotionally. For whatever reason, it does seem hard for us to get in sync with one another around what to talk about in here and maybe how to talk about it. Let's think together about why that may be.

ROSE: OK.

THERAPIST: For me, sometimes I don't have a clear sense of what you need from me because when I do bring up Jordyn, you tend to change the subject, and when I focus on the current pregnancy, you seem uncomfortable. This makes me think that I am missing something important to you and maybe you feel misunderstood when I focus on one baby over another. Does this resonate with you at all? *[Therapist discloses her difficulty collaborating on the goals and tasks of treatment and invites the client's feedback as to what may be transpiring in their relationship.]*

ROSE: Yeah, I can see why that would be confusing. I *do* want to be able to enjoy this pregnancy—you know, get excited for the baby to come, have the baby shower, decorate the nursery, do all the things I once dreamed of doing. But when I start to think of the future with a baby and feel a little excitement or hope, I get panicked, like this could all be ripped away from me again. And, this may sound crazy, but I also feel like it's a betrayal to Jordyn to just move on and replace him with another baby.

THERAPIST: You don't sound crazy at all. Not that I think you would ever betray him, but I understand why you would feel that way *[normalization helps to decrease feeling of shame and inadequacy related to the loss]*. This is really helpful information, because if I understand you correctly it's like, within you, there is this conflict, or struggle, between wanting to hold on to Jordyn, and wanting to look forward to a future with this baby, and it feels like you must choose between two children—which is a horrible feeling. *[Therapist uses normalization, empathy, and validation to build the alliance, as she tries to join or align with the client's understandable ambivalence, which is perhaps one factor that hinders their agreement on tasks and goals.]*

ROSE: Yes, definitely. I guess when you bring up Jordyn, I'm like, wait, I don't want to focus on that because, well, it's painful, and I want to be able to be happy about this baby, but when you bring up this pregnancy, I'm like, wait, what about Jordyn?

THERAPIST: So, this inner conflict gets played out between us, almost like we are working toward competing goals, when really maybe our goal here is to hold both these experiences together so it doesn't feel like such a tug of war inside. Do you think that is a goal that feels right to you, for us to hold both the loss of Jordyn and your hope and connection to this baby? *[Collaboration around the goals and tasks of therapy with a sense that the therapist and client are in this together]*

ROSE: Yes, that would be nice. I just don't know how to do that?

THERAPIST: Sure, that's something we need to figure out together. The other thing, though, is that I don't think you need to feel pressure to feel excited about this pregnancy.

ROSE: I worry about not bonding to this baby. I felt so bonded to Jordyn at this point in the pregnancy.

THERAPIST: I think you will feel bonded to this baby when you are ready. The loss of Jordyn was just so incredibly devastating and traumatic that of course you would approach this pregnancy with a great deal of caution and fear of yet another loss. I don't think you need to feel pressure to feel a certain way about this pregnancy, but I do think there is so much sadness and loss there that needs to be worked through, and I hope we can do some of that work together. *[Collaboration around goals of processing trauma and grief]*

ROSE: [CRYING] I know that is what I need, but how do I do that?

THERAPIST: I think by talking about it when you feel comfortable. *[Establishing task of therapy as client disclosing honestly her experience in order to process trauma and loss]*

ROSE: I don't know where to start?

THERAPIST: If you feel comfortable, maybe start by telling me about that powerful and intense image you described earlier of holding Jordyn in your arms?

ROSE: I'm afraid. I don't know if I can. I've been so alone in my thoughts. I haven't even talked about this with my husband. I'm afraid if I start talking about it, I will fall apart, and I can't for this baby.

THERAPIST: Your feelings and experiences have been very private. Maybe it feels more contained or in your control that way? That's understandable. But I think that if we hold these feelings and memories together, you won't feel so alone, and you will, over time, start to feel better. Is that something that sounds like it would be helpful to you? *[The repair of the rupture and establishment of a stronger therapeutic bond helps the client to feel less alone and isolated and allows the client to feel safe enough to work on other therapy goals, mainly the processing of trauma and loss.]*

ROSE: *[crying]* Yes, well, it all started when I felt a pain in my side . . .

Couple's Session

THERAPIST: Welcome. Can you tell me a little bit about what you hope to accomplish here together today?

ROSE: I want us to be able to communicate better. You know I've been struggling with Jordyn's death and every time I try to talk to Roger about how I feel, he gets very dismissive, and he will say things like, "We just need to focus on the future, and there's no point staying in the past." I feel like he is critical of my depression and anxiety and wants me to just snap out of it, but I can't.

THERAPIST: OK, so let me just ask some questions so I can better understand and then I'll check in with you, Roger. Sound OK to you both? *[Couple nods.]* What do you want or need from Roger in those moments?

ROSE: For him to listen and validate how I feel and share what he is feeling too.

THERAPIST: That's helpful information. You have a clear sense of what you need from Roger. And when you feel he instead dismisses or invalidates you, which of course, Roger, I know is not your intention, how does that make you feel, and how do you then respond to him?

ROSE: Well, it makes me feel guilty that maybe I'm ruining this pregnancy experience for him and like maybe I should be stronger and just more grateful for this pregnancy. It also makes me feel alone. Jordyn was our son. I know he must have feelings about his loss, but he won't talk about it. So, I guess I'll try to get some reaction out of him, but when I don't get anything from him, I'll get frustrated and just go to my room and sleep all day.

THERAPIST: It sounds like you are really looking for more connection with Roger, but when you feel kind of rebuffed by him, you start to criticize yourself and withdraw and feel more depressed. *[Client nods.]* OK, for you, Roger, let's start with what your goal is for today?

ROGER: I'm just here to learn how to better help her. I obviously don't know the right thing to say or do, but I just don't want her to be so sad all the time. We have waited so long for this. I just want her to be able to enjoy it. Rose has talked about having a baby for as long as I've known her, and I don't know how to help her.

THERAPIST: It's hard for you to see her in pain and to feel helpless to do anything about it. I get the sense that comes from a very loving place. *[Therapist uses empathy to "pull in" Roger and to start to build an individual-level alliance with him.]*

ROGER: Yes, I obviously don't want to see her hurting and I feel like I should know what to say to make her feel better, but everything I try just seems to backfire.

THERAPIST: You care about Rose and want to comfort her. It's clear you hate seeing her in pain. So, what do you think gets in the way? Because it seems like you both, on the surface of things, have compatible goals. Rose, you want to receive comfort, and Roger, you want to give it. *[Through empathizing with both partners' experience and highlighting their shared goal, the therapist avoids a split alliance. Framing the problem as an "external" third force that gets in the way of their shared purpose helps to build the within-couple alliance and sense of safety for no one person is to blame.]*

ROSE: I think he wants to comfort me by talking me out of my feelings, but it only has the opposite effect.

THERAPIST: My guess is, Roger, that your intention really is to comfort Rose and that it is very hard for you to see her hurting, so what do you think goes on for you when she wants to talk about her feelings about Jordyn's loss?

ROGER: I guess, I get kind of panicked, like if I say or do the wrong thing, I'm going to let her down and fail her once again.

THERAPIST: "Once again"?

ROGER: *(Choking up)* You know, it was awful being there. Rose had to be induced knowing that Jordyn was, you know, and it was hard, not as hard for me as it was for Rose, but hard to just watch her go through that physically and emotionally and not be able to do anything about it. I should have listened to Rose when she said something didn't feel right. I let everyone down.

THERAPIST: I get the feeling, Rose, that you can connect with Roger around blaming yourself for this devastating loss. *[Therapist highlights shared experience.]*

ROSE: Yes, I had no idea you felt that way. I feel like I failed you and Jordyn. It was my body. I was his mother. He was inside of me, and I lost him *[tearing up]*.

THERAPIST: You both are carrying such guilt and sense of responsibility over Jordyn's death, and it sounds like that guilt or sense of failure has really been eating the both of you up inside. Yet, the two of you have been so alone in these feelings, instead of working them out together. *[Therapist highlights common struggle—i.e., damage to self-esteem and feelings of guilt, shame, and inadequacy left behind by the trauma of loss.]*

ROGER: I just don't want to make her feel worse with my feelings?

THERAPIST: I don't want to speak for you, Rose, so correct me if I'm wrong, but I don't think that will make her feel worse. I think talking about your feelings with each other, in the long run, will make her and you feel better and less alone?

ROSE: I agree, and I think maybe part of the reason it hurts so much when I feel Roger won't talk about Jordyn with me is that I'm afraid he's angry with me and blames me for Jordyn *[sobbing]*. Because I couldn't do anything to pro-tect our baby.

THERAPIST: Is that true, Roger?

ROGER: No, never, not once.

THERAPIST: Can you tell Rose that and look at her?

ROGER: *[Looking at Rose]* Never, in no way have I ever blamed you. If I blame anyone, I blame myself.

ROSE: *[Moving closer to Roger]* There was nothing you could have done. You were the one who sprang into action to plan the funeral and take care of all those details when I was too depressed to even open my eyes, and I can't even imagine how hard that must have been for you. But what you can do for me now is just let me be sad and be sad with me.

ROGER: I can try, but I don't know how to do that exactly. I've always dealt with bad things by moving forward and not dwelling on the past. That's how I was raised.

THERAPIST: It's a real struggle for you to sit with Rose's feelings, but it also seems like you have very strong feelings of loss that maybe you don't always know what to do with.

ROGER: Yes, I think that's true.

THERAPIST: Maybe, Rose, it's easy to miss how Roger is really struggling to manage his own painful feelings and keep it all together right now?

ROSE: Yeah, I always thought he just doesn't feel as deeply as I do, but now I'm beginning to see he is hurting too.

ROGER: Of course I'm grieving Jordyn too. It hurts me that you think I'm not. I just don't know how to express it the way you do.

THERAPIST: We have two people here that are hurting and feel so alone in profound feelings of grief and self-blame. Maybe our goal in here is to help you both feel safe enough in this relationship to come to each other with these feelings, so you aren't so alone in them? *[Therapist frames treatment goal in terms of common experiences and struggles. Roger becomes more invested in therapy, as his goal moves from supporting Rose to processing the loss together.]*

COMMON CHALLENGES TO ESTABLISHING AND MAINTAINING A STRONG ALLIANCE

In early sessions, the most common challenge to establishing an alliance with clients who have suffered a pregnancy loss often lies in the therapist's ability to frame the therapeutic goals in a way that validates the client's loss as real and grief as legitimate. The therapist rushing to "fix" the client's grief, perhaps through solely focusing on action-oriented interventions or disputing "irrational" thoughts, will likely, unintentionally, leave the client feeling as if once again she is alone in her distress, misunderstood, and invalidated. Similarly, "passing over" or ignoring instances of loss altogether will most likely also be experienced as invalidating (Markin, 2016). At the same time, the therapist focusing on client historical insight, personality reconstruction, or early life experiences unrelated to the client's conscious experience of loss will also likely be experienced by the client as unempathetic. When the therapist is either too action-oriented or too insight-oriented, the therapist inadvertently fails to frame the goals and tasks of treatment to meet the client's needs in a way that acknowledges and validates the client's concerns and level of distress. In couples therapy, it is often challenging to establish an alliance with the partner who did not physically lose the pregnancy. The therapist must frame the therapy goals in such a way that helps each partner to feel personally invested in the work of therapy.

CLINICAL IMPLICATIONS

- Build and maintain the alliance throughout therapy. This involves a warm, safe, and trusting emotional bond in which the client feels safe to approach and process feelings of trauma and loss, and in which the client feels understood, decreasing feelings of shame and inadequacy.
- Early on, establish agreement on therapy goals and associated tasks because they reliably predict therapeutic success. In the case of

pregnancy loss, these goals most often involve processing trauma, grieving, and repairing self-esteem. In couples work, helping the couple to better communicate, understand, and validate each other's unique way of coping with trauma and loss is an important goal.

- Therapists should be open to client feedback, especially pertaining to alliance ruptures, and actively collaborate with clients around the goals and tasks of treatment. This empowers clients and helps them to feel a sense of agency and control, contrary to prior experiences.
- In couples therapy, while in some ways it is natural to focus on the woman (or in lesbian couples the partner who "carried") because the loss most often involved her body, therapists should avoid split alliances by focusing on shared purpose and common experience. The goal is not to eradicate grief, but to help the couple talk about it in such a way that makes them feel as if they are in this together and not alone.

4

Empathy in Psychotherapy for Pregnancy Loss

Undoing Aloneness, Healing Narcissistic Wounds, and Processing Trauma and Grief

Psychotherapy for pregnancy loss and other reproductive traumas is all at once incredibly complex and surprisingly simple. The seeming simplicity of this kind of work lies in the fact that, typically, the therapist is not called to "fix" some chronic client problem, or even to "cure" a diagnosable mental disorder, but rather to facilitate the normal and adaptive process of grieving the loss of an attachment object (Bowlby, 1980). The process of grieving, or mourning, is inherently interpersonal (Littlewood, 1996) and can only unfold within a supportive and caring relationship in which empathy is felt and expressed by a caring other, and experienced and internalized by the bereaved person. Unfortunately, grieving parents often experience a famine of empathy from society at large (Markin & Zilcha-Mano, 2018), and thus come to therapy with an aching hunger for therapist empathy, devouring even crumbs of understanding (Diamond & Diamond, 2017). In one sense, the fact that an empathic relationship appears to be fundamental to the success of treatment (Leon, 2015, 2017) suggests that the process should be relatively straightforward; after all, empathy is supposedly fundamental to all good therapies (Frank, 1971; Rogers, 1957). Empathic understanding of the loss of a loved one is not necessarily something that even requires special training. Yet, it is anything but straightforward or easy to truly empathize with a bereaved parent's experience of trauma and loss; to see real-life pictures of a mother's stillborn baby, so small he could fit in the palm of her hand; to hear the horrific physical details of her miscarriage and to not turn away in disgust, as she describes to you bleeding out her baby; to feel all the longing and desperation she carries to hold a baby she never even had the chance to meet; or to grasp the complexities involved in a couple's decision to terminate a wanted pregnancy due to the diagnosis of a genetic anomaly, as they tentatively share with you their experience of signing on the dotted line to have

Psychotherapy for Pregnancy Loss. Rayna D. Markin, Oxford University Press. © Oxford University Press 2024.
DOI: 10.1093/oso/9780197693353.003.0004

a procedure that will rid them of a baby they would do anything to protect; all while the client's very self is at its most fragile, broken apart by overwhelming guilt and shame. From this, a deceptively simple task of psychotherapy for pregnancy loss is to provide an empathic relationship in which the naturally adaptive process of mourning can unfold.

This chapter begins with a brief empirical review of empathy in psychotherapy. Evidence-based relationship principles derived from research on empathy in psychotherapy are then applied to the treatment of clients who have specifically suffered a pregnancy loss. Based on theory and research, the author describes how various aspects of empathy can help undo the client's sense of aloneness, heal narcissistic injuries that resulted from the loss, and process trauma and grief. Therapist–client vignettes derived from an amalgamation of real-life clinical experiences are given to demonstrate the application of these concepts. Finally, common challenges to empathy in therapy for pregnancy loss and clinical implications are discussed.

CASE VIGNETTE: EMPATHY

Emily is a 32-year-old married female with no living children who presented to treatment after losing three consecutive pregnancies for unknown reasons. She expressed a great deal of caution and hesitancy in starting treatment, rescheduling sessions several times before coming in for an initial session. She explained that she already tried two previous therapists to help cope with her multiple losses. Emily stated,

> The first therapist seemed like he was trying to get me to see that my baby was just a bunch of cells [tearful and angry], and that if I could think about it more logically that way I wouldn't feel so sad. Then, the second therapist . . . it felt like all she wanted to do was go back to my childhood and see what other bad things my miscarriages reminded me of. I know she was probably trying to be helpful, but it just felt so irrelevant to me, like she didn't get how devastated I was feeling right then.

The lack of understanding and empathy that Emily experienced from these previous therapists may have been the result of several factors, including a lack of therapist experience and training with these issues, the widespread cultural denial of the significance of pregnancy loss, and/or the personal anxiety that tends to be triggered by traumatic loss in many people, including therapists, which can lead to defensive minimization. It could have also been the case that Emily's own self-critical voice filtered whatever these therapists were actually saying, distorting the intention of the message. While a combination of *interactional factors* most likely led to Emily feeling misunderstood in these prior therapy relationships, the important point is that she did not *feel* empathized with and thus dropped out of treatment. Further, the lack of empathy she experienced with these prior therapists rubbed salt on a pre-existing wound because it mirrored the lack of understanding and support that she experienced from family, friends, and certain medical providers, who told her that miscarriages happen all the time, that she should relax, and that she will get pregnant again, leaving her to feel alone and misunderstood.

With all of this in mind, the therapist began treatment by acknowledging that it would make sense to her if it felt hard for Emily to be vulnerable and to trust her in the therapy, given Emily's prior experiences feeling misunderstood and dismissed in relationships. The therapist validated that while these situations and interactions are often complicated, it is typically difficult for grieving parents to feel understood and supported by important others, which can make it hard to grieve the loss of a pregnancy/baby. The therapist explicitly acknowledged Emily's losses as real and her grief as legitimate. These initial acknowledgments and validations helped to build trust and rapport. One important event in the therapy occurred when Emily disclosed that she underwent a D&E procedure after her last miscarriage. She stated that while she believed this was the right healthcare decision, the experience of the procedure left her feeling out of control and violated. The therapist empathizing with how scary that must have been ultimately helped Emily to feel safe enough to disclose that as a teenager she was raped by a stranger in a parking lot. Emily never told anyone about the assault and just pretended like nothing happened for fear that others would blame her. The therapist tried to understand Emily's experience of pregnancy loss in context of this aspect of her personal history. She suggested that Emily's experience of feeling ashamed (Emily's fear of being blamed for the rape and later for her miscarriages can be seen as both a projection of her feelings of shame and as a response to social stigma around rape and pregnancy loss being the "woman's fault"), and alone and misunderstood after the loss of her unborn babies, and of feeling out of control and violated during the D&E, perhaps resurrected similar feelings connected to the sexual assault. This gave Emily a new perspective on her present experience.

Over the course of treatment, with the help of the therapist's moment-to-moment empathic attunement, Emily was able to process the trauma and grieve the losses associated with both her past assault and more recent miscarriages, through telling her story and having it acknowledged, understood, and validated. Within 12 sessions, Emily reported feeling sad, but not depressed, and less alone. She reported feeling less defective, or as if there was something shameful or wrong with her that caused these bad things to happen. Emily experienced her therapist as someone who genuinely liked, valued, and understood her, which counteracted her feelings of shame and helped her to grieve. As Emily explained,

> Beating myself up about all the things I could have done to cause or prevent my miscarriages was taking up all the space in my brain. When I stopped listening to that self-critical voice for just a second and heard the understanding in my therapist's voice, I realized just how sad I really was. I thought, "It's not that I am bad, I just feel bad."

EMPATHY: AN EVIDENCE-BASED RELATIONSHIP PRINCIPLE

Empathy and Outcome

Like other relationship principles, research has yet to examine the association between empathy and therapy outcome with pregnancy loss clients specifically. However, there is an impressive body of literature on empathy and therapy outcome with other client populations from which to draw. Several meta-analyses suggest that empathy is a consistent predictor of outcome (Bohart et al., 2002; Elliott et al., 2011). A recent meta-analysis found that empathy is a moderately strong predictor of outcome for 82 independent samples and 6,138 clients, regardless of therapist experience level, length of treatment, and client presenting problems (Elliott et al., 2019). While results from this meta-analysis found that empathy generally predicts outcome across theoretical orientation, empathy was found to be a little more important in CBT treatments. This finding is surprising given that client-centered and psychoanalytic theories (particularly contemporary relational psychoanalysis) have historically emphasized empathy as a central change mechanism (Kaluzeviciute & Walla, 2020), whereas CBT has focused on using empathy to build rapport as a basis for the rest of the work (Elliott et al., 2019). Still, the experience of feeling understood appears to be a universal relationship principle that is important to outcome across theoretical orientations and client populations (Elliott et al., 2019).

Although research is sparse in this area, some studies lend more direct evidence that empathy is important to the process and outcome of therapy specifically for pregnancy loss. For example, qualitative results from a single case study of psychodynamic therapy for a client pregnant after loss suggest that the therapist's empathy and validation of the client's grief as real, and of her experience of isolation and loneliness post-loss, were curative factors in psychotherapy, perhaps contributing to diminished pregnancy-specific anxiety, trauma, and grief (Markin & McCarthy, 2020). Similarly, empathic support by medical providers seems important to the resolution of grief and improved self-worth after pregnancy termination due to a fetal anomaly (Geerinck-Vercammen & Kanhai, 2003; Lafarge et al., 2014), perinatal loss (Gold, 2007), and miscarriage (Swanson-Kaufman, 1986). Empathy may be especially important to pregnancy loss clients because of the lack of understanding these clients may experience in relationships outside of therapy and because of the damage to self-esteem brought about by a pregnancy loss.

A related concept to that of empathy is positive regard. Invoking Rogers' conceptualization of positive regard, Farber et al. (2018) define it as the "therapist's affective attitude toward his or her clients" that is characterized by "warmth, liking, affirmation, nonpossessive love, and affection" (p. 292). In their meta-analysis of 64 studies and 369 effect sizes, comprising 3,528 clients, an aggregate effect size of $g = .28$ between positive regard and outcome was found, suggesting a moderate yet significant contribution to outcome. Positive regard may be particularly important for clients who have suffered a pregnancy loss. For these clients, experiencing their therapist as liking and affirming them may counteract feelings of shame and inadequacy brought about by a pregnancy loss. This is exemplified in the case vignette above in which Emily's feelings of shame and inadequacy decreased as she came to experience her therapist as someone who genuinely liked and accepted her, which helped Emily to see her miscarriages as something "bad" that happened to her and not because of her.

Empathy Defined

Despite the notable body of research on empathy, researchers have long struggled with how to best define it (Elliott et al., 2019). Recently, research in the field of neuroscience has led to a more sophisticated understanding of empathic processes. In general, neuroscience research suggests that empathy can be separated into three major subprocesses, each involving specific parts of the brain (see Elliott et al., 2019). These subprocesses range from a relatively automatic and intuitive, body-based emotional mirroring, which takes place in the limbic system (Decety & Lamm, 2009; Goubert et al., 2009), to a more conscious, conceptual, and cognitive perspective-taking process that is localized in the prefrontal and temporal cortex (Shamay-Tsoory, 2009). While research has found that the conscious-conceptual aspects of empathy do not highly correlate with the intuitive-emotional elements of empathy (Duan & Kivlighan, 2002; Hein & Singer, 2010), skilled therapists probably coordinate both (Elliott et al., 2019). Thus, from neuroscience research, we know that empathy is not a single and uniform concept, but one involving multiple subprocesses that are both emotional and intuitive, as well as conscious and verbal, which may operate independently of each other or work in concert.

Empathic Modes and Type of Understanding

Consistent with this, Elliott and colleagues have derived a more concise and evidence-based definition of empathy, arguing that empathy is a higher-order category under which different subtypes, aspects, and modes can be nested (Elliott et al., 2019). Specifically, they distinguish between three main modes of therapist empathy: *empathic rapport* (the therapist shows a benevolent compassionate attitude toward the client and tries to show understanding of the client's experience [Elliott et al., 2019]), *communicative attunements* (active efforts to stay attuned on a moment-to-moment basis with the client's communications and unfolding experience [Elliott et al., 2019]), and *person empathy* (a sustained effort to understand the historical and present context or background of a client's current experiencing [Elliott et al., 2004]). Additionally, each one of these three empathic modes may involve emotional and/or cognitive aspects. In the pregnancy loss literature, Irving Leon has written extensively about the role of empathy in psychotherapy (Leon, 2010, 2015, 2017). Like the types of empathic understanding (affective and cognitive) suggested by Elliott et al. (2019), he argues that empathy involves *emotionally resonating* with the client's affective experience, as well as *cognitively* seeing the world from another's perspective (Leon, 2010, 2015, 2017).

Empathic Interventions

The therapist's cognitive and/or affective understanding can be viewed as an intrapsychic variable that may or may not be outwardly expressed or communicated by the therapist. There are many ways of expressing empathy (explicitly and/or implicitly), including therapist nonverbal behaviors (e.g., head nods, tone and rhythm of voice, body language) and therapist techniques or interventions. Some of these empathic interventions include *empathic reflections* (conveying understanding of the client's experience), *empathic affirmations* (attempts by the therapist to validate the client's perspective), *empathic questions, experience-near interpretations, nonverbal expression, evocative reflections* (attempts to bring the client's experience alive in session using rich, evocative, concrete language), and *process reflections and empathic conjectures* (going beyond exploratory reflections in that these interventions guide or infer what clients might be feeling but have not stated out loud) (Elliott et al., 2019). These are examples of therapist interventions that have been used in popular empathy training programs (see Elliott et al., 2004, and Johnson et al., 2005, for more information).

Empathy as a Relational Concept

Empathy can be understood as an interactional variable to which both the therapist and client contribute (Elliott et al., 2019). For example, therapists who demonstrate more cognitive complexity and are more open to conflictual countertransference feelings have been found to be perceived by clients as more empathic (Henschel & Bohart, 1981; Peabody & Gelso, 1982). Many therapists are attracted to infertility and pregnancy loss work because of their own experiences with loss. Thus, the ability to identify and manage countertransference feelings when working with pregnancy loss clients is imperative to utilizing these shared experiences to enhance empathy without overly identifying with the client (Leon, 2017). At the same time, clients who are more open to communicating their inner experience will be easier to empathize with (Elliott et al., 2019). For instance, clients who are securely attached have been found to self-disclose more (Shechtman & Dvir, 2006), whereas clients with an insecure attachment self-disclose less and engage in less adaptive self-disclosures (Mikulincer & Nachshon, 1991; Shechtman & Dvir, 2006), perhaps making these clients more difficult to empathize with. Referring to pregnancy loss clients specifically, Leon (2015) suggests that clients with an adverse attachment history may struggle with experiencing and internalizing therapist empathy because of their insecure internal working models. It is critical in such situations that the therapist remains responsive and flexible to what a given client perceives as empathic (Hatcher, 2015; Owen & Hilsenroth,

2014). For instance, clients with an anxious attachment might perceive therapist soothing, mirroring, and validation as empathic, whereas clients with an avoidant attachment may experience more concrete and structured interventions as empathic (see Chapters 8 and 9 in this book). Supporting this, one study found that more anxious clients rate the alliance higher in interpersonal-dynamic groups but not in CBT groups (Tasca et al., 2007).

CLINICAL APPLICATION: EMPATHIC GOALS AND INTERVENTIONS FOR PREGNANCY LOSS

Below, how the various aspects of empathy can be used to undo aloneness, heal narcissistic wounds (i.e., restore self-esteem and self-worth), and resolve grief and trauma is discussed and illustrated in hypothetical vignettes that are derived from an amalgamation of clinical experience. These goals generally occur in tandem and should not be thought of as completely discrete. Additionally, processing trauma and grief/loss and restoring self-esteem are distal outcomes to treatment, while undoing aloneness is a proximal outcome. For each of the three therapeutic goals, types of empathic understanding (affective/cognitive), empathic modes (empathic rapport, communicative attunement, personal empathy), and empathic interventions are demonstrated in therapist–client vignettes and identified in italics, using the following codes: type of empathic understanding, EU; empathic mode, EM; empathic interventions, EI).

EMPATHY: THE UNDOING OF ISOLATION AND ALONENESS

Clients who have suffered a pregnancy loss typically enter treatment accustomed to family and friends minimizing and/or avoiding their grief (Covington, 2005; Diamond & Diamond, 2016; Leon, 2015). Although grieving parents look to family and friends to understand and share their sadness, support persons may respond with such clichés as *it wasn't meant to be*; *just think positive*; *time heals all wounds*; *don't worry, you'll get pregnant again*; or *you just need to relax*. Such comments, although well meaning, minimize or deny parents their experience of grief and invalidate their loss as real (Lang et al., 2011). Miscarriage in particular is seen as a "non-event" and the fetus as a "non-person" (Frost & Condon, 1996). Consistent with this, perinatal grief, or a parent's emotional reaction following a pregnancy loss, has been likened to Doka's (1989) concept of *disenfranchised grief*, which is used to describe an experience of loss not openly acknowledged, publicly mourned, or socially supported. In Western society, pregnancy loss is not typically viewed as a legitimate type of loss and expressing feelings of perinatal grief is considered taboo (Layne, 2003; Markin & Zilcha-Mano, 2018). Without culturally defined and accepted mourning rituals for the loss of a pregnancy, as there are for other losses, parents feel they have no outlet through which to mourn

(Lang et al., 2011; Layne, 2003). The fact that a parent's grief reaction is not only misunderstood but also actively discouraged complicates the mourning process and leaves parents feeling isolated and alone (Lang et al., 2011; Layne, 2003; Markin & Zilcha-Mano, 2018).

Empathy, from a caring and trusted other, undoes isolation and aloneness and facilitates the grieving process (Leon, 2015). According to attachment theory, it is a universal human response to turn toward others during times of grief and loss for support and comfort (Bowlby, 1980). From this perspective, when close others are not available to mirror and understand our overwhelming affective experiences, then these feelings and experiences are denied or distorted. Thus, the process of mourning is thwarted without close relationships in which we can share, contain, and make sense of our experience (Bowlby, 1980). *Affective empathy*, or the therapist emotionally resonating with the client's sadness, helps clients feel safe to approach feelings of grief and loss, for they no longer feel as if they are carrying their overwhelming pain alone (Leon, 2015, 2017). *Cognitive empathy* is believed to help bereaved parents to feel understood, genuinely "seen," and less alone (Leon, 2017). The therapist understanding and validating the client's loss as real and grief as legitimate facilitates mourning and heals the scars of social exclusion (Leon, 2017). What is understood and accepted is no longer shameful, threatening, or taboo (Diamond & Diamond, 2017; Leon, 2017). Cognitive empathy and validation of the client's perspective is vitally important to bereaved parents. Essentially, cognitive and affective empathy, through different avenues, lessens the client's sense of isolation and aloneness, which is a desirable outcome in itself and a means to other important treatment goals, such as processing trauma and grief and restoring self-esteem (Leon, 2017).

The vignette below demonstrates how therapist empathy can undo feelings of isolation and aloneness for a client who is seeking treatment due to feelings of loss, guilt, and depression after a PTFA. Leon (2017) discusses how social stigma around PTFA makes empathy particularly difficult to come by for these clients, as this kind of loss is usually misunderstood and stigmatized because it has no clear category. It is sometimes linked to elective abortion because it is the same medical procedure, but it is different in that it is defined as the termination of a much-wanted yet unhealthy child. Other times, PTFA is linked to miscarriage, yet it differs in that PTFA involves additional tasks, including deciding whether or not to terminate the pregnancy (Leon, 2017).

EVE: I want you to know I would never choose to have an abortion. I am completely pro-choice. I would never judge anyone who decided to do that. But I wanted this baby. Her name was Elyse.

THERAPIST: *[speaking slowly and softly]* As we talk today, it's going to be important that I really understand and keep in mind how much you wanted and loved Elyse. She was your little baby.

EVE: Yes, yes.

THERAPIST: I also hear some question or concern over whether you will be judged in here; is that right? *[Therapist attempts to build empathic rapport*

(EM) and to communicatively attune (EM) to Eve's unfolding experience in the room. On one level, the therapist demonstrates cognitive empathy (ET) through reflecting back to the client her experience from her perspective. At the same time, through doing so, the therapist begins to connect with the client on an emotional, nonverbal level, and to emotionally resonate (ET) with her sadness and loss. For example, the therapist holds in mind the lost baby as a person, as "Elyse," as the client does in hers, so that the client is not entirely alone in remembering the lost baby.]

EVE: Yes, I think that's true. It's hard for me to find anyone to talk to about this because it doesn't feel like anyone understands. It's really frustrating to me when other people assume that I didn't want Elyse because she wasn't developing right, because that's not true! In our situation, the doctors said there was very little chance of her surviving full term. I did consider carrying to full term, but the thought of giving birth to a baby that wasn't alive—I just couldn't. Maybe that makes me weak, but I just couldn't.

THERAPIST: I don't think that makes you weak at all. As I was listening to you, I was thinking how difficult it must have been to struggle with such a serious and difficult decision. *[EI; empathic affirmation and validation; self-disclosure to communicate empathy. The therapist empathizing with and validating the client's struggle that is often stigmatized and misunderstood in society helps the client to feel less alone and ashamed.]*

EVE: Thank you.

THERAPIST: I also hear that it's been difficult to feel so misunderstood *[client nods]. [EI; empathic reflection]* What has been the hardest part about that? *[EI; empathic question]*

EVE: I think probably just feeling so alone. I miss Elyse. Sometimes when I first wake up in the morning, for a second, I forget. I reach down to rub my belly only to remember she's not there anymore and it hits me like a ton of bricks all over again. I tried to tell my sister this the other day, to explain to her what it's like. We are very close and usually she gets me, but not this time. I know she was trying to comfort me, but she was like, "I know how you feel. I had a miscarriage." I wanted to scream, "No, you don't know how I feel! I wish I had a miscarriage, then I wouldn't have had to make that awful decision!" I just wanted to shake her! Like, "Why don't you understand? Where are you? Open your eyes!" I know my sister is trying her best to understand and support me; it's just hard to understand what it's like to go through something like this until you are forced to go through it yourself.

THERAPIST: I hear such longing and desperation in your voice. *[EI; empathic conjecture]* Like you really want to reach out for your baby, to touch her, to connect with her again, and, in the same way, to reach out and grab your sister, to bring her back to you so she can understand so you won't feel so alone. *[EI; evocative reflection; EM; communicative attunement; EU; affective empathy]*

EVE: Yeah, you could say I'm pretty sad and lonely, but I kind of brought that on myself. I mean, I do kind of push my sister away when I feel she doesn't understand me; I just feel so angry that she gets the luxury of not under-standing what it's like to be in this awful position—not just her, but people in general.

THERAPIST: So, yeah, you are angry, angry over being forced to be in this ter-rible situation and angry that other people don't have to experience this the way you have, and it seems like that anger makes you feel even more isolated? *[EI; experience-near interpretation]*

EVE: I think so, like sometimes when I am feeling especially sad and want to call my sister, I stop myself because I'm like, "What's the point? She won't understand anyway," and then I'm back to being angry. Like I know it sounds awful, but why me? Not that I would want this to happen to someone else, but why me?

THERAPIST: It sounds like it has been hard to process your loss through all the feelings of anger and isolation.

EVE: Yes, but do I deserve to grieve? It was me who went into that hospital room and saw the heartbeat on the monitor. It's awful. You go in and you hope for a heartbeat because that's instinct. At the same time, you hope you don't hear it, so you don't need to make such an awful decision. But I heard it, and I still told the doctor to go ahead with the procedure. Then they put me to sleep, and I woke up with no baby. I didn't even need to see it happen. I got out of it.

THERAPIST: Given all you've struggled with, I would hardly say you got out of anything.

EVE: But what kind of mother am I?

THERAPIST: The kind who loves her baby very much and was faced with a pro-foundly difficult decision. You were forced to make a decision not that you wanted, but to avoid something that was even worse. *[EU; cognitive empathy, or understanding of the client's experience of terminating a much-wanted child, which helps the client to feel less alone and ashamed; affective empathy, or resonating with the torment of making such a difficult decision]*

EVE: *[Sobbing and looking straight at the therapist with almost pleading eyes]* It just hurts so much!

THERAPIST: The pain of losing Elyse feels so heavy, like a ton of bricks. *[EI; evoc-ative reflection, using client's language from earlier]* I think, though, that we can look at that hurt together and then it won't feel quite as heavy. Maybe you can even give some of those bricks to me to hold. *[Therapist attempts to emotion-ally resonate (EU; affective empathy) and share the client's sadness to undo her sense of aloneness and process trauma and grief]*

HEALING NARCISSISTIC WOUNDS: COUNTERACTING SHAME AND RESTORING SELF-ESTEEM

Parents who experience pregnancy loss almost always feel defective or inferior, unable to do what it seems like everyone else in the world can do: have a normal pregnancy and a healthy child (Diamond & Diamond, 2017). A woman may feel as if she has failed to do the one thing she was made or born to do and is not really a woman (Diamond & Diamond, 2016, 2017). These women may question who they are and how they fit into the world since society does not yet recognize them as a mother, but they no longer feel like a single woman (Côté-Arsenault & Brody, 2009; Layne, 2003; Markin & Zilcha-Mano, 2018). Valued parts of their identity as a parent and as a "real" woman may feel stolen. Because of the massive blow to self-esteem and identity brought upon by a pregnancy loss, clients often present to treatment in a narcissistically fragile condition, meaning that they have little self-esteem to buffer feelings of shame and inadequacy, are highly self-critical, and experience others as similarly attacking, critical, and wounding (Leon, 2010). Grieving parents are forced to rebuild the self at the same time they are grieving the loss of a baby (Diamond & Diamond, 2017; Leon, 2015). In psychotherapy for pregnancy loss, healing narcissistic wounds and restoring the client's self-esteem is a therapeutic goal in itself, as well as a means to facilitate the grieving process (Diamond & Diamond, 2017; Leon, 2010, 2015). The client feeling understood, validated, and cared for by the therapist helps her to internalize and solidify a more benign and compassionate sense of self (counteracting shame and restoring self-esteem). It is from this more stable and compassionate sense of self that the client can then grieve the loss (Leon, 2010), as demonstrated in the vignette below.

Empathic Modes

The therapist's empathic attunement, validation, and affirmation help to heal narcissistic wounds left behind by the loss of a pregnancy (Diamond & Diamond, 2017; Leon, 2015, 2017). Below, the author theorizes how different empathic modes (Elliott et al., 2019) increase client self-esteem and solidify the client's sense of self and identity, while regulating shame and inadequacy, following pregnancy loss, in specific yet related ways. First, *empathic rapport*, or the therapist's attitude of compassion and benevolence and of a genuine desire to understand the client's perspective, serves as a counter to the client's harsh internal self-critical voice and constant sense of inadequacy. Because these clients are temporarily in a narcissistically fragile state, even benign comments made by the therapist may "sting" and feel like an attack on the client's self. There is often an interaction effect that occurs wherein these clients feel especially sensitive to criticism and attack from others because they themselves feel so fundamentally inadequate and broken, and, at the same time, because of the widespread societal invalidation of perinatal loss, even well-intentioned others are indeed unknowingly insensitive and perhaps dismissive or minimizing of their feelings and experiences.

The therapist's benevolence, compassion, and curiosity about the client's subjective experience, once internalized by the client, supports her self-esteem and sense of self (Leon, 2010). Empathic rapport may be particularly important at the beginning of treatment to the establishment of an alliance, allowing the client to engage in the work of therapy despite her sense of shame. Once the client feels as if someone can understand and feel compassion for her, it becomes difficult to feel as if she is entirely defective or abnormal.

Second, the therapist's moment-to-moment empathic attunement to the client's emerging experience over time, or *communicative attunement*, ultimately repairs the self, reducing shame and empowering and validating the client (Leon, 2010, 2017). This process unfolds in the space between client and therapist, as the therapist reflects back to the client an image of the client that is more realistic, internally derived, and less shame-induced. And, the client internalizes the therapist's empathic attunement, replacing self-criticism with self-understanding or insight, judgment with compassion, and a sense of worth that is derived from what one can accomplish (in this case, the birth of a healthy child) with a sense of self that is internally derived (for example, the fact that one is a loving and a committed parent, irrespective of one's reproductive capacity). Communicative attunements are particularly important when clients tell their story of reproductive loss. The therapist listening to the details of the client's loss experience with genuine interest, holding and tolerating both the pain and the horror without judgment, fear, or disgust, helps the client to feel less "defective, abnormal, and ashamed" (Diamond & Diamond, 2017, p. 375). What the client thinks is unspeakable, un-understandable, and intolerable becomes speakable, relatable, and tolerable, and therefore less shameful and threatening (Diamond & Diamond, 2017). Lastly, *person empathy* helps to understand how the client characteristically maintains self-esteem and how this has been disrupted by pregnancy loss. Therapists need to have empathy for the fact that the typical ways in which a client maintains self-esteem may no longer work after a pregnancy loss because of the magnitude of the trauma.

Affective and Cognitive Empathy

Healing narcissistic wounds probably involves aspects of both affective and cognitive empathy. On an affective level, when the therapist emotionally resonates or connects with the client without feeling overwhelmed or disgusted, then the client feels less *overwhelming* because someone else was able to hold and tolerate her feelings; she feels less *disgusting*, for a trusted other has taken in her deepest feelings and experiences without rejection or hesitation. Sometimes fully understanding a client's experience of loss involves "tuning in" to the music behind the lyrics and grasping dimensions of the client's experience that they have not yet verbalized or acknowledged but that the therapist intuits (Leon, 2015, 2017). On a cognitive level, when clients feel as if the therapist understands their experience or perspective, then they feel worthy of being understood. A conceptual or cognitive understanding of the client's perspective can lead to normalizing and validating the client's experience, which can bolster self-esteem. Importantly, both affective and cognitive understanding lifts clients out of their sense of aloneness, mitigating shame and improving self-esteem (Diamond & Diamond, 2017; Leon, 2010). The vignette below demonstrates how these different aspects of empathy can be used to heal narcissistic wounds for a client who, after multiple losses via IVF, is considering egg donation.

DIMIRA: I can't believe this happened to me again. I guess I should expect it by now. I'm so stupid.

THERAPIST: You aren't stupid at all. Of course you are in shock. No matter how many times a mother loses a child, it never hurts any less or is any easier to grapple with. *[EI; empathic affirmation; the therapist normalizes and validates to regulate the client's shame. Through doing so, he maintains an empathic rapport (EM), offering a benign and compassionate voice to counter the client's self-critical one.]*

DIMIRA: I just feel so embarrassed!

THERAPIST: It must be so hard to feel that way right now when you just suffered such a devastating loss. *[EI; empathic conjecture]* What's the most embarrassing part? *[EI; empathic question]*

DIMIRA: I guess that I thought I could actually do this. Who was I kidding? I feel like everyone is laughing at me. Like, "See? We always knew there was something wrong with you!" What kind of woman can't have a baby? I can't even look my husband in the eye anymore. I feel so guilty that he got stuck with me. But I can't stop. I keep pressing him for another round of IVF, even though in my gut I know it's not going to work. Even the doctor is now saying we should really consider egg donation.

THERAPIST: It sounds like the doctor advising egg donation really hurt you. It really stung. *[client crying]* It feels devastating. *[EI; empathic conjecture; EU; affective empathy (therapist resonates with narcissistic wound inflicted by medical advice to consider egg donation)]*

DIMIRA: It felt like he was punching me in the gut. I couldn't breathe. I feel so defective.

THERAPIST: There is so much shame there and such a strong self-critical voice that really takes some big punches at you when you are at your most vulnerable. There is also so much hurt and loss right behind that. *[EI; empathic conjecture; EM; communicative attunement]*

DIMIRA: *[crying]* You don't understand. It's my fault. The reason we can't conceive is because of my defective eggs.

THERAPIST: This feels so personal. It doesn't feel like there is something wrong with your reproductive system; it feels like there is something wrong with *you* that cuts right to the core of who you are. *[EM; communicative attunement; EI; experience-near interpretation]*

DIMIRA: Yeah, I don't feel like myself anymore. I'm a person who has always worked hard and been successful. Every goal I've ever had for myself I've reached because I worked until I reached that goal, no matter what. That hasn't happened with this, and I don't even know who I am anymore.

THERAPIST: You are incredibly hard-working and persistent and that's really served you well in life. I think your work ethic and capacity to persist despite the obstacles have given you the strength to endure through all these traumatic losses and medical procedures. When a lot of other people would have given up, you are still fighting to have a baby because you are at your core a fighter. *[EM; person empathy; the therapist understands that being "successful" is an important way in which the client has historically maintained self-esteem and that this part of her identity is currently threatened due to infertility and loss. He attempts to reframe her experience of loss not as proof of her failure but of her persistence and resilience.]*

DIMIRA: Yeah, I guess I didn't think of it that way. I know rationally I should not do another round of IVF, but it's so hard for me to give up and agree to egg donation.

THERAPIST: It makes complete sense to me that emotionally it is hard to let go of the dream of having a genetic link to your child. It is another loss on top of all the other losses you have suffered that needs to be grieved. *[EI; experience-near interpretation; EU; cognitive empathy]*

DIMIRA: It really is a loss for me. I didn't think of it that way before *[getting teary-eyed]*.

THERAPIST: Try and stay with those feelings of sadness coming up for you. *[EU; affective empathy; therapist emotionally resonates with client's sadness and attempts to deepen her emotional experience]*

DIMIRA: *[crying]* I just feel so ungrateful. Shouldn't I just appreciate having a baby no matter how that baby is conceived?

THERAPIST: You can feel grateful for your baby and sad that it didn't happen the way you hoped or dreamed. It's not an either/or.

DIMIRA: You don't think it would make me a phony or like less of a mother?

THERAPIST: No, I don't. But what's important is how *you* define being a mother.

DIMIRA: I guess to love your child no matter what, to accept them and care for them.

THERAPIST: And would you do that for a baby that wasn't genetically linked to you?

DIMIRA: Of course I would!

THERAPIST: You didn't even hesitate there.

DIMIRA: Because I guess it's still a part of me, like that mom part that loves your baby no matter what; that's kind of nice to know that part is still there.

THERAPIST: There is nothing wrong or "defective" *[therapist uses client's language to describe her eggs from earlier in the session]* with the quality of your love as a mother; that can't be taken away from you. *[With the client's self-esteem and identity now more intact, the therapist and client can turn toward helping her grieve the loss of a genetic link to her future child as well as the loss of prior pregnancies.]*

Of note, the progress that the client in the above vignette demonstrates may in many cases take longer in therapy to achieve than displayed here. This is partly because, initially, the client's sense of self is often in a state of disorganization and fragmentation that disrupts her capacity to "take in" or "hear" therapist empathy and/or multiple or different perspectives. Often, empathic interventions in the beginning of therapy serve mostly to repair the client's overall fragmentation and consolidate the client's sense of self. Later in treatment, more restorative empathic interventions can be made and tolerated by the client (D. Diamond, personal communication, February 23, 2020).

PROCESSING TRAUMA AND GRIEF: HEALING AND GROWING FROM THE HORROR OF LOSS

Perinatal grief is complicated by the fact that the loss is often experienced as a traumatic event by bereaved parents (see Chapter 2). Because of this, perinatal grief has been conceptualized as a type of *traumatic grief*, which generally involves an abrupt or unexpected loss that is so devastating that it overwhelms or surpasses the mind's usual ways of coping with distress and of making sense of the world (see Neria & Litz, 2004, for a review). The experience of a pregnancy loss is often so shocking, devastating, and overwhelming that the mind does not possess adequate resources (coping mechanisms, defenses) to process and integrate the experience. Trauma theory (Herman, 1992) suggests that when the amount of stress engendered by some traumatic event exceeds one's ability to cope or to integrate the emotions involved in the experience, the mind, to survive, splits off the emotions from the experience. Overwhelmed, the mind cannot tolerate, process, or think about the emotions related to the trauma in an organized and coherent manner (Herman, 1992). This complicates the grieving process for bereaved parents who are challenged with the task of mourning just as their usual capacity to process and integrate experience is compromised due to trauma (Markin, 2018). It is important for clinicians to have empathy into the fact that the overwhelming distress surrounding the loss may surpass the client's usual ways of coping, causing much anxiety and disorganization (Leon, 2010, 2015). An empathic therapy relationship can help bereaved parents to process trauma and loss through (a) building narrative coherence, (b) providing a safe base to process traumatic affects, and (c) facilitating post-traumatic growth (see Markin, 2023).

Cognitive Empathy and Narrative Coherence

In the author's clinical experience, *cognitive empathy* facilitates the processing of trauma and grief through building *narrative coherence*, as the therapist steps into the client's chaotic and disorganized frame of reference and empathically organizes, articulates, and integrates the client's experience of loss (Markin, 2023). In the trauma literature, *narrative coherence*, or narratives with more complexity, elaboration, and articulation, are associated with fewer symptoms of post-traumatic stress and anxiety (Amir et al., 1998; Beaudreau, 2007; Brown & Heimberg, 2001; Suedfeld et al., 1998). Moreover, successful treatment of traumatic stress symptoms is associated with improved insight and narrative coherence and decreased disorganization (van Minnen et al., 2002). Although these studies have looked at other types of traumatic events and not pregnancy loss specifically, Engelhard et al. (2003) found that a lack of *a sense of coherence* was a significant risk factor for poor maternal outcomes after perinatal loss.

For the therapist to help the client articulate and organize a coherent and meaningful narrative of her loss, the therapist must first have an empathic understanding of the client's "story." From this, clients telling their story of reproductive loss is an integral part of treatment (Diamond & Diamond, 2016, 2017; Leon, 2015, 2017). Often, the story must be told repeatedly, each time with a little less disorganization and a little more elaboration and articulation. Narrative coherence is facilitated as the therapist conveys empathic understanding of what happened and what the experience meant to the client, making sense of and clarifying her reactions (Leon, 2010, 2015, 2017). The therapist's moment-to-moment empathic understanding and mirroring (i.e., *communicative attunements*) helps to organize what may feel like a confusing, disjointed, and overwhelming experience to the client (Leon, 2015). This is a collaborative process, as the client actively participates in clarifying her internal experience, validating or modifying the therapist's understanding (Leon, 2010). In this sense, cognitive empathy helps the client to reflect upon her experience of the loss, rather than continually reliving it as if it were occurring in the present, which helps to process trauma.

Of course, it goes without saying that clients should never be pressured into telling their story and clinical intuition and skill is needed to ascertain "timing." For example, clients with a history of early trauma may need more time in treatment before they can feel safe to talk about and process their story of reproductive trauma and loss. Further, the client merely retelling their horrific story of loss may only serve to retraumatize the client, perhaps explaining why psychological debriefing interventions following other kinds of traumatic events have been found not be effective, or even harmful, in the long run (Rose et al., 2002). Instead, clients need to tell their story within a safe, trusting, and empathic relationship that helps them to understand and process traumatic events, not just merely relive them.

Affective Empathy and Processing Traumatic Affect

Affective empathy is an important function of any secure attachment relationship. Not unlike what transpires within the caregiver–infant dyad, in the therapy relationship, emotional resonance and connection provide a holding environment in which the therapist can share and co-regulate the client's sadness, which helps the client to feel less alone and facilitates grieving (Leon, 2010, 2015, 2017). Attachment theory (Bowlby, 1969, 1980) suggests that clients will feel safe to approach and process traumatic affects when they experience the therapist as a *secure base* from which it is safe to explore new feelings, thoughts, and experiences, and a *safe haven* to which they may return when feelings and experiences become too overwhelming or painful (Leon, 2010; also see Chapters 8 and 9 in this book). As clients recount their story of loss to the therapist, they often experience much of the same emotions that were present at the time of the event because these emotions were too traumatic and overwhelming to process at the time (Leon, 2015, 2017). The therapist intuitively sensing and connecting with the client's sadness, terror, shock, despair, and/or rage allows the therapist to vicariously be there with her during the loss to comfort, understand, and co-regulate her affective experience, just like a secure attachment figure (Leon, 2010, 2015). This way, the client can relive the traumatic experience of loss on an emotional level, but this time with more support, comfort, and sense of control or agency (Leon, 2017). The therapist empathically connecting and joining with the client's pain and sense of horror or helplessness on an implicit-relational level helps to calm and contain the client's overwhelming and disorganized experience of loss and to process and make sense of it.

Empathy and Post-traumatic Growth

Parents who have lost a pregnancy/baby frequently feel as if a great struggle has been forced upon them. The loss of a baby challenges a parent's basic assumptions about the world as a fair, just, and predictable place. Therapists need to have empathy into the fact that many of the client's core beliefs and basic assumptions have been challenged (Leon, 2015). This can make it difficult for bereaved parents to find meaning in their loss and to make sense of events, which is a fundamental aspect of processing traumatic loss (Krosch & Shakespeare-Finch, 2017).

Despite all this, many bereaved mothers report growth or positive changes in themselves after a pregnancy loss (Büchi et al., 2007). *Post-traumatic growth* refers to positive changes that people may experience following a struggle with challenging events, including bereavement (Calhoun & Tedeschi, 2006). Studies suggest that post-traumatic growth following a pregnancy loss is related to the amount of grief and traumatic stress the mother experiences (Engelkemeyer & Marwit, 2008; Krosch & Shakespeare-Finch, 2017; Tian & Solomon, 2020). Bereaved parents often feel an increased sense of compassion and appreciation for life, develop closer relationships with others, and gain a greater sense of personal strength (Krosch & Shakespeare-Finch, 2017; Tedeschi & Calhoun, 1996). Through a process of cognitive reappraisal, bereaved mothers tend to find meaning in three main areas: *sense making* (e.g., following the birth of a healthy baby after a prior loss, parents often make sense of events by reasoning that without this prior loss, they would not have their current baby), *benefit finding* (e.g., bereaved parents often reprioritize family and meaningful relationships over money, success, or external rewards), and *identity change* (e.g., many parents learn their inner strength and resilience as well as their deep capacity to love) (Gillies & Neimeyer, 2006; Tian & Solomon, 2020). In essence, while the trauma of loss can shatter a person's core beliefs and assumptions, it also provides an opportunity to re-evaluate these assumptions, as people struggle to make sense of the loss and search for meaning (Krosch & Shakespeare-Finch, 2017). Elisabeth Kübler-Ross (1975) best captured this when she wrote:

The most beautiful people we have known are those who have known defeat, known suffering, known struggle, known loss, and have found their way out of the depths. These persons have an appreciation, a sensitivity, and an understanding of life that fills them with compassion, gentleness, and a deep loving concern. Beautiful people do not just happen. (p. 96)

Therapist empathy can help bereaved parents to find meaning in their loss and to process and grow from the trauma that follows. Supporting this, one study found that grief and trauma best facilitated post-traumatic growth for bereaved mothers following a pregnancy loss when in the context of an empathic and supportive partner relationship (Tia & Solomon, 2020). In this study, partner supportive communication, which moderated the relation between grief and post-traumatic growth, consisted of multiple aspects, including *elicitation of thoughts and emotions, effective listening, displaying care,* and *empathy.* Therapists can similarly provide clients with this kind of empathic supportive communication in several ways. First, as the therapist explores the client's thoughts and feelings and comes to grasp an empathic understanding of the client's frame of reference (i.e., cognitive empathy), the therapist can then accurately reflect back the emerging belief or meaning system of the client in a more organized manner. This crystallizes and supports the client's developing schemas and beliefs. Second, the therapist's display of genuine care, concern, and acceptance builds empathic rapport and facilitates the process of rebuilding one's core beliefs and assumptions. Finally, finding meaning from tragedy is a formidable task, and the therapist emotionally resonating (i.e., affective empathy) with the client's struggle makes her feel a little less alone to do this (Leon, 2015, 2017).

In the vignette below, the therapist uses cognitive empathy to build narrative coherence, affective empathy to process traumatic affects surrounding the loss, and empathic understanding to facilitate post-traumatic growth with a client traumatized by a recent miscarriage.

THERAPIST: If you feel comfortable, it might be helpful to tell me more about your miscarriage?

FRANCESCA: I don't know why I'm so depressed all the time? It's not like it was a real baby.

THERAPIST: Hmm, the tears in your eyes suggest that it *was* a real baby to you. Parents can often be surprised how attached they get early on in a pregnancy. *[Therapist emotionally resonates with Francesca's unspoken sadness and normalizes her feelings of loss. ET; affective empathy; EM; communicative attunement and empathic rapport; EI; process reflection and empathic affirmation]*

FRANCESCA: *[crying]* It's just the whole thing was kind of traumatic.

THERAPIST: Miscarriage is often a very scary experience. Can you tell me more about what happened? If we talk about what happened together, maybe it won't feel as scary. *[Therapist again normalizes Francesca's experience and introduces the idea that the relationship can help to regulate fear and distress.*

ET; cognitive empathy; EM; empathic rapport; EI; empathic reflection, empathic question, process reflection]

FRANCESCA: OK. I was at a gas station of all places! I thought I felt something, so I went to the bathroom. I had a bad feeling at the time, like I knew something wasn't right. When I checked there was a lot of blood. I just remember being very shocked by the amount of blood, and it lasted for days. Later, my doctor told me it was normal, but at the time, I was scared.

THERAPIST: That must have been very frightening and so hard not to know that everything you were feeling and experiencing was completely normal. *[The therapist validates and normalizes, subtly organizing Francesca's overwhelming experience through stepping into and reflecting back her frame of reference. Through emotionally holding the client, the therapist begins to establish himself as a safe base from which she can process her trauma. ET; cognitive and affective empathy; EM; communicative attunement; EI; empathic reflection and affirmation]*

FRANCESCA: What's weird is that in the moment I didn't feel sad or worried about the baby. I was mostly panicked that when I left the bathroom everyone would see it all over me and my insides would be on display. I was embarrassed, I guess. Without thinking, I flushed everything down the toilet. Later, I read posts online from women saying you shouldn't flush your baby down the toilet. I have so much regret now. I replay that in my mind over and over. I just discarded my baby. I should have been more focused on the baby instead of myself.

THERAPIST: I understand you wanting to remember your baby, but certainly there is more than one way to do that. *[The therapist validates Francesca's wish to remember her baby without reinforcing her guilt. The therapist also senses Francesca's deep feelings of shame but senses that directly addressing these feelings at this time will further humiliate her.]*

FRANCESCA: I'm embarrassed to admit this, but maybe there is a part of me that doesn't want to remember?

THERAPIST: How so?

FRANCESCA: When I came out of the bathroom, I was sure everyone would know what happened, but when no one did, I acted like nothing happened. I didn't tell my husband or doctor for 2 days. Isn't that strange?

THERAPIST: Sometimes when we experience something very devastating and shocking, we do things that otherwise we wouldn't do because we are overwhelmed and trying our best to cope. Maybe you had an understandable wish that nothing happened, and it was comforting to live in that fantasy for a bit. *[Therapist helps to build narrative coherence through helping Francesca to make sense of and articulate her experience of trauma and loss. ET; cognitive empathy; EM; communicative attunement; EI; experience-near interpretation]*

FRANCESCA: Yeah, I think that is it. Now I'm scared to go to the bathroom because it gives me panic attacks.

THERAPIST: Of course, the bathroom must be a reminder of how frightening the experience was for you—a tangible reminder that the loss did happen and how caught off guard you felt. I think, though, that the more we talk about your feelings, the less anxiety you will feel. *[The therapist senses that Francesca is not ready to directly process feelings of grief and loss, but first must deal with the horror or trauma of the loss. The therapist indirectly suggests that other feelings are at play here that may feed into her anxiety. He continues to reflect back and make sense of her experience of loss, validating and normalizing, to help Francesca feel safe enough to continue to explore her traumatic experience. ET; cognitive empathy; EM; communicative attunement; EI; empathic conjecture]*

FRANCESCA: I've never watched anyone die before. I know it's not the same as seeing a person who is already living die, but to see something dead come out of me was just very scary.

THERAPIST: Oh, Francesca, that's just horrific. You must have felt so out of control and vulnerable. *[ET; affective empathy, as therapist joins with the client's feelings of trauma]*

FRANCESCA: Yeah, the whole thing felt very exposing because it's not like it happened in the privacy of my own home, where I have control over what I share with whom. I've always been a private person. I don't share personal things with people easily, but it felt like that choice was taken away from me. I had no choice but to be exposed in a very public situation.

THERAPIST: That must have been a very vulnerable feeling. *[ET; cognitive empathy; EM; communicative attunement; EI; empathic reflection]*

FRANCESCA: It was. I hate feeling that way. I like to be in control of what I share.

THERAPIST: Sure, you want to feel like vulnerability is on your terms, it's your choice. Maybe there is something there about trust or wanting to feel safe with someone before you open up. Have you always felt that way?

FRANCESCA: I think so. As a kid my mom was depressed and everything was always about her, so I never really felt I could talk about me, ya know? I learned to keep my feelings to myself and deal with it on my own.

THERAPIST: Yes, of course, that makes sense you would learn to do that as a child. No wonder it was hard feeling like your insides were on display in a very public way after your miscarriage. *[The therapist understands the client's experience of loss within her personal history and uses her language from earlier. Connecting this aspect of her personal history to her current loss experience helps to build narrative coherence. ET; cognitive empathy; EM: personal empathy, EI; empathic conjecture]*

FRANCESCA: Yeah, I never thought of that, but that makes sense. But you know, for some reason, I told my mom about the miscarriage, which is weird because like I said I don't tell her anything really. I guess I just needed a mom, and it was actually a really great conversation. She told me something she never told me before, that she had several pregnancy losses when I was a kid, which precipitated her depression. For the first time, I felt less angry with her, and I could understand why she was so depressed and unavailable to me. After all these years, I forgave her a little and felt closer to her. It's not that everything is perfect now between us, but understanding that about my mom's history gave me a new perspective.

THERAPIST: Wow, that sounds very healing and important. For the first time you felt you could relate to her and feel connected in a way you wanted but didn't get growing up. You were able to see her from a different perspective, as a person struggling with loss like you are now. Maybe that understanding released some of the anger you were feeling and made room for new feelings. *[The therapist reflects back Francesca's changing core beliefs and assumptions about her mother, and how this new understanding gives meaning to the trauma of loss for Francesca. ET; cognitive empathy; EM; communicative attunement; EI; empathic reflection and conjecture]*

FRANCESCA: Yeah, and obviously I would rather not have gone through the miscarriage, but it did bring my mom and I together in a way I never thought possible and made me more understanding of the disappointing things people sometimes do when they are hurting inside.

THERAPIST: I see. So while of course you would rather not have gone through this experience to get here, it sounds like going through the loss experience has opened up more compassion and understanding within you for others, particularly your mother.

FRANCESCA: Yes, I think so, and I never thought that would be possible with my mother.

THERAPIST: So, from that place of compassion and understanding, what would you tell the you who was going through this loss, feeling so scared, vulnerable, and exposed in that public bathroom? *[The therapist senses that this new and more compassionate part of Francesca that has developed as a result of her personal growth from the trauma can help heal the traumatized shame-laden part of self.]* Maybe we can even go back to that moment together and, together, feel what she was feeling in that overwhelming moment? *[Therapist is vicariously there with Francesca at the time of the loss, supporting her affectively in the way she did not have at the time of the loss, and perhaps as a child with her mother when depressed. ET; affective empathy; EM; communicative attunement; EI; evocative open question)*

FRANCESCA: I guess that she did the best she could in a difficult situation. Maybe she wasn't ready to let other people see what happened because she wasn't even ready to acknowledge it herself. *[Francesca's narrative of her loss experience is now more coherent, reflecting the fact that she has begun to process the trauma and grow from it.]*

COMMON CHALLENGES TO THERAPIST EMPATHY IN PSYCHOTHERAPY FOR PREGNANCY LOSS

For clinicians to fully immerse themselves into the client's experience of loss is to vicariously live through the death of a baby sometimes every hour, on the hour, every day of the week. This kind of empathic immersion can easily lead to therapist burnout and emotional fatigue (Leon, 2017). It is important for therapists to know their limits and boundaries so that they do not become emotionally taxed and unintentionally withdraw from the work of therapy, as this will feel like yet another loss or abandonment to the client (Diamond & Diamond, 2017). Additionally, the therapist's own experiences with pregnancy loss, or other types of loss, may help him or her to empathize with the client, but also may easily lead to distortions or projections (Leon, 2017). To effectively empathize without overly identifying with the client, the therapist needs to find a way to focus on the client and enter into her internal world, without losing the therapist's own perspective or experience. All this requires an impressive capacity for self/other differentiation, insight, and affect regulation. Because of this, it is important for the therapist to engage in ongoing personal reflection and perhaps supervision and/or personal therapy (Leon, 2017).

Another challenge to therapist empathy is the client's own ambivalence or difficulty experiencing the therapist's care and understanding. While most clients genuinely want to feel understood and cared for, accepting empathy is often not as easy as it sounds. For pregnancy loss clients, accepting an empathic relationship in which they could mourn and move on is, on one hand, what they need to feel better, and, on the other hand, the end of what feels like the last fragile connection they have to the lost baby. It is important for the therapist to empathize with this struggle and to understand it, rather than attempt to solve or get rid of it. Therapists can explore with their clients other ways in which they can honor their attachment to the lost baby, such as a memorial, letters to the deceased baby, artwork, etc.

Lastly, perhaps the greatest challenge to therapist empathy is that it requires the therapist to defy every human inclination to avoid the realities of death, the horrors of loss, and the meaninglessness and injustice of a world in which innocent babies die and mothers mourn. Like our clients, as therapists we must also find a way to make meaning from the trauma of loss in order to approach painful and overwhelming feelings and experiences that otherwise are typically avoided.

CLINICAL IMPLICATIONS

- Empathy involves a conceptual understanding of the client's experience of loss as well as an emotional resonance with the client's feelings of trauma and loss, including sadness and despair, and horror and powerlessness.
- Just the therapist empathically listening and validating the client's loss as real and grief as legitimate undoes aloneness and facilitates grieving.
- Therapist empathy helps to heal clients' chronic sense of inadequacy and failure, as what is understood is no longer shameful or threatening.
- The processing of trauma and grief occurs within a relationship where the client's traumatic experiences are understood and organized by an

empathic other and in which she can feel supported and safe to tolerate
and process traumatic affects.
- Therapist empathy can help bereaved parents to find meaning in the
  horror of loss and to re-evaluate priorities, assumptions, and beliefs,
  which often leads to personal change and growth.

5

Emotion in Psychotherapy for Pregnancy Loss

Mourning as an Affective-Relational Process

In psychotherapy for pregnancy loss, grief is almost always the third person in the room, and whether overtly acknowledged or not, it finds a way of making its presence known. Grief can look like a loud and aching longing for the baby that died and the future that was lost, so intense that it leaves parents desperate and broken apart into a million agitated pieces. Other times, it can be more elusive and look like a quiet yet powerful jailor that has confined and silenced the overwhelming pain a grieving parent holds inside. Despite all this, somehow, most grieving parents manage to mourn and move on but are forever changed by the experience. Yet, because of the intensity of emotion and the profound sense of loss, bereaved parents simply cannot do this alone. Grief is given a voice when someone else can hear it, a face when someone else can see it, and a rest when someone else can help hold the weight of it. Though bereaved parents need a relationship in which they can experience, express, and co-regulate overwhelming feelings of sadness and loss in order to mourn, perinatal grief is often invalidated, avoided, or dismissed in Western society (Markin & Zilcha-Mano, 2018). Therapy can offer bereaved parents an empathic and affect-regulating relationship in which to mourn.

This chapter begins with a brief empirical review of different aspects of emotion work in psychotherapy, particularly emotional expression due to the availability of research in this area. Evidence-based relationship principles derived from research on emotion in psychotherapy are then applied to the treatment of clients who have suffered a pregnancy loss. Based on theory and research, the author describes how therapy can help bereaved parents to overcome avoidance of, and more deeply experience and express, productive emotions, co-regulating them within a secure attachment relationship with the therapist. Hypothetical therapist–client vignettes that are derived from an amalgamation of real-life clinical experiences demonstrate the application of these concepts. Finally, common challenges to emotion work in psychotherapy for pregnancy loss and clinical implications are discussed.

Psychotherapy for Pregnancy Loss. Rayna D. Markin, Oxford University Press. © Oxford University Press 2024.
DOI: 10.1093/oso/9780197693353.003.0005

CASE VIGNETTE: EMOTIONAL EXPRESSION

Jenny was a 28-year-old married female with no living children who sought therapy after giving birth to a stillborn baby girl named Hope. Two weeks before her estimated delivery date, Jenny called her doctor several times reporting lack of fetal movement. Finally, Jenny's doctor suggested she come in for an ultrasound for "peace of mind" but stated it was probably "just nerves." Much to Jenny and her husband Pete's horror and surprise, the ultrasound technician could not pick up a heartbeat. The couple soon learned that this was due to an extremely rare and random occurrence of the umbilical cord wrapping itself around Hope's throat. Jenny then went through induced labor and delivery knowing she would give birth to a stillborn baby, an experience that Jenny describes as so devastating and traumatic that she does not remember most of it. The hospital staff encouraged Jenny and Pete to hold Hope and to take pictures that they could keep, along with a copy of Hope's footprints and baby blanket. However, when Hope was placed in Jenny's arms, she started to experience extreme anxiety and suffered a severe panic attack, during which she felt as if someone was suffocating her. These panic attacks and associated feelings of anxiety have continued since Hope's death and have interfered with the grieving process, as Jenny explains that she can't even think about how sad she is to have lost Hope without feeling overcome by anxiety and panic. Jenny berates herself for "squandering" the one opportunity she had to hold her baby. She now has such a strong longing to hold Hope in her arms that it physically aches. Jenny reports extreme feelings of shame and inadequacy. She feels as if she should have known something was wrong earlier on and could have saved her baby. Jenny feels betrayed by her body and like her womb is no longer a safe place but a "baby graveyard."

During their initial meeting, the therapist encourages Jenny to tell her story of loss in as much detail as she feels comfortable, sending the implicit message that Jenny's feelings of trauma and loss are not too overwhelming or threatening but, rather, will be accepted, tolerated, and contained within the therapy relationship. Early on in treatment, Jenny and her therapist agree on the goal of therapy being to help Jenny experience and process her feelings of trauma and grief, together, without associated feelings of shame, guilt, and anxiety that all seem to get in the way of Jenny effectively grieving. As Jenny retells her traumatic experience of loss, she relives the experience all over again and all the emotions she felt at the time come up as if they were happening for the very first time— except this time, Jenny does not feel alone in her chaotic and intense emotional experience, as the therapist listens, empathically responds, tolerates, shares, and emotionally holds Jenny's sadness, despair, and horror over the trauma of loss. As Jenny approaches previously avoided feelings of grief and loss, she starts to feel the familiar anxiety and panic. The therapist, through nonverbals and tone of voice, soothes and comforts Jenny's anxiety, which allows her to more deeply experience and express her profound sadness and despair. As the therapy progressed, it was important for the therapist to help Jenny process not only feelings of sadness and loss, but also the horror she felt around the traumatic nature of the loss. For instance, as Jenny came to trust her therapist, she felt safe to share her private and hidden fantasies related to the loss, which included a horrific image of Hope suffocated in utero that constantly replayed in her mind. Jenny reflected that unlike her relationship with the therapist, in her family of origin no one ever talked about sad feelings; instead, they put on a smile and looked at the bright side of things. As a result, Jenny tends to feel selfish and guilty when experiencing sadness and has learned to suppress these feelings and focus on the positive. However, the death of Hope was so devastating that she simply could no longer suppress her sadness, and she needed soothing from an empathic other. As Jenny experienced, expressed, and better understood her feelings with the therapist, she found herself expressing her feelings more to her husband and mother. Eventually, Jenny and Pete decided to have a memorial service for Hope with close friends and family, an experience she described as emotionally cathartic. The night after the memorial service, Jenny had a dream in which she was having a panic attack, feeling as if hands were wrapped tightly around her throat. She suddenly realized that the hands were her own and slowly brought them down to her chest to cradle Hope. The therapist asked Jenny, "Now that you are free to speak, I wonder what words or sounds might come out?" Jenny responded, "I would tell Hope, 'You will always be with me. I'm sorry I couldn't keep you safe, but you were always loved.'" "What was that like to say?" the therapist inquired, to which Jenny replied, "Very sad, but I also feel lighter and like I can breathe a little bit more, this sadness now feels right, and I don't feel as anxious and panicked anymore."

EMOTIONAL EXPRESSION: AN EVIDENCE-BASED RELATIONSHIP PRINCIPLE

Peluso and Freund (2019) define *emotion* as a feeling state that has a well specified object, unfolds over seconds to minutes, and involves coordinated changes in subjective experience, behaviors, and physiology, as consistent with the definition proposed by Suir and Gross (2016). With perinatal grief, the specified object is most often the lost baby, but can also be more diffuse and involve the loss of one's reproductive capacities, loss of identity, loss of future hopes and dreams, or loss of one's *reproductive story* (Jaffe et al., 2005). Subjective changes associated with grief may include a general feeling of malaise, depression, panic, or despair, and associated behavioral changes typically include withdrawal to mourn one's losses or social support seeking. There are also physiological correlates of bereavement, including increased production of stress hormones, changes in heart rate and blood pressure, and immune imbalance (Buckley et al., 2012). Other emotional experiences that accompany perinatal grief include sadness, horror or fear, anxiety, depression, shame and guilt, longing, and anger (Diamond & Diamond, 2016).

Most experts agree that in any therapy for pregnancy loss, a bereaved parent's emotions related to the loss need to be experienced and expressed as well as processed for parents to effectively mourn (Covington, 2006; Leon, 2015). While studies have yet to examine the association between emotions and therapy outcome with pregnancy loss clients specifically, there is an emerging body of literature on how emotions, particularly the expression of emotions, relate to the process and outcome of therapy with other client populations from which to draw (Peluso & Freund, 2019). Productive *emotional expression* in psychotherapy refers to overcoming avoidance of, and strongly experiencing and expressing, emotions that were previously suppressed or restricted (Greenberg, 2016). For instance, the full affective range of a bereaved parent's grief is often avoided, suppressed, or minimized because it is experienced as too unbearable to fully tolerate and because it is typically invalidated by society (Markin, 2017). From this, the goal of therapy is to overcome the avoidance of emotions related to the loss and to experience and express them in an adaptive manner that allows the bereaved to mourn and move on with a greater sense of meaning and acceptance. Previous meta-analyses that have examined emotional expression or emotional experiencing and therapy outcome have found a significant medium effect size (Diener et al., 2007; Pascual-Leone & Yeryomenko, 2017). Peluso and Freund (2019) have conducted the most comprehensive meta-analysis to date. They looked at the relation between both therapist and client emotional expression and the therapy process and treatment outcome, albeit over a relatively small number of studies ($N = 6–42$), and in all cases found a significant medium to medium/large effect size.

Emotional processing, on the other hand, refers to how "individuals experience, organize, make meaning of, and resolve emotional episodes" (Peluso & Freund, 2019, p. 425). Emotional processing has been found to positively correlate with treatment outcome and positive change within a session (Stalikas & Fitzpatrick, 1995; Town et al., 2017; Whelton, 2004). Because the loss of an unborn baby is often a traumatic loss, grieving parents typically need help organizing and making sense of the chaotic, undifferentiated, and overwhelming affect associated with the event. Furthermore, making meaning from the loss is often an important part of resolving perinatal trauma and grief (Leon, 2015; see Chapter 4 in this book). There is probably a reciprocal relationship between emotional processing and emotional expression. Emotions that are experienced and expressed can then be better understood and organized. Once processed, these feelings become more tolerable and less overwhelming, which may increase the client's capacity to experience and express them.

Emotional Expression and the Therapy Relationship

Although it is not known exactly how emotions facilitate a positive therapy outcome, some evidence suggests that emotions relate to outcome through the therapy relationship (Beutler et al., 2000). In particular, the working alliance (defined as agreement on bonds, tasks, and goals) has been found to be a significant factor in whether emotional expression is productive for therapy (see Peluso et al., 2019). This may be because the tasks and goals of therapy can be framed around emotion work, such as the task of facilitating emotional expression and the goal of emotional resolution or meaning making (Beutler et al., 2000; Greenberg & Pascual-Leone, 2006; Iwakabe et al., 2000). Consistent with this, the meta-analyses, in which Peluso and Freund (2019) found significant effects for therapist and client emotional expression and the therapy process, largely included studies that defined "therapy process" as the working alliance. Peluso and Freund (2019) suggest that there is a reciprocal relationship, in which emotional expression facilitates the bond dimension of the alliance and a strong bond enables more productive emotional expression in therapy. For example, in therapy for pregnancy loss, a strong bond characterized by the therapist's emotional resonance with the client and sharing of her sadness presumably facilitates the processing of trauma and grief (Leon, 2015). As Leon (2015) observes, "Grieving does not occur in an interpersonal vacuum" (p. 234). It is not just the expression of grief and loss that is therapeutic, but moreover the experience of having a caring and trusted other understand, share, and soothe one's sadness.

In addition to the bond dimension of the alliance, emotional expression is also intricately tied to the tasks and goals of therapy when the goal of treatment is focused on the client's underlying feelings and emotional pain (Greenberg, 2014). It is important that the therapist and client agree that the focus of therapy will be on feelings, that feelings give us information, and that the client will not be alone in experiencing painful or overwhelming feelings because the therapist and client are in this together (Greenberg, 2014). With pregnancy loss clients who often feel as if their feelings of loss are dismissed or minimized, it is especially important for the therapist to validate their feelings of grief and loss as legitimate, and to emphasize that grieving is a normal and adaptive process that, though painful, leads to a greater sense of resolution and meaning. The goal of therapy is not to take away the client's feelings of grief and loss, but to better tolerate and understand these feelings, together.

Emotional Expression Across Theoretical Orientations: Changing Attachment Schemas

Emotional expression is most likely important to all therapies for pregnancy loss and, in fact, appears to similarly predict the therapy process and outcome across different theoretical approaches (Peluso & Freund, 2019). Therapies of disparate theoretical orientations have progressively moved from a left-brain focus on verbal and conscious experience to a right-brain focus on nonverbal, affective, and unconscious processes (Schore, 2014). As such, emotional experiencing is a common unifying theme across all relationally oriented therapies of different theoretical orientations (Markin, 2014). These approaches have in common the overarching belief that the ability to experience and express emotions is rooted in early attachment relationships and replicated within the client's attachment relationship with the therapist (Peluso & Freund, 2019). This replication provides the opportunity in therapy for corrective emotional experiences that repair a client's neglectful or traumatic experiences with early attachment figures, fostering change on an attachment or schema-based level (Peluso & Freund, 2019; Schore, 2014). The brain appears to be particularly malleable to rewiring insecure internal working models during affect-laden moments in therapy (Schore, 2014). The loss of a wanted pregnancy/baby may be one such affect-laden moment, in which a therapist who sensitively responds to a client's emotional distress not only facilitates the grieving process but also rewires affect-regulating attachment internal working models (also see Chapters 8 and 9 in this book). For example, in the case vignette above, Jenny learned to suppress feelings of sadness and loss within early attachment relationships because such feelings were experienced as selfish, giving rise to feelings of guilt that interfered with the grieving process. However, as Jenny's feelings of sadness and loss were accepted, soothed, and sensitively responded to by the therapist, unlike in early attachment relationships, Jenny felt safe to experience, express, and process these feelings.

Emotion Regulation and Attachment

Emotion regulation refers to how individuals manage the experience and expression of emotion (Peluso & Freund, 2019) and is learned within early attachment relationships (Bowlby, 1969; Schore, 2014). Securely attached infants learn that their distress will be consistently understood and regulated within a safe and supportive relationship with the caregiver, and, over time, internalize this interpersonal soothing as self-soothing capacities (Bowlby, 1969; Greenberg, 2014; Mikulincer & Shaver, 2003; Schore, 2014). In particular, securely attached individuals are believed to have had caregivers who helped them cope with and repair early experiences of separation and loss (Bowlby, 1980). As adults, they are thus equipped with various tools for emotion regulation that they can use to cope during stressful experiences such as loss, including turning toward others for interpersonal soothing as well as turning inward for self-soothing (Bowlby, 1969; Schore, 2014). Securely attached clients have positive internal working models of self and other and so are more readily able to experience and internalize the therapist as an empathic and soothing presence to whom they can turn when affectively overwhelmed. From this, therapy with securely attached clients who have suffered a pregnancy loss is usually primarily supportive, as these clients possess the skills to effectively cope with or regulate distress in general, and separation and loss in particular, but have had their usual coping resources taxed by the trauma of loss and often by the lack of available and understanding support persons. Consistent with this, attachment security has been associated with a more favorable bereavement reaction after other kinds of losses (Waskowic & Chartier, 2003) and with fewer symptoms following a perinatal loss (Scheidt et al., 2012).

Conversely, when a secure attachment figure is not available to mirror, sensitively respond to, and co-regulate the infant's emotional experience, these feelings and experiences are denied or distorted (Bowlby, 1969). As adults, these individuals lack effective emotion regulation skills and either under- or over-regulate emotional experiences (Greenberg, 2014; Mikulincer & Shaver, 2003;

Schore, 2014). For instance, insecurely attached individuals often have difficulty regulating grief and loss and are at risk for complicated grief reactions (Schenck et al., 2015), presumably because they once lacked a caregiver to help them cope with and repair early experiences of separation and loss (Bowlby, 1969, 1980). Specifically, individuals with an avoidant attachment learned to suppress feelings of sadness and loss upon separation from a caregiver to avoid rejection, humiliation, or criticism. From this, bereaved parents with an avoidant attachment may deny feelings of grief and loss, as they have learned to overly self-soothe or down-regulate emotional experience at the expense of interpersonal soothing and connection. Although these individuals have learned to distance themselves from their feelings to cope, they are left with suppressed distress that is unresolved and interferes with their ability to deal with adversity (Luyten et al., 2017).

On the other hand, individuals with an anxious attachment learned to cope with separation and loss in early attachment relationships by escalating their distress and clinging to an inconsistent and preoccupied caregiver for fear of abandonment or rejection. Overwhelmed by the intensity of their emotional distress, these individuals have difficulties processing and regulating affect and crave interpersonal soothing and connection at the expense of autonomous self-soothing. Their preoccupation with abandonment and overwhelming anxiety tend to get in the way of mourning the loss of a pregnancy and processing grief (Bowlby, 1980; Scheidt et al., 2012; Schenck et al., 2015).

Given this, psychotherapy for perinatal grief with insecurely attached clients may require the rewiring of affect-regulating attachment internal working models to more secure before grief and loss can be fully processed. Internal working models are believed to shift through co-regulating emotional distress within the therapist–client dyad in ways that repair early attachment trauma (Bowlby, 1988). Therefore, theoretically, clients with an avoidant attachment need a therapy relationship in which it feels safe to approach previously avoided emotions and to accept the empathy and soothing offered by the therapist, without feeling alone in their distress, overwhelmed, or ashamed. Clients with an anxious attachment, on the other hand, may need a relationship in which it feels safe to downregulate emotional distress and more autonomously self-soothe, secure in the knowledge that the therapist will be available for comfort and containment when truly needed. In other words, through the therapist–client attachment relationship, avoidant clients learn emotional regulation strategies related to interpersonal soothing that involve more comfort with intimacy and closeness, whereas anxious clients learn self-soothing strategies that require more comfort with autonomy and separateness.

PRODUCTIVE AND UNPRODUCTIVE EMOTIONAL EXPRESSION FOR PREGNANCY LOSS

Primary Versus Secondary Feelings

Fundamental to emotion work of any kind, and to pregnancy loss therapy specifically, is the fact that not all emotions are alike, with some being more productive to the therapeutic work and adaptive than others (Peluso & Freund, 2019). It is essential for therapists to be able to differentiate productive emotions that should be encouraged or "up-regulated" in therapy from unproductive emotions that should be downregulated. In EFT (Greenberg, 2015), more productive or adaptive emotions are called *primary emotions*, defined as a discrete number of universal emotions that are experienced and expressed the same regardless of culture, race, or developmental background; these include sadness, fear, surprise, disgust, and anger. These feelings are our first response to a specific trigger and motivate us to take some adaptive action (Greenberg, 2014; Peluso & Freund, 2019). From a bioevolutionary perspective, primary emotions serve a critical survival role for the species by providing information about personally meaningful situations (Ekman, 2007; Peluso & Freund, 2019) and encouraging some adaptive action that benefits the self (Greenberg & Safran, 1989; Rottenberg & Gross, 2007). After the loss of a pregnancy, the primary emotion is often sadness or grief, which tells us that we have lost something or someone personally meaningful and moves us to either seek support or withdraw to reflect and mourn. Grieving is thus an adaptive process that allows the bereaved to accept the loss, mourn, and move on with a greater sense of meaning. Other primary emotions, such as fear or terror around the horror of losing a child and even of the physical experience of pregnancy loss, or anger as a normal protest against loss, are often present alongside sadness and need to be experienced and processed as well. It often surprises therapists that through the exploration of very traumatic and difficult feelings related to grief and loss, other more positive and primary emotions arise as well—for instance, a mother, who despite her sorrow over the loss of her stillborn baby boy, experiences pockets of pure joy when recalling the few precious moments that she spent with him post-delivery.

One way in which therapists can help clients experience and process primary emotions related to grief and loss is by helping them to design personally meaningful mourning rituals. Mourning rituals provide clear and customary rules and procedures for grieving and for expressing feelings of loss, while also providing the bereaved with emotional containment from family, friends, and the community (Markin & Zilcha-Mano, 2018). These rituals help parents to express their grief, in part, through transforming the lost baby into a specific child so that the parent has someone tangible to grieve (Leon, 2015). From an attachment perspective, it is important for mourners to internalize and transform their relationship with the deceased, rather than severing all ties (Frost & Condon, 1996). Rituals like creating a gravesite, having a memorial service, and writing letters to the deceased baby help the parent to internalize the lost baby and transform the relationship (Frost & Condon, 1996). Therapists can collaborate with clients to design personally meaningful rituals relevant to the client's cultural and religious context that serve as an avenue for expressing grief and loss (Markin & Zilcha-Mano, 2018).

On the other hand, unproductive or maladaptive emotions are our subsequent reaction to our initial primary emotions. These feelings are called *secondary emotions* in EFT and serve to avoid or inhibit primary emotions. They include anxiety, guilt, and shame or embarrassment (Greenberg, 2015). Following a pregnancy loss, women often report chronic and severe feelings of anxiety, depression, guilt, and shame (Diamond & Diamond, 2016). These common symptoms can be conceptualized as secondary emotions that are maladaptive in that they prevent the client from grieving and experiencing other primary emotions. Recall the primary goal of therapy from an emotion perspective is to overcome avoidance of and deeply experience and express primary emotions, while downregulating secondary emotions. In most cases of pregnancy loss, this involves downregulating shame and guilt, as well as depression and anxiety, while encouraging the experiencing and expression of primary feelings such as sadness and loss.

Secondary feelings arise in the context of pregnancy loss for several reasons. First, as troubling as these secondary emotions are, they are often experienced by the client as a more bearable alternative to fully experiencing and expressing painful and traumatic feelings of grief and loss, especially when the client feels as if she must go through these overwhelming feelings alone. Second, the lack of culturally prescribed mourning rituals, death certificates, flowers, or sympathy cards make it difficult for bereaved parents to recognize or accept primary feelings of grief and loss, which are instead avoided or suppressed through secondary reactions or feelings. Third, because the loss of a pregnancy is a narcissistic loss and an assault on one's self-esteem and identity, parents must grieve at the same time they are rebuilding the self (Leon, 2015). This leads to a pervasive sense of shame and inadequacy that covers up one's grief and loss, as the parent focuses on criticizing the self instead of mourning who and what has been lost. Lastly, pregnancy loss involves *prospective grieving*, wherein fantasies, hopes, and an imagined future must be mourned, as opposed to *retrospective grieving*, wherein the mourner has actual memories of the deceased that are shared by others (Covington, 2005). Especially for early pregnancy loss, the lack of concrete memories associated with the dead baby (such as ultrasounds, quickening, or "showing") may make the child and the loss seem less "real," leading to minimization or denial of feelings of sadness. Unfortunately, when grief is not recognized and expressed, it often manifests as depression, which, unlike grief, does not carry an adaptive action tendency and cannot be transformed into something healing and new.

Activating Versus Inhibiting Affects

Like Greenberg's (2015) conception of primary and secondary emotions, Malan's (1995) triangles of conflict and of person provide a useful way of conceptualizing maladaptive versus adaptive emotions, and how maladaptive emotions or conflicts originated and are maintained in relationships. The three points on Malan's triangle of conflict represent (1) adaptive feelings or *activating affects* (e.g., anger/assertion, sadness/grief, closeness/tenderness, sense of self, enjoyment/joy, interest/excitement, sexual desire, fear/terror); (2) *inhibitory affects* that stop the adaptive action tendency of underlying activating affects (anxiety/fear/terror, shame/guilt/

humiliation, emotional pain, suffering, contempt, disgust); and (3) *defenses* (any thought, feeling, or behavior that arises to avoid uncomfortable feelings as expanded by McCullough et al., 2003). Inhibitory affects are *why* the activating affect is avoided, while defenses are *how* the adaptive affect is avoided (McCullough et al., 2003). For example, grief that is avoided because it is paired with unbearable emotional pain might be avoided through obsessive ruminations about what one could have done to prevent the loss, or grief that is inhibited by self-contempt and shame might be avoided through attacking the self.

After the loss of a pregnancy/baby, some clients will develop emotion conflicts that are situation-specific and not characteristic of the client in general (at least to that degree). Emotion conflicts specific to perinatal grief often arise because of the traumatic and overwhelming nature of reproductive loss, which often occurs amidst a lack of supportive and understanding relationships. However, other clients enter treatment with a more chronic and characteristic fear of affect and have developed characterological defenses to avoid the feared affect. These *affect phobias* (McCullough et al., 2003) are believed to originate within early attachment relationships, are maintained (or changed) within relationships with current persons and the therapist, and impact the client's ability to effectively grieve. For example, expressing sadness or grief over the loss of one's unborn baby will be harder for clients with a chronic phobia or fear of sadness and loss. As children, these clients may have learned from attachment figures that loss is too unbearable to speak about or acknowledge. Similarly, expressing anger over the loss of yet another pregnancy will be more difficult for clients who have learned in past relationships that anger leads to even more relational loss and thus perpetually avoid it. Lastly, while it is almost a universal phenomenon that pregnancy loss assaults a woman's self-esteem (Diamond & Diamond, 2016), when the woman chronically avoids any positive feelings about the self because, perhaps, as a child, she learned that to do so would spark competitive feelings in and rejection from attachment figures, then feelings of shame and inadequacy will be even more pervasive after loss. Whether situation-specific or a chronic affect phobia, the treatment objective when adaptive affects are avoided is to gradually expose the client to the feared affect(s), while regulating the inhibitory affects and preventing the defenses, within an empathic and soothing therapy relationship (McCullough et al., 2003).

CLINICAL APPLICATION OF WORKING WITH EMOTION IN PSYCHOTHERAPY FOR PREGNANCY LOSS: GOALS AND INTERVENTIONS

Below, interventions for self-restructuring, emotional soothing and alliance building, downregulating inhibitory affects and defense relinquishing, and deepening affective experiencing and expression are offered, within the context of a safe, empathic, and affect-regulating secure attachment relationship with the therapist, as demonstrated in hypothetical vignettes.

SELF-RESTRUCTURING: REBUILDING SELF-ESTEEM
AS A NECESSARY FOUNDATION FOR EMOTION WORK

A relatively solid and integrated sense of self and self-esteem are needed to tolerate a wide range of affective experiences. When instead the client possesses a negative sense of self, then *self-restructuring*, or working with the client's representation of herself and the aversive affects that are triggered (McCullough et al., 2003), may be necessary before productive emotion work can occur. Pregnancy loss is often experienced as a violent attack on one's self-worth and sense of self, leading to intense feelings of shame and inadequacy (Leon, 1996). Yet, the ability to grieve effectively requires a stable sense of self so that one can separate oneself from that which was lost (Diamond & Diamond, 2017). Healthy self-esteem serves as a buffer against feelings of shame and inadequacy and allows individuals to tolerate a wide range of emotions, without shame and self-criticism interfering. Bereaved parents are often forced to rebuild their sense of self and self-esteem at the same time they are grieving (Leon, 2015). Consequently, these clients need the therapist to support their tenuous self-esteem and depleted affect-regulation capacities until these functions can be internalized or restored (Leon, 2010).

Below, interventions (see Table 5.1) offered by McCullough et al. (2003) for promoting self-esteem, self-compassion, and a positive image of self are applied in a hypothetical vignette with a client who recently discovered that her recurrent miscarriages were due to poor egg quality.

Table 5.1. EMOTION GOALS IN THERAPY FOR PERINATAL GRIEF
AND ASSOCIATED INTERVENTIONS

Emotion Goal	Interventions
Self-restructuring	• Therapist self-disclosing
	• Highlighting strengths
	• Psychoeducation
	• Normalization, validation, and empathy
	• Acting as good parent to self
	• Internalizing therapist compassion (McCullough et al., 2003)
Emotional soothing and alliance building	• Repeating phrases
	• Using images and simple words
	• Slow pacing, soft voice, and facial tone
	• Reflecting client words
	• Validation and empathic reflection
	• Therapeutic presence (Johnson, 2004)

(*continued*)

Table 5.1. CONTINUED

Emotion Goal	Interventions
Downregulating inhibitory affects and defense relinquishing	• Pointing out defenses that have developed to avoid uncomfortable feelings • Validating that these defenses made sense within a certain time and place, particularly in early attachment relationships, but no longer are working • Speculating on what feeling is being avoided and why • Regulating inhibitory affects so that the activating affect can be experienced in small doses without the inhibiting affect present (McCullough et al., 2003)
Deepening affective experiencing and expression	• Evocative and experiential questioning and reflection • Empathic conjecture and inference (based on what attachment theory tells us about emotions) • Slowly increasing the client's tolerance of intense emotions by co-regulating them • Exploring the information that feelings give us and what they motivate us to do • Processing the experience of affect regulation within the therapist–client dyad (Johnson, 2004)

These interventions are suggested in McCullough et al. (2003) or Johnson (2004) and applied within the context of therapy for pregnancy loss here.

MARY: After the last miscarriage, which was our fifth one, I needed to have answers, so we finally went to the fertility clinic and had a workup done. We should have done it a long time ago, but I kept dragging my feet and making excuses. I didn't want confirmation of what I already knew: Something *is* wrong with me and that's why we can't have a baby!

THERAPIST: Mary, that sounds incredibly painful to walk around feeling so responsible and so damaged. *[Mary starts to tear up.]* It's OK, try to stay with those feelings; there is a lot of hurt there, maybe shame too. *[Therapist offers empathy, validation, and emotional soothing.]*

MARY: There is. I feel so deficient in the most basic biological way possible, it's like primitive. This is just something that my body was supposed to know how to do. Wait, I should explain, sorry. The tests showed that I have poor egg quality, and this is likely the cause of our miscarriages. When the doctor told me that I literally felt like he was stabbing me in the gut. I mean, am I even a real woman anymore?

THERAPIST: It feels like this isn't just a problem with your reproductive system, but a problem with your very self that cuts to the core of who you are like a sharp knife. *[Therapist expresses empathy and subtly separates Mary's reproductive system from her sense of self.]*

MARY: Yes, yes *[crying]*! I feel so betrayed by my own body and so angry with myself. What is wrong with me?

THERAPIST: Oh, Mary, I don't think anything is wrong with you. I think you are coming to grips with yet another major loss. *[Therapist self-discloses to validate the client and build self-esteem.]* In my experience, many women who are going through similar situations feel as if they have failed some test of their own self-worth and even of their womanhood. *[Therapist provides psychoeducation to normalize Mary's experience and reduce shame.]*

MARY: That's not my feeling, it is a fact. The tests confirmed it. *[Mary's self-criticism interferes with her taking in the therapist's empathy and compassion.]*

THERAPIST: Wow, there is that really powerful self-critical voice! *[Mary nods in agreement.]* So, why is this voice so determined on punishing you for this, even after all you have already suffered? *[Therapist externalizes the self-critical voice to help Mary get some distance from it and separate it from her sense of self.]*

MARY: I think the fact that I probably won't be able to use my own eggs to gets pregnant brings up a lot for me. Growing up, I wasn't exactly the most "ladylike." My mother would always chastise me for not being more like other girls, but I just wasn't into what other girls were into, and I always got along better with my brothers and their friends. I knew my mother did not approve. I tried to please her by wearing more dresses and things like that, but that just wasn't me. I think I had a lot of shame about it when I was younger. I thought I was just a freak. I mean, in my small town, I didn't know anybody like me until I went away to college and met people who were not as gender conforming as the people I grew up with. I think that's why now, as a school counselor, it's important to me to support kids who are going through something similar and feel like they don't fit in these narrow gender boxes, ya know? So, they don't feel alone.

THERAPIST: You've really been through a lot, and I can see why these fertility struggles would bring this all up again for you at this time.

MARY: Yeah, it feels like this is yet another way, but a really big way, that I have failed at being what a woman is supposed to be, even though intellectually I know that's not true. I can so imagine what my mother would say if she knew!

THERAPIST: Well, I want to come back to that, but first I really wanted to say how amazing I think it is that you have used what must have been a very confusing and isolating experience growing up to help other kids who are similarly struggling now, so they don't feel alone and inadequate the way it sounds like you did growing up. *[Therapist self-discloses and highlights Mary's personal strength.]*

MARY: Thank you, I appreciate that.

THERAPIST: You said you can imagine what your mother would say? Can you elaborate?

MARY: Oh, you know, probably something about how if I dressed in pink, grew my hair long, and crossed my legs then my eggs would be better, probably something ridiculous like that.

THERAPIST: On an intellectual level you know those kinds of comments are absurd, yet, at the same time, I imagine they still sting emotionally and are not what you would want to hear *[Mary nods]*. If it feels OK to you, let's try something kind of different together. Imagine it is 30 years from now and you have a daughter who is similarly experiencing fertility problems. How would you respond to her? How would you feel toward her? *[This exercise helps Mary to imagine herself as her own compassionate parent.]*

MARY: I would just want to be there for her, so she didn't feel alone or like a failure.

THERAPIST: What would you want to say to her, or do?

MARY: I would probably give her a hug, tell her I loved her and that this isn't her fault.

THERAPIST: Can you try to really picture yourself hugging her in your mind and try to hear yourself saying those words to her. How did that feel to do? *[Client acting as good parent to self]*

MARY: It felt bittersweet. I mean, it feels good because it feels like I'm giving that to myself in a way but also sad because obviously I wish it was my mother doing that for me.

THERAPIST: Of course, yes, that makes sense. Tell me more about how it felt "good"?

MARY: It's kind of like telling a younger version of myself, "You are OK just the way you are, even if that's different."

THERAPIST: What did it feel like to hear?

MARY: Validating. It sounds like you saying this *[smiling]*, but if I wouldn't think less of my own child for experiencing fertility problems, then why am I doing that to myself? *[Mary internalizes compassion of therapist.]*

EMOTIONAL SOOTHING AND ALLIANCE BUILDING

Before the emotional experience of perinatal loss can be deepened and processed, it must first be regulated by the soothing presence of the therapist. Emotional soothing, or the therapist containing, holding, and regulating overwhelming and traumatic affects associated with the loss, goes hand in hand with alliance building in EFTs (Greenberg, 2014; Nødtvedt et al., 2019; Timulak et al., 2017). As the therapist soothes and comforts the client in her moment of distress, the therapist becomes a trustworthy and dependable figure from which the client can seek comfort and containment when needed, thereby strengthening the bond. Over time, the therapist's affect-regulating presence is internalized by the client as self-soothing capacities (Greenberg, 2014).

The therapist's way of being and nonverbal communications are probably more soothing than anything the therapist says or does (Diamond & Diamond, 2017).

As reported in Greenberg (2014), the type of implicit affect regulation and emotional soothing that is experienced within a good therapeutic relationship occurs through right-hemispheric processes. It is not verbally mediated, but emotionally communicated within a relationship, through nonverbal affective-relational means such as facial expression, vocal quality, and eye contact (Schore, 2003). This is similar to the kind of right-brain, nonverbal-affective communication that occurs between caregivers and their infants, which serves to soothe the infant's distress while also strengthening their bond, which in itself is soothing (Schore, 2014). Below, right-brain interventions for emotional soothing and alliance building (often used in EFTs [see Johnson, 2004]) are exemplified in a hypothetical vignette with a client seeking therapy after losing a twin during pregnancy (see Table 5.1).

GIANNA: They call it "vanishing twin syndrome," like my baby just—*poof!*—disappeared, like a cute magic trick. She didn't vanish, she died. She wasn't a trick, she was real.

THERAPIST: What was her name? *[Therapist validates the loss as real by asking the baby's name, which intensifies the personhood of the unborn baby and the associated affects.]*

GIANNA: *(sniffling)* Sadey.

THERAPIST: Sadey was a real little person *[therapist uses imagery by making a cradling motion, looking down as if she were gazing at a newborn]*. She was your little person. It feels awful when others don't see that. *[Empathic reflection and validation]*

GIANNA: Yes, exactly. It makes me so frustrated. Once I found out we were carrying twins, I loved them both. I started making all these plans to be a mom to two babies. Now, people will say things like "try and focus on the fact that you are still pregnant" or "most people don't even know they were carrying a twin."

THERAPIST: Ouch *[therapist facial expression signals physical pain]*, that must sting! *[Use of imagery]*

GIANNA: It really does. Then I start to feel guilty, though, because maybe I should just feel happy over the baby I still have, and I am happy and grateful, but I'm also sad.

THERAPIST: Of course, it's profoundly difficult to welcome one baby and lose another. One baby does not replace another *[empathic reflection and validation]*. *[Gianna is then silent, but the therapist sees tears in her eyes that she is holding back.]*

THERAPIST: What feelings are coming up for you right now? I see so much emotion in your eyes. *[The therapist's tone of voice is warm and comforting.]*

GIANNA: It hurts so much.

THERAPIST: It's so painful; try to stay with that pain. *[Use of simple words, slow pacing. The therapist leans forward to signal she is present emotionally with Gianna.]*

GIANNA: *[sobbing]*

THERAPIST: It's OK, let it come, just try and make space for your feelings, that's the pain of losing your Sadey. *[Therapist pauses, giving Gianna space to experience her sadness while nonverbally "holding" Gianna.]* It's OK *[slow pacing and repetitive words]*. It's all coming up *[pause]*. We can just make room for your feelings together. *[The therapist's tone of voice is warm, calm, and soothing.]*

GIANNA: *[crying]* She's really gone.

THERAPIST: She's gone. She's really gone *[therapist uses Gianna's words and repetitive, simple, phrases]*. There's so much longing in your voice *[empathic reflection]*.

GIANNA: Yes, I just want her back. I feel so empty inside.

THERAPIST: You feel empty, incomplete *[reflecting client's words]*. Just try and stay with that feeling. *[The therapist is fully present and joining Gianna's sadness and loss.]*

GIANNA: I'm afraid that I'm going to fall apart, and I can't do that to this baby.

THERAPIST: The sadness feels so heavy that it could break you apart. I understand. Maybe, for a little bit, you can give me some of the weight to hold so it doesn't feel so overwhelming? *[Use of images; therapist communicates they are in this together]*

DOWNREGULATING INHIBITORY AFFECTS AND RELINQUISHING DEFENSES: APPLYING MALAN'S TRIANGLE OF CONFLICT AND OF PERSON

When underlying activating affects (or primary emotions), such as grief and loss, are chronically avoided and inhibited, then, before they can be deeply experienced and expressed, clients must first feel safe enough to relinquish defenses and to experience previously avoided activating affects without inhibitory affects (or secondary emotions) present (see McCollough et al., 2003, conceptualization of affect phobias). From an attachment perspective, clients will approach previously avoided emotions when they feel safe enough to express these emotions in relationships, without fear of additional relational loss, neglect, or rejection. Thus, the most fundamental "intervention" for downregulating inhibitory affects and relinquishing defenses is not actually an intervention at all per se, but the establishment of a safe and trusting therapist–client relationship. However, within a safe and trusting therapeutic relationship, specific interventions (first proposed in McCullough et al., 2003) can be used to downregulate inhibitory affects and relinquish defenses (see Table 5.1). These interventions are demonstrated in a hypothetical vignette below with a client who is avoiding sadness/grief (*activating affect*) related to a prior miscarriage because her experience of sadness is associated with intense feelings of guilt (*inhibiting affect*). She then avoids the guilt by attacking herself and focusing on others (*defenses*). The client's avoidance of sadness in general, and in relation to the pregnancy loss specifically, with important others (*current persons*) originated within early attachment relationships, after her mother abandoned the family when the client was just 9 years old and the father's drinking worsened (*past figures*), a loss that has been re-evoked by the pregnancy loss (see McCollough et al., 2003, conceptualization of affect phobias). As demonstrated below, unresolved losses from a grieving parent's past may become fused with the loss of an unborn baby and complicate the grieving process. In this case, the unresolved past loss must first be grieved before the parent can process her grief over the lost baby (Leon, 2015).

ESTHER: This past Saturday was supposed to be my due date. I couldn't help but think about it all day. We still went to my dad's house for his birthday. I didn't want to cancel on him just because I was feeling down, but I ended up feeling guilty the entire time because I think I ruined his birthday with my bad mood. My husband kept asking me if I was alright, and I was like, "Yes, yes, I'm just tired." I felt awful that I was making him worry.

THERAPIST: It makes sense to me that that was a hard day for you, anniversaries and due dates can really bring about another wave of grief, yet it sounds like you were kind of hard on yourself for feeling that way? Almost as if you felt guilty for grieving? *[Labeling the inhibitory affect (guilt) and speculating about what emotion lies underneath (grief/sadness)]*

ESTHER: Yeah, I just don't want to bring anyone down with my bad mood or make them worry about me. I mean, it feels selfish to make my dad's birthday about me and show up to his celebration crying, and my husband is already worried enough about me.

THERAPIST: Is there a feeling attached to that statement?

ESTHER: I guess guilt.

THERAPIST: Is there a "story" that the guilt tells you about what might happen if you were to share your feelings with others? In this example, with your husband or your father, but you've talked about a similar feeling with close friends and even in here with me? *[Exploring the function of the inhibitory affect]*

ESTHER: I mean, I think what I said before, that if I just mope around depressed all the time, then that's going to make them feel sad too and they are just going to worry about me even more. I remember every date, you know? The date we were supposed to get our 21-week ultrasound, the date the crib was supposed to arrive, the date I was supposed to have my baby shower, and I feel devastated when each date comes around. I can't go crying to them every single time I'm sad! How could I do that to them knowing it would just upset them?

THERAPIST: Right, so there is a part of you that wants to protect them from further pain, and it seems like that comes from a very loving place. At the same time, it sounds like the guilt makes it very difficult for you to feel your grief and show your sadness because if you do, then the guilt sort of gets louder and tells you that you are a bad person because you're doing so knowing it could hurt the people you care about—does that sound right? *[Speculating on what feeling is being avoided and why]*

ESTHER: I mean, yes, I know they wouldn't see it that way, but I just feel like it's selfish to burden them with my feelings all the time, especially on my dad's special day.

THERAPIST: What would be the most selfish part about sharing with your husband, for example, before you left for your dad's, that you were feeling sad today and thinking about what this day was supposed to look like? *[Regulating inhibitory affect so that the activating affect can be experienced in small doses]*

ESTHER: The most selfish part? Well, knowing that saying that would make him feel sad too, and knowing that I could have chosen to spare him the pain.

THERAPIST: And you, when you don't talk about your feelings of sadness and loss and keep them to yourself, are you spared the pain?

ESTHER: No *[sniffling]*, that's why I come here so I can get it out without feeling guilty about hurting someone else, no offense. *[A tolerable dose of sadness can now be tolerated with the guilt somewhat more regulated.]*

THERAPIST: No offense taken. This is something that keeps coming up for you in different ways, this caution around expressing your feelings of grief and loss for fear that they will somewhat hurt the other person. It's only when you really trust that someone can "take it" that you feel safe to let at least some of your feelings out. Do you have a sense of how that started?

ESTHER: Well, I've already told you about my mom leaving when I was young. When she left, I was completely confused and scared and very lonely, but my dad really fell apart. His drinking got worse. Sometimes he would leave me with my aunt for days, and I wouldn't know when he would come back. So yes, of course I was sad when she left, but I couldn't add what I was going through to his plate, he couldn't have handled it. He needed me to be strong.

THERAPIST: That sounds devastating, Esther. I can understand why that child would feel almost terrified of her own sadness. To a child in that situation, it must have felt like needing her dad emotionally would destroy him. So, of course, as a child you would learn to stuff or dismiss your sadness and focus on your dad instead, because you needed him whole and intact. The problem is that I don't know if that's working anymore for you? When your mom left you didn't have anyone you felt you could rely on to share your grief, so of course you learned to dismiss it and focus on others instead, but the problem with that as an ongoing strategy is the grief never gets worked through. *[Validating that defenses made sense within a certain time and place, particularly in early attachment relationships, but no longer work]*

ESTHER: Yeah *[sniffling]*, it's all kind of related, isn't it? This might sound crazy, but I remember pinching myself very hard when I was a kid when I would start to cry and telling myself not to be a crybaby. I didn't want my dad to see me cry, and for the first time in like 15 years I caught myself pinching my hand to hold back tears at my dad's birthday party, and like berating myself up in my head for being sad.

THERAPIST: Wow, there is so much pain there that you are holding all alone.

ESTHER: Yes [sniffling].

THERAPIST: This is kind of what your mind does when you feel sad: You start to beat yourself up and focus on others because feeling sad doesn't feel good, it feels selfish to you, and I think very risky because you don't feel safe that people close to you can handle your feelings without falling apart. [Pointing out defenses that have developed to avoid uncomfortable feelings]

ESTHER: I think that's exactly it. As much as I hate her for leaving, I really wish my mom was here. I just have a sense that as a woman she could understand what I am going through right now and I could go to her with my feelings about this.

THERAPIST: Yeah, yeah, it makes complete sense that you would really want or need a mom right now and really feel that loss very acutely. In some ways, it sounds like at the same time you are grieving the miscarriage, you are also grieving the loss of your mom again.

DEEPENING PRIMARY AFFECTIVE EXPERIENCING AND EXPRESSION

The deepening of primary affective experiencing and expression is a principal goal in psychotherapy for pregnancy loss. This usually occurs after secondary emotions have been downregulated and the therapeutic relationship has evolved into a secure attachment relationship in which the client can seek comfort and containment from the therapist when affectively overwhelmed. The overall treatment goal is for the client and therapist, together, to approach, in tolerable doses, previously avoided emotions, and to co-regulate these feelings within the dyad, as the therapist and client work toward better understanding them. The objective is not to take the client's grief away, but for the client to be able to turn toward others for support and comfort, and, over time, to develop self-soothing capacities (Greenberg, 2014).

To deepen affective experience in a productive way, it is essential that clients experience their feelings and not just talk about them in an abstract or intellectual manner (which can be a defense against affective experiencing). Moreover, it is not just affective experiencing and expression that is healing, but the relational experience of the therapist accepting, understanding, validating, and sharing in the client's emotional experience (Greenberg, 2014). Experiencing and expressing primary emotions related to the multiple losses associated with pregnancy loss, within a secure attachment relationship with the therapist, is often corrective because it undoes the isolation that many parents felt after the loss of an unborn baby (Leon, 2015). Below, interventions for deepening emotional experience and expression often used in EFTs (see Johnson, 2004) (see Table 5.1), within a secure affect-regulating therapy relationship, are illustrated in a vignette with a client who is pregnant 10 years after giving birth to a stillborn baby and currently experiencing flashbacks, dissociation, and hypervigilance. This vignette also demonstrates how affect-laden moments in therapy can lead to corrective emotional experiences that rewire attachment schemas.

SHEETAL: We had our ultrasound this week. I knew it would be difficult, but I wasn't prepared for just how difficult it actually was. I tried to breathe through it, but the second they lied me down on the table and I felt the cold jelly on my stomach, I could feel my throat tightening, my heart racing, and my chest, like, constricting. I could see the ultrasound tech fiddling with equipment and there was something about that absent look in her eye that brought me back to the delivery room when Viva was born, and it was as if those nurses and doctors from Viva's birth were there with me in that moment, with that look that they all get when they have bad news but don't want to tell you. I can feel my palms getting sweaty right now just talking about it with you. Ten years later and it's like it happened yesterday. Will I ever not feel this way?

THERAPIST: Sheetal, that sounds so incredibly painful and overwhelming. I can really sense how out of control and powerless you felt, now and then.

SHEETAL: Yes, exactly.

THERAPIST: Of course being pregnant again and going through these kinds of medical procedures are going to bring up feelings around Viva's death. It's not that it's always going to feel this way, but this specific situation just brings it all up. Maybe, though, as hard as these feelings are, they are trying to give us some important information? It might be helpful for us to slow down and better understand these intense feelings, together, so they don't feel so overwhelming and out of control? *[Exploring the information that feelings give us and what they motivate us to do]*

SHEETAL: I know I need to work through these feelings so that I can be a better mom to this baby, but honestly, I just want to run away, like I even feel antsy as we talk about this.

THERAPIST: That's understandable; these are really devastating and overwhelming feelings. Of course you would want to run from them as a form of, like, self-preservation, but as long as you keep avoiding them, as understandable as the wish to do so is, they will keep catching up to you. *[Slowly increasing the client's tolerance of intense emotions by co-regulating them]*

SHEETAL: I know, I know. How do I do that, though?

THERAPIST: If it's OK with you, let's try focusing in on that feeling you had on the table during the ultrasound. It sounds so important. You couldn't breathe, your heart was racing, your chest and throat were closing up. Just try to focus in on that feeling, knowing you are not alone and I'm in the room with you, and let's just see what comes up for you. You can close your eyes if you feel comfortable. *[Evocative and experiential questioning and reflection]*

SHEETAL: OK. *[Pause]* Well, an image comes up for me.

THERAPIST: Good. Can you describe it to me? *[Evocative and experiential questioning]*

SHEETAL: I'm in the delivery room.

THERAPIST: Good. Who is there with you? *[Evocative and experiential questioning]*

SHEETAL: I just pushed Viva out. It was a difficult and confusing labor. I know she's out, but I don't hear her. The nurses and doctors are there, and they are rushing around sort of urgently, but they don't look or speak to me.

THERAPIST: Good. Is it OK to keep going?

SHEETAL: Yes, it's OK.

THERAPIST: What do you hear? *[Evocative and experiential questioning]*

SHEETAL: Sort of rumblings that I can't make out from the doctors, and I hear myself screaming, "What's going on? What's going on? Is the baby OK?" But no one is answering me.

THERAPIST: I know this is hard; you are doing a great job. What are you feeling now as you tell me this? *[Evocative and experiential questioning]*

SHEETAL: Scared, just so scared and helpless, like no one will tell me what's going on, no one will help or listen to me!

THERAPIST: Let's check in with your body. What are you feeling in your body right now? *[Evocative and experiential questioning]*

SHEETAL: My chest feels tight, like it did during the ultrasound. I think it's really my heart that hurts.

THERAPIST: What does the hurt feel like? *[Evocative and experiential questioning]*

SHEETAL: Like I just want to die, I'm so devastated. It's like this throbbing ache in my chest that travels up my throat but can't come out of my mouth.

THERAPIST: What does it want to say? If the words could come out? *[Evocative and experiential questioning]*

SHEETAL: I think it wants to scream for someone to give me answers, like, "Look at me, damn it! What is going on with my baby!"

THERAPIST: Yes, you were so confused and frightened. You were dependent on the doctors to help you and your baby, and you felt very alone and confused. *[Empathic conjecture and inference]*

SHEETAL: Yes, exactly.

THERAPIST: Is there more to the image?

SHEETAL: *[crying]* Yeah, me holding Viva. I was in shock at the time; I couldn't process what was going on. It all happened so fast. No one was, like, explaining things to me as we went along. I couldn't even process she was gone before they put her in my arms and told me I should say goodbye. She was so blue, so lifeless *[sobbing]*. I wasn't prepared. I wasn't ready.

THERAPIST: It's OK, just make space for these feelings, this very deep and intense grief you've been carrying inside. Of course it was traumatic, you were in shock. Of course you couldn't process what was going on or your feelings at the time. It was so horrific and unfathomable that it was hard to make sense of *[empathic conjecture and inference]*. Is there something you want to say to Viva right now, as you hold the memory of holding her in your mind? *[Experiential questioning]*

SHEETAL: That I love her. I always will remember her, and I'm sorry I couldn't protect her.

THERAPIST: All these feelings need to come out. It's OK, just make room for them, so much grief there. *[Increasing client's tolerance to intense emotions by co-regulating them; therapist and client pause as they both sit in the client's feelings of sadness and loss, horror, and helplessness]* What has it been like to share these profound feelings of grief with me today? *[Processing experience of affect regulation within the therapist–client dyad]*

SHEETAL: It was hard. I feel very drained, but I feel less agitated. I do feel really sad, though.

THERAPIST: Yes, that makes a lot of sense. And it is OK to feel sad; your grief is a signal that you've lost someone important to you and that you need to mourn. In a way, the panic or anxiety you have been feeling, particularly during the ultrasound, may be was a sort of clue that there are other feelings there that needed our attention *[exploring the information that feelings give us]*.

SHEETAL: Yeah, I think so. I never talked to anyone, not even my husband, about the details of that day. I was in grief counseling for 2 years after Viva's death, and we never talked about those details. I've told you before how we just don't talk about feelings in my family. If I were to go to my mother with this or any of my aunts, they would find a way to make it about them and I would end up feeling guilty for something, but with you I felt like you were listening to me.

THERAPIST: So, what was it like to feel listened to in that way by me? *[Processing the experience of affect regulation in the therapist–client relationship]*

SHEETAL: I felt less alone, safer, I guess, to go back to that awful day.

COMMON CHALLENGES TO EMOTION IN THERAPY FOR PREGNANCY LOSS: PERSONAL REFLECTIONS

As a clinician, to step inside and fully immerse myself in the client's profound sense of loss and all the trauma that so often surrounds it, I hold on to a set of firm beliefs that anchor me in what can be a chaotic sea of emotion. I believe that grief, though devastating, will not destroy me or the client, and will ease and evolve into something else with time. I understand the pain and vulnerability of finally allowing oneself to express the grief one carries inside to another but believe that grieving alone is a much more painful fate. I truly believe that the client and I can contain the longing, the despair, the horror, and the sadness. I trust that mourning is an intrinsically adaptive process that will help to heal the client's wounds over time, although surely scars remain, and I believe that it is our scars in life that shape and transform us as people, but also as parents. Clinicians working with the effects of pregnancy loss have the monumental challenge of finding a way within themselves to tolerate feelings of trauma and loss, and not just of any loss, but that of a baby. Yet, if the clinician is frightened of these feelings and avoids them, then it is unlikely that the client will feel safe approaching them. In other words, the most difficult challenge that therapists often face when doing this work has little to do with the client and more to do with the therapist's capacity to manage personal emotional reactions.

Therapists' unintentional avoidance of client affect in this clinical context often goes unrecognized and unchecked because it reflects society's dismissal, rationalization, and minimization of perinatal grief in general (Layne, 2003; Markin & Zilcha-Mano, 2018). This may look like the therapist leaning toward left-brain interventions when a right-brain solution is needed for a right-brain problem (i.e., one having to do with emotions and trauma), such as over-focusing on action-oriented interventions, or prematurely encouraging bereaved mothers to "move on" (Markin, 2016). It may also look like the therapist and client never, not once, talking about the horrific details of the actual loss experience, something that clients rarely bring up without first being invited to by the therapist. In conclusion, clinicians working with bereaved parents will often report feeling overwhelmed by the client's emotions, unsure of what to say, and fearful of saying the wrong thing. Yet, it has never been my experience that bereaved parents necessarily need you to know what to say, but rather, how to say it, with an attitude of care and compassion, a soothing presence, and a willingness to join in their emotional experience.

CLINICAL IMPLICATIONS

- Overwhelming feelings of grief and loss are best experienced, expressed, and co-regulated within a secure attachment relationship with the therapist.
- For clients with past attachment trauma, the experience of having the therapist support, understand, and co-regulate overwhelming emotional experiences, during the stressful and affect-laden experience of losing a pregnancy/baby, may have the dual effect of helping the client to resolve grief, while also rewiring attachment internal working models.
- It is important that the therapist and client agree that the tasks and goals of therapy have to do with overcoming avoidance of and deeply experiencing feelings, together, to facilitate the process of grieving.
- Emotional resonance with the client's sadness helps the client to feel less alone and facilitates grieving (Leon, 2015). This kind of emotional resonance, or sharing of sadness, is probably not best achieved through the nonverbal, intuitive, and affective language of the right brain.

6

Alliance Rupture and Repair Episodes in Psychotherapy for Pregnancy Loss

An Attachment Perspective

Central to the rupture experience in any important relationship is the very human struggle of how we are to engage in the pleasure of love when that love often comes with the pain of loss. Humans arguably grapple with this enigma from "cradle to grave," as infants first learn in early attachment relationships how to withstand the experience of separation and loss in order to ultimately stay connected (Bowlby, 1982, p. 127), or how to trust that after moments of rupture, disconnection, or separation from a caregiver, the dyad will come back together for reunification and repair. Moments of physical separation and/or affective disconnection from attachment figures conjure a unique kind of pain—one that can only result from the loss of another who is experienced as a part of the self, making the repair process especially important. Similarly, when that infant, now a mother herself, is forced to mourn the loss of her unborn baby, she grieves not just the loss of a separate person in the world but of a precious and vulnerable part of self. The intense distress that results from this unique kind of loss, combined with the lack of comfort and support that grieving parents typically receive, often resurrects early attachment experiences for the mother in which, as an infant, she similarly felt alone in her despair over disconnection and in the pain of separation.

In this chapter, it is proposed that in psychotherapy for pregnancy loss, early attachment issues related to a lack of repair after moments of separation and/ or affective disconnection are often triggered and reenacted within the therapy relationship, particularly for clients with a history of inadequate or adverse attachment experiences. Furthermore, these reenactments commonly precipitate alliance ruptures in which the client once again feels alone, unsupported, overwhelmed, and misunderstood in her feelings of separation and loss. These

Psychotherapy for Pregnancy Loss. Rayna D. Markin, Oxford University Press. © Oxford University Press 2024.
DOI: 10.1093/oso/9780197693353.003.0006

alliance ruptures present the opportunity to repair old attachment wounds and to facilitate the grieving process. Ultimately, we somehow learn to relish in the joy of love when we are no longer afraid to approach the pain of loss, for we trust that even in moments of separation we are not alone.

This chapter begins with a brief empirical review of how alliance rupture and repair episodes in the therapy relationship relate to the process and outcome of therapy, with a specific emphasis on understanding the rupture-repair process through an attachment framework. Evidence-based relationship principles derived from research on rupture and repair episodes in psychotherapy are then applied to the treatment of clients who have suffered a pregnancy loss. Unique dynamics specific to the experience of pregnancy loss are proposed to contribute to alliance ruptures, including (a) narcissistic injuries brought about or exacerbated by the loss of a pregnancy, (b) the tendency to invalidate or minimize pregnancy loss grief in Western societies, and (c) past attachment issues related to a lack of emotional containment, support, and understanding that have been resurrected by the experience of pregnancy loss. Resolution strategies for repairing these alliance ruptures are suggested and demonstrated in hypothetical therapist–client vignettes. Finally, common challenges to identifying and repairing ruptures in psychotherapy for pregnancy loss are discussed and clinical implications are offered.

CASE VIGNETTE: ALLIANCE RUPTURE AND REPAIR

Shelby was a 25-year-old married female with no living children who entered therapy for feelings of depression, anxiety, and low self-esteem, following multiple early-term miscarriages. Blaming herself for the miscarriages, Shelby felt like a complete failure and disappointment to her husband, whom she described as supportive and understanding. In general, Shelby reported a lack of social support. Family and friends often told Shelby to focus on the positive—that she was young and still had plenty of time to have children. Though well-meaning, these comments left Shelby feeling misunderstood, alone, and as if she should be "over this by now." Similarly, Shelby explained that her mother, who was a labor and delivery nurse, overly focused on the medical aspects of pregnancy loss at the expense of her feelings and reactions. When Shelby tentatively expressed the need for more emotional comfort and support, her mother stated that it was too painful for her to focus on Shelby's losses, and she preferred not to "wallow" in the past. In response, Shelby felt incredibly guilty and kept her feelings and needs to herself even more than before. As a result, Shelby felt disconnected from her mother, making her feel even more alone and anxious. As therapy progressed, Shelby would come to understand that, perhaps because of her mother's own traumatic history of loss, this dynamic reflected a longstanding pattern in their relationship in which her mother would reject or criticize Shelby's need for emotional understanding and support (or repair) after moments of separation, disconnection, or loss, resulting in Shelby blaming herself for having these needs and wants in the first place.

Interpersonally, Shelby seemed very young and emotionally fragile to the therapist, pulling for a maternal caregiver countertransference. Shelby was, in many ways, deferential to the therapist and appreciative of the therapy, stating that therapy was the one place she could let out her feelings without fear of hurting others or burdening them and experience empathy and understanding, contrary to other relationships. At the same time, she was ambivalent about experiencing painful feelings of grief and loss. She would sob one session and want to talk about superficial topics the next. She even became mildly combative when the therapist attempted to reflect on what was transpiring for her internally during these less deep sessions. To empathize with the client's ambivalence, the therapist commented that it is a natural human inclination to avoid pain. Much like we automatically remove our hand from a flame after burning it, we instinctively avoid emotions that are experienced as too painful to bear. Just like one would need a pretty convincing reason for keeping one's hand on the fire, perhaps Shelby needed a reason for staying with these painful feelings? Much to the therapist's shock, in response, Shelby seemed to panic. She turned red, became short of breath, and suddenly felt hot and sweaty. The therapist inquired as to what was going on for Shelby, who explained that what she heard the therapist "really" saying is that she is a "bad" client and is "kicking her out" of therapy. The therapist reflected on Shelby's powerful self-critical voice, which seemed to cause her a lot of hurt and anxiety in relationships. Shelby disclosed that she has always worried that others would discover her "badness" and reject her, an experience that was confirmed and exacerbated by the experience of pregnancy loss, as Shelby reasoned that there must be something fundamentally wrong with her for pregnancy after pregnancy (or baby after baby) to physically reject her and her body. In response, the therapist disclosed that she was not aware of feeling angry or wanting to reject Shelby, but rather felt overprotective of her. She wondered out loud if her overprotective feelings may have, in some way, made it difficult for Shelby to directly express what she needed to feel safe in their relationship? Shelby replied that perhaps she needed more reassurance from the therapist that she is "doing a good job," but did not want to anger or hurt her. The therapist validated Shelby's need for more affirmation and disclosed that rather than feeling hurt, as Shelby expected, Shelby's authentic disclosure made her feel more connected to her. After this "rupture and repair" episode, Shelby's feelings of sadness and loss seemed to flow freely in the therapy. With the therapist, she explored and processed feelings of grief and loss over her miscarriages and over the loss of not having important others available for support and comfort during these losses to help process and emotionally contain her experiences. The rupture-repair process left Shelby feeling safer to approach painful feelings of grief and loss, for she trusted that the therapist would be available for emotional comfort and containment when needed and would sensitively respond to her separation distress, unlike past attachment figures. Shelby's self-esteem also increased as she began to experience her sadness upon separation and loss and her need for repair not as negative aspects of self, but with understanding, appreciation, and compassion.

ALLIANCE RUPTURE AND REPAIR: AN EVIDENCE-BASED RELATIONSHIP PRINCIPLE

The therapeutic alliance literature highlights the importance of building a strong working relationship with clients (Flückiger et al., 2018). In some therapeutic approaches, the alliance is most often in the forefront, the central focus of treatment, and a key mechanism of change (Safran & Muran, 2000). Breakdowns in the alliance are believed to represent "critical junctures" in psychotherapy and opportunities to revisit and revise dysfunctional interpersonal and attachment patterns (Safran & Kraus, 2014, p. 381). In other approaches, the alliance most often lies in the background, as a necessary precondition for other therapeutic tasks that are believed to lead directly to successful outcomes (Beck, 2011). Yet, even in these approaches, the therapist must directly address the alliance when something goes awry and a rupture occurs (Eubanks et al., 2018). In fact, alliance ruptures have been found to be relatively common, and more frequent than therapists often realize (Safran & Muran, 2000).

Although research on rupture-repair events in therapy for pregnancy loss is sparse, there is a growing body of research supporting the importance of these events with other client populations. A recent meta-analysis of 11 studies (1,314 clients) examined the relation between rupture-repair episodes and client treatment outcomes and found a significant-moderate relation between rupture/resolution and positive client outcomes (Eubanks et al., 2018), consistent with a prior meta-analysis (Safran et al., 2011). The relation between rupture-resolution and client dropout was also significant (Eubanks et al., 2018). Consistent with this, pregnancy loss clients may be at risk for premature dropout due to ruptures that result from misunderstanding events with the therapist in which feelings of perinatal grief and loss are unintentionally not acknowledged or understood (Markin, 2016). Furthermore, in their meta-analysis, the rupture-repair and outcome association did not significantly differ depending on client personality diagnosis, therapist experience level, or theoretical orientation (CBT vs. psychodynamic) (Eubanks et al., 2018). Because studies suggest that alliance ruptures are important to the therapy process and outcome across theoretical orientations, identifying and effectively repairing ruptures is likely relevant to all therapists (Safran & Kraus, 2014). It is argued below that there are certain aspects of the experience of pregnancy loss that precipitate certain rupture experiences across theoretical approaches and thus are relevant to all therapists.

A few initial studies provide some evidence that alliance rupture-repair events occur in therapy for pregnancy loss and relate to outcome in complicated ways. Markin and McCarthy (2020) found qualitative evidence that alliance ruptures were common in a case study of psychodynamic therapy for a client pregnant after loss, and that unrepaired ruptures may have contributed to dissatisfaction with treatment and lack of change on psychiatric symptoms. These unrepaired ruptures occurred mostly later in treatment and were relational in nature, having to do with the client's conflictual wish for emotional containment and nurturance from the therapist. On the other hand, early treatment ruptures had to do with misunderstandings related to the experience of infertility and pregnancy loss and were largely repaired, which facilitated the client's experience of feeling understood and supported. Similarly, a small qualitative study involving interviews about the therapeutic relationship with therapists who completed treatment with a pregnancy loss client found that ruptures that were successfully repaired were associated with successful outcomes (i.e., a stronger alliance and clients feeling safer to express feelings), while unrepaired ruptures were associated with poor outcomes (i.e., premature termination and increased client ambivalence toward treatment) (Gosai & Markin, 2019). Although these studies are preliminary, their findings reflect what is commonly observed in the larger psychotherapy literature. The relationship between alliance rupture-repair and therapy outcome is complex in that failure to repair a rupture most likely predicts a poor outcome, whereas the successful resolution of a rupture likely facilitates a successful outcome (Eubanks et al., 2018).

Theoretically, pregnancy loss clients may be especially vigilant and reactive to moments of misunderstanding or tension in the therapy alliance. Understandably so: The recent traumatic experience of a pregnancy loss often leaves these clients sensitive to experiences of separation or disconnection in relationships. Ruptures with the therapist, which represent an affective-relational separation or disconnection, may compound the client's already profound sense of aloneness and loss. The emotionally injurious effect of alliance ruptures for these clients may be understood in context of the fact that a woman's attachment needs for nurturance, understanding, and support are believed to be heightened during pregnancy in preparation to empathically nurture and care for her own vulnerable infant (Leon, 1990, 2015), and may further intensify after a pregnancy is lost, when she finds herself dependent on the support and comfort of others in order to cope and grieve. With the bereaved mother's attachment needs for support and nurturance, as well as her sense of loss and loneliness, all heightened, even relatively minor ruptures, which at other times in her life may have gone unnoticed, may be experienced as deeply injurious to the self and to the relationship.

Definitions

Most of the research on alliance ruptures is based on Bordin's (1979) conceptualization of the alliance, which consists of (a) agreement between client and therapist on the goals of treatment, (b) collaboration between client and therapist on the tasks of treatment, and (c) an affective bond between the client and therapist. From this, a rupture in the alliance is defined as a deterioration in the alliance, or a disagreement on the tasks or goals of therapy, or a strain in the emotional bond between the therapist and client (Eubanks-Carter et al., 2010; Safran & Muran,

2000). Safran, Muran, and colleagues (Muran et al., 2005) view the development and breakdown of the alliance within a contemporary relational framework, wherein ruptures are never any one person's "fault," but a mutual dyadic process to which both participants contribute (Safran & Krauss, 2014). A rupture is typically thought to be *resolved* or *repaired* when the client and therapist resume their collaboration on the work of treatment with a strong affective bond (Eubanks et al., 2018). Ruptures can vary in intensity from very dramatic moments of conflict or misunderstanding to more subtle moments of misattunement and tension in the therapeutic relationship (Eubanks et al., 2018). Several other terms have been used in the psychotherapy literature to describe problems in the alliance, such as empathic failures, transference–countertransference enactments, resistance and ambivalence, and misunderstanding events (Safran & Krauss, 2014; see Muran, 2017, for a review).

Withdrawal and Confrontation Ruptures

Ruptures are typically organized into two main subtypes: *withdrawal* and *confrontation* ruptures (Harper, 1989a, 1989b; Muran & Eubanks, 2020; Safran & Muran, 2000), each having a unique resolution process (Safran et al., 1990; Safran & Muran, 2000).

In withdrawal ruptures, the client moves away from the therapist and the work of therapy and deals with difficulties or misunderstandings in the therapy relationship by falling silent, offering minimal responses to questions, shifting topics to an unrelated matter, or becoming overly compliant to the therapist's requests or interventions (Eubanks et al., 2018). Clients who withdraw during moments of tension in the relationship are usually struggling with interpersonal fears and internalized criticisms that inhibit the expression of negative feelings (Safran & Kraus, 2014). As seen in the earlier case of Shelby, pregnancy loss clients typically feel inadequate and as if they have failed to do the one thing they were born or made to do (Diamond & Diamond, 2016). Fearing that the therapist will attack or criticize them, as they attack and criticize themselves, they may suppress negative affect and competing wishes or needs during a rupture and withdraw. From this, the repair process typically involves providing clients with the interpersonal safety needed to express feelings and experiences that are typically suppressed (Safran & Kraus, 2014).

In confrontation ruptures, the client moves against the therapist by expressing anger or dissatisfaction with the therapist or treatment in a blaming or demanding way, or by trying to pressure or control the therapist (Eubanks et al., 2018). With pregnancy loss, confrontation ruptures may occur out of a place of desperation, as the client presses the therapist to "fix" her overwhelming suffering. The repair process involves the therapist's empathic engagement with the client to help her express disowned feelings of disappointment, hurt, shame, vulnerability, lack of control, and/or the need for nurturance (Safran & Kraus, 2014; Safran & Muran, 2000).

STRATEGIES FOR REPAIR OR RESOLUTION OF ALLIANCE RUPTURES

Strategies for resolving alliance ruptures include *direct strategies*, which involve the therapist and client explicitly acknowledging the rupture, and *indirect strategies*, whereby the rupture is resolved without being explicitly acknowledged (Eubanks et al., 2018). Because clients who have suffered a pregnancy loss often feel inadequate and self-critical, directly addressing ruptures is sometimes too shameful to tolerate in the moment (Diamond & Diamond, 2017). In this case, the therapist must find more indirect ways to repair the rupture and validate the client without minimizing the importance of the rupture and repair process. Whether the therapist chooses to directly or indirectly repair the rupture depends on the strength of the alliance, the nature and intensity of the rupture, and whether the client can tolerate the shame and/or anxiety associated with exploring relationship problems in the here and now.

Repair strategies also range from *immediate* strategies, which aim to repair the rupture quickly so that the client and therapist can return to or change the task that they were working on before the rupture occurred, to *expressive strategies* that aim to shift the focus of the therapy session to exploring the rupture and the client's needs or concerns that underlie it (Eubanks et al., 2018). A delicate balance between immediate and expressive strategies is often needed for pregnancy loss clients who most often seek therapy for help with the resolution of grief and trauma and not for personality reconstruction or interpersonal change per se. At the same time, from a relational-attachment perspective, directly addressing ruptures in the therapeutic relationship could help the client process past unresolved attachment issues related to separation and loss that are interfering with the grieving process. These strategies are exemplified in the therapist–client dialogue under the "Clinical Application" section of this chapter.

Table 6.1 lists the specific rupture subtypes and resolution strategies (and provides an example of each) included on the Rupture Resolution Rating System (3RS; Eubanks-Carter et al., 2015), an observer-based measure of alliance rupture-repair events. These can be a helpful heuristic for therapists to use to identify different kinds of in-session ruptures and specific resolution strategies.

Table 6.1. Types of Withdrawal Ruptures, Confrontation Ruptures, and Resolution/Repair Strategies

Withdrawal Rupture	Client Example
Denial	I don't know why you keep asking me about the miscarriage. It really was not a big deal. It happens all the time and we will get pregnant again.
Minimal response	*Therapist:* Miscarriage can be a pretty traumatic experience for some people. Do you want to tell me about it, as much as you feel comfortable? *Client:* Yeah, it was hard.
Abstract communication	You ask if I'm feeling sad? Well, these things are generally hard for people. I mean a lot of women go through depression after a loss.
Deferential and appeasing	Yeah, I mean, you're the expert. If you think my feelings about my miscarriage are related to my feelings about my brother's death, then you would know.
Content/affect split	We went in for a routine ultrasound and the ultrasound technician wouldn't look me in the eyes, so I knew something was not right. I saw the baby on the screen, and he even seemed lifeless to me. Turns out there was no heartbeat. Afterward, I really didn't feel much of anything. I went to Burger King and back to work.
Self-critical and/or hopelessness	I just feel like I'm not doing this right. I'm not a good mother. I couldn't protect my baby. I'm not a good client. I can't even grieve the right way!

Confrontation Rupture	Client Example
Complaint about therapist	I just feel like you are not giving me what I need, and it's frustrating. I need some strategy for dealing with my mother when she says insensitive things to me. I need some concrete steps, a plan for how to change. It's frustrating that I keep telling you this.
Client rejects therapist intervention	No, learning that poor egg quality was the reason behind my miscarriages didn't make me feel any kind of way about myself or my body. I'm not sure why you would suggest that.
Complaints/concerns about the activities of therapy	*Therapist:* It sounds like it's hard to talk to your husband about the loss because he wants to make you feel better and you want to talk about your feelings. Do you think it would be helpful to role-play a little? You could be your husband and I could role-play you? *Client:* No, I don't think that would be helpful. We aren't here to talk about my husband.
Complaints about the parameters of therapy	This just isn't helping me. I'm still anxious. I'm still depressed. I constantly worry about losing this pregnancy like all the ones before. Maybe if we met more frequently it would help.

(continued)

Table 6.1. CONTINUED

Complaints about progress of therapy	I'm still not feeling better. I'm still crying all the time and frustrated with everyone for not understanding me. It takes a lot of effort for me to get here, and the therapy is just not helping me the way I need.
Client defends self against therapist	You said I had an abortion. I did not have an abortion. I mean, medically I did, but I wanted my baby. I just couldn't do it. I couldn't imagine taking care of a sick child and a sick mother. I feel like you are judging me and not understanding, just like everyone else.
Efforts to control/ pressure therapist	I need you to tell me what to do! I can't sleep. I can't eat. I can't be around any of our friends with babies. My family has had enough of me and tells me it's time to move on, and my husband is worried. I need you to help me figure out what's wrong with me and how to fix it!

Resolution/Repair Strategy	Therapist Example
Therapist clarifies misunderstanding	Let me see if I understand this correctly. You left here last week feeling like I was judging you for trying to get pregnant again so quickly after your last loss. Let me think about that. *[Pause]* I was not aware of feeling judgmental, but maybe what you were picking up on is my concern. Maybe what you needed in that moment, though, was my understanding and support and not my concern. Can we talk more about that?
Therapist changes tasks/ goals	OK, I hear you saying that talking about the pregnancy loss per se isn't what you need right now because it's the feeling that you've lost your wife, or some part of your connection with her, that is most distressing for you in this moment. So, it sounds like we need to switch gears and talk more about that?
Therapist illustrates tasks or provides rationale for treatment	You've talked about feeling profoundly emotionally abandoned by others, especially your mom, after Josh's death *[stillborn baby]*. I could be off here, but it feels to me like this is both an old and a new feeling. That is why I asked how your parents coped with your sister's death when you were young. I'm sorry if it felt like I was changing the subject.
Within context of rupture, therapist invites client to discuss thoughts and feelings with respect to therapist or some aspect of therapy	*Client:* Last week after our session we both were pulling out of the parking lot at the same time. I saw an infant car seat in the back of your car, and I had a very strong reaction. I know it sounds crazy, but I felt so mad at you! *Therapist:* I bet! Tell me more about what you were feeling in that moment?

Table 6.1. CONTINUED

Within context of rupture, therapist acknowledges own contribution to rupture	I think you are right. I think I did change the subject when you started talking about how purple Abby *[stillborn baby]* looked after delivery. I'm sorry. I can see why you would feel abandoned by me in that moment.
Within context of rupture, therapist discloses own internal experience of the client–therapist interaction	I feel a lot of pressure right now to take away your sadness, your grief. And, on one hand, I really want to be helpful and make you feel better, but, at the same time, in my experience there really is nothing I can do to take away feelings of grief. It's more of a process we must go through together, but I'm feeling very hesitant to tell you this for fear of disappointing you and making you angry.
Therapist links rupture to larger interpersonal patterns between client and therapist	We are in this place again where you are needing something from me and I'm not giving it to you, which leaves you feeling so alone in your pain and loss.
Therapist links rupture to larger interpersonal patterns in client's other relationships	Once again you find yourself in this familiar place of feeling overwhelmed by your sadness and not knowing what to do. So, you look to me, your mom, your sister to know what to do to help you, and we aren't quite getting it either, and you are left feeling very alone and like, what's wrong with me that no one (including yourself) knows what to do with my feelings?
Therapist validates client's defenses	It's only natural to be on guard in here with me if you don't feel safe. If you feel like I would somehow judge you for being an inadequate woman, somehow compare myself to you and look down on you for your fertility struggles, then why would you feel safe to be vulnerable with me?
Therapist responds to rupture by redirecting or refocusing client	Talking about the details of your loss feels like too much right now, and that's OK. Can you tell me more about what you imagined your pregnancy would be like?

Types of withdrawal and confrontation ruptures and repair strategies are taken from Eubanks-Carter et al. (2015).

Metacommunication

Repairing ruptures may be less about what the therapist says and more about the therapist's capacity to sensitively attune and respond to the client's internal experience during the rupture and repair process, as well as to the therapist's own experience (Safran & Kraus, 2014). Much like the kind of nonverbal, affective, moment-to-moment tracking that occurs on an implicit level between caregivers and their infants as they negotiate ruptures or moments of misattunement, what is affectively and nonverbally communicated during rupture and repair moments in the therapy relationship may be just as, if not more, important than any particular strategy (Safran & Kraus, 2014). *Metacommunication*, or the process of communicating with the client about the implicit transactions taking place in the therapeutic relationship, plays an important role in working through ruptures in the alliance (Safran & Muran, 2000). The ability to observe and then verbalize what is being affectively and nonverbally communicated in the relationship during ruptures is particularly important to working through attachment trauma and other transference-like reenactments (see Muran & Eubanks, 2020; Safran & Kraus, 2014).

RUPTURE AND REPAIR: AN ATTACHMENT PERSPECTIVE

Parallels have been drawn between the affective coordination seen in mother–infant dyads and the moment-to-moment negotiation that occurs within therapist–client dyads (Safran, 1993; Safran et al., 1990). In both these relationships, there is a constant oscillation between moments of affective attunement or synchrony, and misattunement or miscoordination, often occurring on an implicit, affective, and nonverbal level (Safran & Krauss, 2014; Tronick, 1989). Adaptive infant–caregiver relationships are, in fact, not defined by unilaterally synchronous or "perfectly timed" interactions, but by repeated cycles of misattunement and repair (Beebe & Lachmann, 2013; Tronick, 1989). Similarly, it has been argued that what is ultimately important to the outcome of therapy is that the dyad can effectively negotiate or repair ruptures when they occur, not that there are never problems in the alliance (Miller-Bottome et al., 2018). Supporting this, clients with rupture-repair episodes were found to improve more in therapy than clients without such events (Eubanks et al., 2018). Additionally, Miller-Bottome et al. (2019) found evidence to suggest that therapy with securely attached clients is not necessarily associated with an absence of ruptures, or with less intense ruptures, but with the ability to successfully repair them. Perhaps secure clients can draw upon early attachment experiences in which ruptures, or moments of miscoordination, were effectively repaired in order to repair ruptures in the therapeutic alliance.

This cyclical process between misattunement or miscoordination and repair in caregiver–infant dyads may serve an important developmental function of teaching the infant how to tolerate and cope with feelings that arise in moments of relational separation or disconnection, while contributing to the development of attachment internal working models of self and other (Bowlby, 1969, 1973; Tronick, 1989). Specifically, in securely attached dyads, the infant learns that, despite momentary experiences of misattunement or miscoordination, the caregiver is generally available and trustworthy and that the self can negotiate relatedness even in moments of disconnection (Tronick, 1989). Through consistent experiences in which the infant's distress over feeling disconnected from an attachment figure is empathized with and sensitively responded to, infants learn to tolerate feelings of sadness and loss in relationships. They come to trust that others will be generally available for support and comfort when needed, that they are worthy of eliciting such support and comfort, and that the self can hold on to the soothing presence of the caregiver even in the caregiver's absence (Bowlby, 1973). Attachment theory predicts that such early attachment experiences, wherein the infant learns how to tolerate momentary lapses in connection and attunement from a caregiver, lead to the capacity to better tolerate and cope with various forms of separation and loss later in life (Bowlby, 1980, 1988). In fact, similar physiological changes (which are believed to be correlates of affective responses) have been observed in infants' responses to separation from the mother as in adults' responses to bereavement (Hofer, 1984). Perhaps this is why attachment security has been associated with a more favorable bereavement reactions (Meier et al., 2013; see Mikulincer & Shaver, 2013; Schenck et al., 2015) and with fewer symptoms following a perinatal loss (Scheidt et al., 2012).

Tolerating Separation and Loss in Bereavement and Ruptures: The Impact of Attachment

The same capacities that help secure individuals to grieve the loss of a loved one through death may also help them to work through the kind of relational loss that is experienced during moments of misunderstanding or miscoordination in the therapy relationship. Specifically, individuals with a secure attachment have a greater ability to experience and regulate affects, particularly related to separation and loss (Bowlby, 1969; Mikulincer & Shaver, 2003; Schore & Schore, 2008), which facilitates the grieving process (Gupta & Bonanno, 2011). Similarly, affect tolerance and regulation capacities may help securely attached clients to experience and process feelings related to separation or disconnection in the therapy relationship. Supporting this, securely attached clients have been found to reflect upon and disclose their experience of alliance ruptures to the therapist, which contributes to the repair process (Miller-Bottome et al., 2018, 2019). Furthermore, secure individuals have a greater capacity to internalize attachment figures or loved ones, even when that person is not physically present. The capacity of secure individuals to internalize another allows them to transform and continue the attachment bond with a loved one even after death and contributes to the resolution of grief (Bowlby, 1980; see Schenk et al., 2015, for an empirical review). Similarly, clients who can internalize the soothing presence of the therapist and the therapist's overall availability and care, even during moments of misunderstanding or miscoordination, are in a better position to negotiate alliance ruptures because they are secure in the knowledge that such events do not destroy the overall therapeutic bond. Lastly, secure individuals are more likely to seek support when distressed over separation (Bowlby, 1969). Support seeking helps the bereaved to grieve and negatively correlates with PTSD following perinatal loss (Christiansen et al., 2014). Similarly, these clients are more likely to disclose their rupture experience to the therapist in an attempt to seek support and resolution, which facilitates repair (Miller-Bottome et al., 2018, 2019).

In contrast, clients with an insecure attachment may experience more difficulties grieving in general and after a pregnancy loss specifically (Scheidt et al., 2012) because they once lacked a caregiver to help them cope with and repair moments of affective disconnection in the caregiver–infant dyad, and thus they never learned how to tolerate and cope with separation and loss (Siegel, 1999, 2001). Supporting this, a few studies have found an association between a history of insecure attachment experiences in childhood and complicated patterns of bereavement in adulthood (e.g., Silverman et al., 2001; Vanderwerker et al., 2006). For example, in avoidantly attached caregiver–infant dyads, there is typically an absence of repair following moments of separation or affective miscoordination or disconnection. Children thus learn to suppress all feelings of loss and the need for repair and connection, rather than feel separation and loss deeply with no one there to soothe them (Siegel, 1999).

As adults, these individuals are more likely to have complicated bereavement reactions, for they have learned to distance themselves from their feelings of loss to cope with separation (Bonanno et al., 1995; Schenck et al., 2015). Their avoidant strategies put them at risk for maladaptive bereavement outcomes, particularly after a traumatic or sudden loss (Meier et al., 2013; see Mikulincer & Shaver, 2013, for a review), such as the loss of a pregnancy or stillbirth (Turton et al., 2001). Studies suggest that while avoidantly attached individuals attempt to suppress painful thoughts concerning loss, they fail to eliminate distress, and the suppressed material can resurface in experience and action when high cognitive or emotional demands are encountered (see Mikulincer & Shaver, 2013, for a review). In the case of pregnancy loss, subsequent pregnancies, fertility treatments, and/or invasive medical procedures may represent such events that place high cognitive and emotional demands on a woman, leading to previously suppressed feelings and experiences resurfacing and causing additional distress. In this same way, avoidant clients may minimize or suppress feelings of separation and loss associated with therapeutic alliance ruptures and the need for connection and repair with the therapist. These clients typically do not disclose specifics about their rupture experience to the therapist, which serves to evade a deeper understanding of the rupture and to stymie the repair process (Miller-Bottome et al., 2018, 2019). They may push the therapist away with anger or dismissal of the importance of the therapist and/or treatment, as a way of avoiding their need for connection and repair, which they see as a weakness. From this, a repair process, in which the therapist sensitively responds to the avoidant client's experience of separation or disconnection during a rupture and the need for repair, undoes the client's sense of aloneness and makes it feel safer to approach and process feelings of sadness and loss (see Chapters 8 and 9 in this book).

In comparison, in the ambivalently attached caregiver–infant dyad, repair following a rupture is unpredictable and at times overwhelming. These children learn that their caregiver(s) could reject, neglect, or abandon them at any time, so they cling to an inconsistent caregiver to prevent the experience of separation and loss before it can occur. Yet, these infants find little reliable comfort in connection even when they manage to receive it, for connections are unpredictable and/ or emotionally intrusive (Bowlby, 1969; Siegel, 1999). Similarly, as adults, these individuals attempt to compulsively ward off feelings of separation and loss in relationships with chronic hypervigilance to any perceived signs of rejection or abandonment (Fraley et al., 2006). Their intense anxiety over abandonment and rejection tends to get in the way of mourning the loss of a pregnancy and with processing grief in general (Bowlby, 1969; Scheidt et al., 2012; see Schenck et al., 2015, for a review). In essence, anxious individuals go to great lengths to avoid the feeling of separation and loss before it can occur, yet always feel alone. When separation and loss cannot be tolerated, however, it cannot be worked through or resolved, following literal loss through death or relational-affective loss through moments of rupture.

Consistent with this, Bowlby (1980) predicted that anxious individuals develop what he called "chronic mourning." As expected, adult attachment studies have consistently found that self-reports of attachment anxiety are positively associated with complicated grief reactions, characterized by intense separation distress from the deceased for prolonged periods of time (Meier et al., 2013; see Mikulincer & Shaver, 2013, for a review). The poor emotion regulation skills of individuals with an anxious attachment (Mikulincer et al., 2009) lead to overwhelming and un-regulated separation distress or anxiety, which suppresses more adaptive feelings of sadness and loss, and even anger, that are considered to be adaptive emotional reactions to the loss of an attachment object (Bowlby, 1980). Anxious individuals learned to defensively exclude primary feelings and reactions to separation and loss in early attachment relationships from conscious experience because these feelings were not understood or regulated during moments of rupture and repair (Bowlby, 1988). As such, anxious clients may talk about their experience of preg-nancy loss in a hyperactivated and distressed manner that elicits support from the therapist (Mikulincer, 1998), and yet resist the therapist's attempts at genuine empathy or deeper exploration. Similarly, anxious clients have been found to use vague and wordy descriptions of their experience of ruptures and to resist the therapist's attempts to attune to their experience of the rupture (Miller-Bottome et al., 2018, 2019). These clients need a repair process in which it feels safe to assert and express their authentic or primary feelings and reactions related to the rup-ture, without fear that such feelings will destroy the relationship (see Chapters 8 and 9 in this book). The experience of working through feelings of sadness and loss, within the context of an alliance rupture, may help them to feel safer to pro-cess feelings of sadness and loss in other contexts as well, such as bereavement. This process is exemplified below in the case of Kaitlyn under the "Ruptures as Reenactments of Past Attachment Experiences of Separation and Loss."

CLINICAL APPLICATION: RUPTURE AND REPAIR
THEMES IN THERAPY FOR PREGNANCY LOSS

The identification of specific rupture themes and of strategies used to repair them are likely to vary across client populations (Eubanks et al., 2018). Consistent with this, while each therapist–client dyad likely experiences and negotiates ruptures in unique ways, it is argued here that there are common, almost universal, alliance rupture and repair themes in psychotherapy for pregnancy loss. These include alliance ruptures related to clients' (a) feelings of shame and inadequacy that result from the narcissistic nature of a pregnancy loss, (b) experiences in which perinatal grief is invalidated or misunderstood, and/or (c) past attachment experiences having to do with a lack of emotional containment and repair that have been resurrected by the pregnancy loss and reenacted within the therapy relationship. Regardless of the specific theme of the rupture, the repair process with bereaved parents almost always involves meeting the client's heightened need for support, nurturance, emotional containment, and empathic understanding. These common rupture-repair themes are discussed and exemplified below in hypothetical therapist–client dialogue, derived from an amalgamation of real-life clinical experience. Subtypes of withdrawal and confrontation ruptures and of resolution strategies listed in Table 6.1 are identified in italics throughout these dialogues.

RUPTURES RELATED TO SHAME AND
INADEQUACY: HEALING NARCISSISTIC WOUNDS

Pregnancy loss is often experienced as a violent attack on one's self-worth, gender identity, and sense of self, leading to intense feelings of shame and inadequacy (Leon, 1996). As a result, bereaved parents are often intensely self-critical and easily wounded or hurt by the comments of others. As one client once phrased it, "I feel like a walking beehive. Everything stings!" This state of "narcissistic fragility" creates fertile ground for ruptures in the alliance to grow, as vulnerabilities in self-esteem leave these clients sensitive to "injury" from perceived or real criticisms and misunderstandings. Even minor misattunements on the part of the therapist may be experienced as an emotional abandonment by the client, and benign comments as an attack on one's very self, precipitating alliance ruptures in which the client feels alone, misunderstood, self-critical and humiliated, and/ or criticized or attacked. Importantly, it is typically more accurate to understand any narcissistic tendencies of clients who have recently suffered a pregnancy loss as context-specific and not as characteristic of the client's personality, although a pregnancy loss can exacerbate pre-existing narcissistic tendencies. Ultimately, helping grieving parents regain a stable sense of self is important because it facilitates the grieving process, so that they can view the lost baby as someone separate from the self (Diamond & Diamond, 2017).

Because of the narcissistic nature of a pregnancy loss, feelings of shame and inadequacy often lie at the heart of many alliance ruptures that occur with this client population. How a client copes with narcissistic shame likely impacts the specific type of rupture (withdrawal or confrontation) and the repair strategies needed. In a psychoanalytic conceptualization of narcissism, there are essentially two ways (polarities or self-states) in which individuals manage intense feelings of shame and inadequacy. Some clients tend to *internalize* feelings of shame and experience the self, to varying degrees, as "bad," inadequate, and empty, resulting in excessive self-criticism and depression. Alternatively, other clients tend to cope with shame and inadequacy through disowning and projecting, or *externalizing*, these feelings and experiences onto others, including the therapist. This allows the client to experience the self, to varying degrees, as basically "good," and, in the extreme, superior over others (McWilliams, 2011).

Clients who tend to internalize shame and feel self-critical and depressed may be more likely to blame themselves for any conflicts or misunderstandings in the alliance and to withdraw from the therapist and the work of therapy. Some clients may fear that if they were to directly express their feeling (particularly anger), needs, or wants related to a rupture, their therapist would then attack or criticize them in the same manner they attack or criticize themselves, further crushing an already fragile sense of self. In this case, the repair process involves therapist validation and empathy, which provides the interpersonal safety needed for the client to directly express feelings of anger, disappointment, or hurt, as opposed to the client blaming himself or herself for tensions or misunderstanding in the alliance and feeling ashamed and depressed. The therapist's acceptance and empathic understanding of the client's needs and concerns during a rupture contrasts the client's internal critic and helps to rebuild self-esteem. In contrast, clients who externalize and project feelings of shame and inadequacy onto the therapist are more likely to become angry and argumentative (an expression of narcissistic rage) in the relationship, leading to confrontation ruptures. Instead of moving against the self during a rupture and becoming self-critical, these clients move against and become critical of the therapist. Empathic connection during the repair process helps these clients to own previously disowned feelings, with more understanding and compassion (Safran & Krauss, 2014).

In the author's clinical experience, pregnancy loss clients are much more likely to be depressed and self-critical and to withdraw during a rupture than to express anger toward the therapist and confront him or her. This may be due to the violent attack on self-esteem that often accompanies the loss of a pregnancy, which leaves parents feeling depressed and self-critical (Diamond & Diamond, 2016). Gender may also be a factor, as most pregnancy loss clients identify as women, who are typically socialized to suppress competing feelings and needs and to blame the self for conflicts or misunderstandings with others in order to preserve the relationship (Gilligan, 2002). It is more common that flashes of narcissistic rage and more subtle confrontation ruptures occur with pregnancy loss clients when they feel as if their experience of loss has been misunderstood by the therapist. Clients often feel angry and envious that others, even the therapist, get to be ignorant about the trauma and the pain of pregnancy loss. The below vignette demonstrates how feelings of shame and inadequacy, brought on by the loss of a pregnancy, can precipitate withdrawal ruptures, and how therapist validation and empathy help to repair the alliance, rebuild client self-esteem, and facilitate the grieving process.

IZZY: It was my cousin's bridal shower last weekend, and I completely lost it on her. It was like all my anger came pouring out of me as I screamed, over and over, that she doesn't care about me. I mean, there she was, having this perfect bridal shower. Everything went as she planned. It just didn't feel fair. In the moment, I felt so wronged and angry, but now I feel so humiliated that I lost it in front of everyone. *[Izzy felt inferior to her cousin and coped with feelings of shame and inadequacy by projecting her sense of "badness" onto her cousin, "moving against" the cousin. One can see how a similar dynamic might lead to a confrontation rupture with the therapist later on in treatment.]*

THERAPIST: It's very embarrassing to think people could see how out of control you felt.

IZZY: Yes, exactly. I was so angry! I don't want people to think I'm an angry person or to be angry with me for hurting my cousin, which they should be anyway. I would deserve it.

THERAPIST: Well, let's try to understand your anger. *[Therapist attempts to circumvent client's shame and understand her anger, rather than criticize it.]* Sometimes people say hurtful things when they are hurting inside. Does that fit for you?

IZZY: Yes, yeah. I didn't think of it that way before, that I was hurting inside, but I really was. I just felt like such a failure, like I don't measure up. My cousin, who is getting married 4 years after me, will probably be pregnant before I am and on their first try!

THERAPIST: It would make sense to me if you felt kind of envious of your cousin. Like, why do good things seem to come so easily and perfectly for other people, but not for me? What's wrong with me?

IZZY: Yes, it makes me so mad! It's not fair. I was angry that everyone was sitting around happy for my cousin and her perfect wedding without thinking that this might be hard for me.

THERAPIST: Sure, and maybe right behind the anger is hurt *[Izzy gets teary]*. Can you stay with the hurt for a moment?

IZZY: I just felt like nobody cared about me and how I was feeling, which is ridiculous, because everyone has been so supportive of me through all the fertility treatments and miscarriages. But, in that moment, I felt like nobody cared about how I was suffering. I felt so damaged and inadequate compared to my cousin, and like she was rubbing it in my face, but I know that sounds crazy.

THERAPIST: In that moment, you felt so inadequate that you essentially felt invisible.

IZZY: I guess *[looking down, getting red in face]*. *[Nonverbals and minimal response suggests withdrawal rupture marker.]*

THERAPIST: Did you just have a reaction to what I said? *[Invites thoughts and feelings]*

IZZY: No. I mean, I don't know. You are totally right. I was being selfish. I just feel embarrassed. *[Deferential and appeasing; self-critical]*

THERAPIST: Help me understand. It sounds like I said something that made you feel criticized? *[Invites thoughts and feelings; therapist acknowledges contribution to rupture; direct repair intervention]*

IZZY: You didn't do anything wrong. You were right. It was just *one moment*, my cousin's shower of all places, when my family wasn't focused on me. They are so supportive all the time. My cousin deserved to have that moment. I shouldn't have reacted that way. *[Deferential and appeasing; self-critical]*

THERAPIST: So, it felt like I was sort of dismissing or minimizing your feelings as selfish or unimportant, like an overreaction? *[Therapist invites thoughts and feelings]*

IZZY: You were just pointing out the obvious. I'm just very sensitive these days. Even my mom is like, "You need to get it together, everyone is walking around on eggshells around you!" *[Deferential and appeasing; self-critical]*

THERAPIST: *[pause]* So, I'm feeling right now like there are several powerful self-critical voices in the room. Do you sense that too? *[Izzy nods]* The thing about these self-critical voices is that they are so loud, they drown out the very important fact that something I said hurt you. *[Therapist discloses internal experience; invites Izzy's thoughts and feelings; acknowledges contribution to rupture.]*

IZZY: You didn't mean to. *[Deferential and appeasing]*

THERAPIST: No, I don't believe I did, but that doesn't change the fact that I hurt you, and that matters to me. *[Therapist discloses internal experience and encourages Izzy to directly express her feelings associated with the rupture, rather than blaming herself and withdrawing.]*

IZZY: Thanks. I guess my feelings were hurt a little. Something about you saying that my family wasn't supporting me in "that particular moment" kind of stung. But isn't that just me being too sensitive?

THERAPIST: Maybe you were accurately picking up on the fact that, even in a subtle way, I failed to acknowledge that there are actually lots of "mini" moments, not just "that particular moment," that add up over time, in which you are forced to confront situations that feel profoundly unfair, remind you of all that you have lost, and make you feel like you don't measure up to other people who seem to easily have what you want. *[Therapist acknowledges her contribution to the rupture.]*

IZZY: Yeah, that's how I feel a lot with people, not just you.

THERAPIST: I think, with me in here, and with family members, it's the feeling that others aren't acknowledging or fully seeing how painful this experience has been for you that leaves you feeling profoundly hurt. But, somehow, that hurt quickly turns into rage and anger, like with your cousin, or, alternatively, you minimize or dismiss the hurt, like in here with me, and that makes it even harder for people to see how hurt you truly are. *[Link rupture to other relationships; example of expressive repair intervention]*

IZZY: *[crying]* Yes, exactly. But I don't want it to come off like I'm blaming you. I don't want to chase away every person in my life because I need you all right now. It's not realistic to expect people to always understand what I'm feeling or to support me in every single moment.

THERAPIST: Right, but I don't exactly hear it that way. I hear you saying that you are hurting, and you need me to see that, the full extent of it. *[Therapist validates defensive position.]*

IZZY: I guess that's what I didn't do with my cousin, tell her I was hurting. I didn't realize I was hurting until now. I just felt so inferior to her in that moment and jealous. I lashed out. Looking back now, I didn't think she would understand, or if I told her that her shower was hard for me emotionally that she would get mad at me, but now she's mad at me anyway. *[Izzy fears that others will attack or criticize her the way she attacks/criticizes herself, leading to suppression of feelings, needs, and wants.]*

THERAPIST: Is that what made it hard to tell me that I hurt your feelings? You were afraid I would get angry with you? *[Invites thoughts and feelings; links rupture to outside relationships]*

IZZY: Yes, I think so.

THERAPIST: And how did you perceive my reaction? *[Invites thoughts and feelings]*

IZZY: Supportive, understanding.

THERAPIST: And how did that make you feel? *[Invites thoughts and feelings]*

IZZY: It made me feel better about myself, like my feelings are understandable and valid. But, in a way, I guess it also made me feel sad.

THERAPIST: What's the saddest part?

IZZY: I'll never have what my cousin has. Even if I can stay pregnant, it will never be that blissful experience of assuming that a pregnancy is going to equal a healthy baby. She gets to be pregnant and joyful about it. I might get one but will never get the other. *[With Izzy's shame more regulated, Izzy can now explore feelings of grief and loss.]*

RUPTURES RELATED TO SOCIETAL INVALIDATION OF PREGNANCY LOSS: REPAIRING EMPATHIC FAILURES

Although a relatively common occurrence, the raw emotional, psychological, and physical experience of pregnancy loss remains, for the most part, cloaked in mystery and silence (Markin & Zilcha-Mano, 2018). In Western society, grieving parents are actively discouraged from openly acknowledging or publicly mourning their loss (Doka, 1989). In stark comparison to other types of losses, when a pregnancy is lost there are no religious or social gatherings to support the bereaved and to validate their loss as real and grief as legitimate (Frost & Condon, 1996; Keren, 2010; Markin & Zilcha-Mano, 2018). Without clear and customary mourning rituals, parents are left not knowing how to mourn, deprived of their right to mourn, and feeling as if their grief is not recognized by society (Lang et al., 2011; Markin & Zilcha-Mano, 2018). Instead, there is an active culture of denial and rationalization that discourages parents from grieving and invalidates their loss as real (Frost & Condon, 1996). From this, it has been argued that there is a *cultural taboo* against the public recognition and expression of perinatal grief that hinders parents' ability to mourn (Markin & Zilcha-Mano, 2018).

The cultural taboo against the validation and expression of perinatal grief may be recreated within the therapy relationship, as feelings of grief over a pregnancy loss are unintentionally or unconsciously minimized or avoided by the therapist and/or client (Markin & Zilcha-Mano, 2018). Because these clients often feel as if their very traumatic experience of loss is shunned by society, they typically enter therapy feeling alone and misunderstood. Understandably, they are often sensitive to criticism, self-critical of the fact that they have not yet moved on, and reluctant to express their feelings to the therapist for fear they will be dismissed once again (Covington, 2006; Markin & Zilcha-Mano, 2018). When the therapist similarly, although unintentionally, fails to validate, acknowledge, or understand the client's experience of loss, alliance ruptures, characterized by misunderstanding events and empathic errors, are likely to occur (Markin, 2016). Well-intentioned and otherwise empathic clinicians may make empathic errors with pregnancy loss clients simply due to a lack of knowledge, as the experience of pregnancy loss is not something typically talked about in society and clinicians rarely receive training in this area, even though most will work with a client who has lost a pregnancy (Markin, 2018). In addition, clinicians may unknowingly discourage, invalidate, or avoid clients' feelings of perinatal loss because of the very human tendency to turn away in the face of overwhelming trauma in order to cope (Markin, 2018), and/or because, as therapists, we too are products of a society that actively discourages perinatal grief, perhaps because the death of a baby is so traumatic (Markin & Zilcha-Mano, 2018). In particular, therapists with more adverse childhood attachment experiences may be more likely to dismiss the client's attachment to the lost baby and feelings of grief and loss (see Strauss & Petrowski, 2017 for a review of therapist attachment and the process and outcome of therapy).

Repairing alliance ruptures that are characterized by the therapist's lack of empathic understanding or validation of the client's experience of perinatal grief and loss is important to the therapy process because the therapist's empathic support and sharing of sadness helps the client to feel less alone and facilitates the grieving process (Leon, 2010, 2015). Therapist comments about pregnancy loss that are experienced as insensitive or invalidating by the client rub and inflict pain upon a pre-existing and open wound, inflicted by the many similar insensitive comments of others that leave the client feeling alone and misunderstood. The therapist acknowledging the rupture, and one's contribution to it, helps to validate the client's loss as real and grief as legitimate. An effective repair process reduces the shame that results from having one's experience socially excluded and misunderstood, and heals painful disruptions in empathy experienced in outside and inside therapy relationships (Leon, 2015; Markin & Zilcha-Mano, 2018).

The social stigma around acknowledging or validating a parent's experience of pregnancy loss may be amplified for parents who identify as part of a marginalized group, who already have aspects of their experience silenced and excluded. For example, to become pregnant in the first place, LGBTQ+ parents are often forced to navigate a heteronormative system that does not leave room for their experience and invalidates them as parents (Holley & Pasch, 2015). When a pregnancy is then lost, lack of understanding and support may make it even harder for these clients to have their experience of grief and loss acknowledged and validated (Markin, 2023). Alliance ruptures can occur when therapists internalize this heterosexist bias, interfering with their ability to empathize with the parent's experience of loss, as exemplified below.

THERAPIST: Tell me what brings you in today?

CARLY: Well, I don't know how much experience you have with situations like mine? *[pause]* My wife [Sandy] and I have been through a lot this past year trying to have a baby. Having kids was always part of our plan. We decided to go the fertility clinic route. We used Sandy's eggs and agreed that she would carry the baby this time because she is 5 years older than me, and I would do it next time. But the process of IVF was a lot more physically traumatic for Sandy than we realized it would be.

THERAPIST: Was there a problem with Sandy's eggs? Why did she need IVF?

CARLY: No, people ask that a lot. It's kind of annoying. Neither one of us is infertile, we just don't make sperm. We decided to use an anonymous sperm donor. We thought that would be less complicated. *[Carly indirectly "complains" about therapist; first indication that she feels misunderstood and angry, or "annoyed," with the therapist; confrontation rupture marker]*

THERAPIST: I'm sorry, I misunderstood. Thanks for explaining that. Please go on. How did the transfer go? *[Therapist acknowledges contribution to the rupture and redirects client; immediate repair strategy]*

CARLY: The transfer went fine. Everything looked great. Then, at 13 weeks, we miscarried.

THERAPIST: I'm sorry. How is Sandy doing? It often surprises people how hard miscarriage can be.

CARLY: *[in an angry and exacerbated tone]* People always say that, too! They always ask how Sandy is doing; no one ever asks about me. Or, they won't exactly ask how Sandy is doing but say insensitive things to her like "at least it happened early" or "it's for the best." I never know if that means "it's for the best" because this child would have been at a disadvantage being raised by two mothers. But even when people are saying insensitive or hurtful things to Sandy, at least they are talking to her and acknowledging that she was a mother to this baby. From the start, I felt like others didn't see me as a real parent to our baby, so now it would never occur to them that I'm grieving the loss! *[Complaint about therapist, speaking about her in the displacement as yet another person who does not see the client's role as a parent as legitimate or her grief as valid]*

THERAPIST: What do you mean? *[Invites thoughts and feelings]*

CARLY: When we were trying to get pregnant, the doctors and staff at the fertility clinic would always assume I was Sandy's friend or sister when we would go in for appointments. It was like a constant coming-out process: "No, I'm not the sister or the friend. I'm the second mother." I would never know how people would react to that, and it would cause additional anxiety. Then, the doctor would talk directly to Sandy like I wasn't even in the room. I wasn't even invited into the room when the doctor told Sandy she was miscarrying. I was told to wait in the waiting room like I was no one to our baby, just an outsider. And legally, I wasn't considered a mother to the baby, which is insulting, ya know? I was going to adopt her when she was born, and now I'll never get that chance, that validation that I was her mom too. It's hard enough when people you don't really know treat you that way, but when I told my own mother about our loss, her response was, "At least it wasn't *really* your baby."

THERAPIST: Wow, this sounds like a very deep and painful wound that keeps getting reopened. You find yourself in these repeated situations, with the doctors, the clinic staff, your mother, and now, here with me, where you are left feeling completely invisible, invalidated, and excluded. Is that right? *[Link rupture with therapist to outside therapy relationships and experiences; expressive repair strategy]*

CARLY: Yes, exactly.

THERAPIST: I get the feeling that I just picked at that wound and opened the scab and that I hurt you. *[Therapist discloses internal experience and acknowledges contribution to rupture.]* Can you tell me more about what you were experiencing when I asked about Sandy? *[Invites thoughts and feelings]*

CARLY: Look, I don't think this is helpful for me to talk about *[rejects intervention]*. I was really looking for a therapist with experience working with couples in similar situations *[complaint about therapist]*. It took me over 2 hours to get here and the fee is more than I was hoping to spend *[complaints about the parameters of therapy]*. We are already in debt from the cost of IVF, so I just want to make sure I'm getting what I need from this *[complaints about progress of therapy]*.

THERAPIST: OK, I think I'm beginning to understand. Tell me if I'm getting this? I imagine that when a person has repeated experiences with family, friends, and even doctors of feeling misunderstood, invisible, or invalidated, it is of course going to be difficult for that person to come into therapy and trust that a stranger will be able to understand and meet their needs. Given everything you've been through, it would make sense to me if you came in here with a healthy dose of caution about me. When I asked about Sandy, and not specifically about how *you* were feeling, it must have felt like your worst fear come true, like I wasn't really seeing or acknowledging you and your experience. No wonder you are now concerned that I won't be able to understand or help you. *[Therapist validates client's defensive posture.]*

CARLY: Yes, I was very nervous about this. I never know how people are going to react.

THERAPIST: Understandable, and I have to give some real thought to why I asked about Sandy first. I'm sorry I made any assumptions. That's not fair to you. *[Therapist acknowledges contribution to rupture.]*

CARLY: I'm sorry I got so angry.

THERAPIST: I think you had a very healthy sense that something wasn't right in here, that, on some level, I wasn't understanding or acknowledging an important part of your identity as a parent and as a grieving mother. I'm glad you listened to that internal sense and told me how you felt because it's important to me that you feel truly seen in here. *[Validation of client's anger; therapist discloses internal experience]*

CARLY: It's just a very lonely feeling when no one sees your pain or believes it's real.

THERAPIST: That sounds important. Can you say more? *[Invites thoughts and feelings]*

RUPTURES AS REENACTMENTS OF PAST ATTACHMENT EXPERIENCES OF SEPARATION AND LOSS: FACILITATING A SECURE ATTACHMENT AND THE GRIEVING PROCESS THROUGH REPAIR

Because bereaved parents typically feel unsupported, misunderstood, and invalidated during a time of great distress, when the attachment system is activated, early experiences in which they similarly felt a lack of support, understanding, and emotional soothing with important attachment figures after other instances of traumatic loss are likely to re-emerge (Markin, 2018). Past instances of abuse or neglect with caregivers, repeated moments of separation or affective miscoordination or misattunement with no repair, and/or early experiences in which the client felt alone, scared, and overwhelmed in feelings of grief over the loss of an important other may all be activated by and merge with the loss of a pregnancy or baby (Leon, 2015). Supporting this, Hughes et al. (2004) found that although a similar number of women who experienced a stillbirth and control women reported childhood trauma, only women who had a stillbirth were unresolved with respect to this trauma, suggesting that the unresolved state may be evoked by the subsequent traumatic loss of a stillbirth. The authors suggest that the experience of pregnancy loss raises the issue of support and understanding more broadly and of emotional containment (Hughes et al., 2004). As the woman often turns to her own mother for support and comfort after the traumatic loss of a pregnancy or baby and experiences, yet again, a familiar sense of a lack of emotional containment, support, and understanding, similar past experiences in which she felt alone in feelings of sadness and loss upon separation are evoked and need to be grieved.

It is proposed that early unresolved attachment experiences related to a lack of repair after instances of separation and loss are evoked by and may merge with the loss of a pregnancy, and, furthermore, are reenacted within the therapy relationship. Reenactments of early attachment experiences related to a lack of repair may lead to alliance ruptures in which the client experiences the therapist as the unsupportive, unresponsive, overwhelming, or insensitive caregiver who is unable or unwilling to understand and soothe feelings of distress over separation and loss. This is consistent with the theory that alliance ruptures represent a series of reenactments within the therapeutic relationship (Safran & Krauss, 2014; Safran & Muran, 2000). Clients with an insecure attachment, who were more often left alone in their feelings of sadness, fear, anger, confusion, and distress over separation with no repair (Siegel, 1999), are perhaps more likely to experience a lack of emotional containment and understanding from the therapist and subsequent alliance ruptures. Perhaps this explains why it has been observed that pregnancy loss clients with an adverse attachment history struggle to establish a good alliance and to experience therapist empathy (Leon, 2015; Markin, 2018). It is important to recognize that the client's experience of the therapist as insensitive or unresponsive may also be, at least in part, accurate, whether because the therapist is unconsciously participating in the reenactment and/or because of internalized societal taboos against acknowledging perinatal grief.

It has been previously argued that the client's attachment style is activated by or associated with alliance ruptures, and, through the repair process, may be altered to more secure (Bowman & Safran, 2007; Daniel, 2015; Safran, 1993; Safran & Segal, 1990). Bowlby (1988) believed that therapeutic change begins with the emergence of a secure attachment bond with the therapist, in which painful emotions can be tolerated and processed and in which internal working models can be reworked. The beneficial effects of enhanced attachment security have been documented in studies of psychotherapy for several mood-related disorders (e.g., Zuroff & Blatt, 2006). It has been similarly suggested that a secure attachment bond with the therapist has beneficial effects for clients suffering from bereavement disorders (Mikulincer & Shaver, 2013). Consistent with this, a rupture-repair process in which the bereaved parent's feelings related to separation and loss are empathized with, emotionally contained, and sensitively responded to, unlike in early attachment relationships, may help the client to feel safe to approach feelings of grief and loss, while rewiring insecure attachment internal working models to more secure, as exemplified in the vignette below.

THERAPIST: What's on your mind today? You seem more quiet than usual. *[Therapist suspects Kaitlyn's minimal responsiveness is a sign of a withdrawal rupture marker and asks questions to elicit thoughts and feelings.]*

KAITLYN: Oh, nothing, I'm fine. *[Fidgets nervously, shaking leg up and down]* *[Denial]*

THERAPIST: Hmm, I'm wondering if your leg agrees with you? *[Both smile.]* *[Invites thoughts and feelings]*

KAITLYN: I guess I'm thinking about the holiday coming up and the fact that everyone is leaving for vacation. My mom is going away with her new boyfriend and my sister and best friend are both going away with their own families. I think they are relieved to get away from me and all my crying. I guess I don't blame them. I've been asking them when exactly they are coming back and if we can spend time together before they leave and no one is texting me back, and I'm just super-agitated. *[Self-critical]*

THERAPIST: It sounds like there is something about your friends and family leaving for vacation that brings up a lot of feelings for you that may be important for us to understand.

KAITLYN: I just don't understand why they are leaving me now, and I don't know what I'm going to do with myself while they are gone. I think I'll go crazy.

THERAPIST: You feel abandoned and maybe scared about how you will handle your feelings without them.

KAITLYN: Yeah, when they told me about their vacation plans it was all very cavalier, like this is no big deal. *[Perhaps complaint about therapist in the displacement]*

THERAPIST: I'm thinking right now that last week I also told you I was going on vacation for the holidays, and I'm wondering if maybe you had some feelings about that? *[Link rupture to outside relationships and invites thoughts and feelings]*

KAITLYN: It's fine. I don't know why I'm anxious about it. *[Denial]*

THERAPIST: I think sometimes we get anxious when we are having other feelings that we can't quite put our finger on. Maybe it would be helpful for us to think together about what you were feeling or experiencing here with me when I told you I was leaving for vacation because it might give us some clues as to what you were experiencing with your family and friends? *[Invites thoughts and feelings; begins to link therapist–client relationship with outside relationships]*

KAITLYN: I mean, obviously it's not your job to remember this, and I'm not blaming anyone for anything at all, but the holidays will be the 1-year anniversary of Sean's death *[stillborn baby]*, and I just think this is going to be very hard for me *[crying]*. *[Deferential and appeasing]*

THERAPIST: Of course this is going to be a hard time for you; that makes complete sense! It would also make sense to me if you felt angry with me for leaving when you need me and hurt that I didn't remember or acknowledge this. *[Invites thoughts and feelings and validates Kaitlyn]*

KAITLYN: *[sniffling]* Thanks, yeah. I guess I was a little upset. Like with my mom, I just wanted her to think of me when she was making her plans, like I wanted to be a part of her equation, and maybe for her to realize that I would need her support and comfort.

THERAPIST: You felt invisible and maybe unimportant to your mom and maybe with me too. *[Links outside relationships to therapist–client relationship]*

KAITLYN: Yes, exactly.

THERAPIST: What do you suppose kept you from expressing your very healthy need for support and comfort during the anniversary of Sean's death to me, or with your mom? *[Invites thoughts and feelings and validates Kaitlyn's attachment need for support and comfort when distressed]*

KAITLYN: Well, I don't want anyone to be angry with me.

THERAPIST: Because?

KAITLYN: Because then who would I have? I need someone to tell me everything is going to be OK because right now I really don't feel like anything will ever be OK ever again.

THERAPIST: It sounds like you are left feeling as if you can either express your needs and perhaps get some support and comfort, but at the cost of possible rejection, or keep your needs to yourself and feel more secure that others will stick around, but resentful and anxious because you feel so alone.

KAITLYN: That about sums it up.

THERAPIST: Is that a familiar experience?

KAITLYN: With my mom, yeah. After Sean died, I was a wreck. I couldn't eat or sleep. I just slept all day. For days I wanted my mom to call me. I mean, she's my mom. I figured she should be the one to reach out to me as another mother. I didn't hear anything from her for days, then she calls me and tells me that she is going to come over with my favorite ice cream and we could watch soap operas all day. For the first time, I got out of bed and showered. I was so excited for her to come over and just give me a hug. Then, in typical mom fashion, she never showed.

THERAPIST: I can't imagine how you must have felt toward her? That image feels so crushing.

KAITLYN: At first, I didn't feel any way toward her. I felt bad about myself. What did I do to push her away? Why doesn't she want to console her own daughter after her grandchild just died? What is so wrong with me? But I never told her how I felt and how upset I was because I was afraid that if I did, then she would come around even less, and then who would I have? I can't exactly go to my father with this, and my sister and friends all have babies. They don't know how to deal with this, and honestly, I don't think they want to. But I guess I should be used to it by now; this is what she did to me growing up. One day we would be eating ice cream and watching bad TV and the next day she would be gone for days with no explanation. I wouldn't understand what happened or when she would come back. I would just lay in bed, not eating or sleeping, or talking to anyone until she returned.

THERAPIST: There is so much pain and loss there. I imagine that little girl so terrified and alone and so overwhelmed with no one to comfort her or help her make sense of what was going on.

KAITLYN: When Sean died it put me right back in that place of feeling so dependent on her for comfort, but that's not exactly her strong suit, so I end up feeling worse about myself and even more alone.

THERAPIST: It sounds like the experience of losing Sean and of feeling like you couldn't depend on your mom when you really needed her brought up all these old feelings of abandonment, of feeling like she just leaves you in your overwhelming feelings of distress.

KAITLYN: Yes, exactly. But the thing is, you never know what to expect from her because sometimes she is really good at comforting me. So I want her to stay with me and not go on this vacation because sometimes I do find her really comforting.

THERAPIST: What do you want to say to your mom?

KAITLYN: I want to tell her I'm angry with her for flaking on me when I really need her, but I'm afraid she won't care enough to stay.

THERAPIST: And that would really be devastating.

KAITLYN: Yes, completely [crying].

THERAPIST: Your mom isn't here right now, but I am. Is there something you're maybe holding back about how you feel about my vacation? If you were to take a risk right now, what would you say to me? [Invites thoughts and feelings; links outside and therapy relationship]

KAITLYN: I might say that I'm a bit annoyed that you are leaving now of all times.

THERAPIST: Annoyed, yes, I can see why, maybe even angry. Like, "Come on, you're a therapist, you should know that I'm in pain and need you right now!" [Therapist validates Kaitlyn's anger or protest against separation.]

KAITLYN: Maybe, but I understand. [Deferential and appeasing]

THERAPIST: Intellectually, sure. But emotionally, that scared little girl inside of you is so afraid she will be left alone in her distress. I bet she wants to tell me she's angry and maybe kick and scream a little, like, "Hey, where are you going? Come back!" Not the grown-up version of you, of course, but the child inside who needs comfort . . .

KAITLYN: Yes, I think she would be very angry, but too scared to say anything about it.

THERAPIST: What would she say, if she wasn't so afraid?

KAITLYN: How could you leave me? Can't you see how much pain I'm in! I lost my baby!

THERAPIST: Good, keep going.

KAITLYN: I lost my baby, he's gone [sobbing], and I'm so empty without him and so alone. And you are not here for me when you should be!

THERAPIST: I see how much pain you, and that little girl inside, are in, and, no, I do not want to leave you alone in all these feelings of sadness and loss, and I will come back. I hope that I can leave you with a sense that even when I'm not here physically, I am still here with you? *[Therapist discloses internal experience; attempts to provide corrective attachment experience]* Did you have a reaction to what I just said?

KAITLYN: It feels good to hear you say that you are going to come back, but I also feel sad that my own mom can't say that to me.

THERAPIST: You are grieving not just the loss of Sean, but also the loss of not having your mother consistently available to comfort you in the ways that you have wanted and needed.

CLINICAL CHALLENGES

The clinician's ability to identify ruptures when they occur, particularly withdrawal ruptures that may be relatively easier to miss, is often a challenge to treatment (Eubanks et al., 2018). Relatedly, it can be challenging for clinicians to identify moment-to-moment, nonverbal-affective ruptures, or moments of misattunement, in the therapy relationship, as these often require a great deal of sensitivity to recognize. However, because pregnancy loss clients typically have a heightened sensitivity to relational loss due to recent experiences with traumatic loss, they may be particularly sensitive to feelings of separation or affective disconnection within the therapy relationship. Thus, it may be especially important for clinicians to be able to identify subtle shifts, or moments of affective misattunement or miscoordination, in the alliance. The willingness to identify alliance ruptures often requires a fundamental paradigm shift for many clinicians, from viewing ruptures as either personal or treatment failures, to a normal and potentially therapeutic part of the therapy process. Moreover, in the author's experience, repairing ruptures with pregnancy loss clients is difficult to do without prior understanding of the psychological and societal dynamics of pregnancy loss. For example, the knowledge that even benign comments by the therapist may be experienced as an attack by the client suggests that supportive interventions are needed for repair.

It often catches therapists by surprise just how quickly they find themselves in a reenactment, wherein they unknowingly, and often in very subtle ways, play the part of the client's unsupportive or unempathic caregiver in times of traumatic loss, and that their otherwise very compliant and "nice" client, on a more unconscious or covert level, harbors feelings of anger, rage, and disappointment in the therapist as a result. It can be a challenge to recognize this dynamic as it quickly unfolds and to step outside of it in order to sensitively respond to the client in a corrective manner, contrary to past attachment figures. This often requires therapist flexibility to respond to the client in ways that the client needs, and not necessarily in ways that fit a therapist's theoretical orientation (see Hatcher, 2015)—for example, the client who wants her psychoanalytic therapist to "do something" to ease her pain, unlike her parents who she has always experienced as "just sitting on the sidelines and observing," as she becomes engulfed in grief and anguish, or the client who wants her CBT therapist to just listen and normalize her experience, and not to "do" anything to take away or "fix" her pain, as she has come to expect her attachment figures to try and do. Lastly, clinicians need to be able to tolerate feelings of separation or disconnection in the therapy relationship that arise from moments of misunderstanding or tension to directly address alliance ruptures. This sends a message to the client that feelings of separation and loss can be tolerated, that they will not destroy us or the relationship, and that others can be trusted for support and comfort even in moments of disconnection. Therapists must put aside their feelings of inadequacy that a rupture occurred in the first place, to meet the client's need for a rupture *to* occur, so that the client can learn to cope with the pain of separation and loss within an empathic and caring relationship.

CLINICAL IMPLICATIONS

- Therapists need to have knowledge of the psychological, relational, societal, and medical aspects of pregnancy loss to avoid alliance ruptures characterized by misunderstanding events.
- While ruptures due to the therapist's lack of knowledge regarding the various aspects of pregnancy loss should be avoided or quickly repaired, other ruptures, particularly those that are reenactments of early attachment experiences related to separation and loss and a lack of emotional containment and repair, should be considered opportunities to heal old attachment wounds and rewire insecure attachment internal working models to more secure, and not as treatment failures.
- Because pregnancy loss clients have a heightened need for nurturance and support, and because they typically harbor intense feelings of shame and inadequacy and feel invalidated and misunderstood in society, they are typically sensitive to even subtle lapses in therapist attunement, which can be experienced as deeply wounding. Therapists need to carefully track their attunement to the client's experience.
- The successful repair of ruptures leaves clients with experiential knowledge that they can turn to the therapist for emotional containment, support, and understanding when in distress, helping them to feel safer to approach feelings of grief and loss.

7

Managing Countertransference in Psychotherapy for Pregnancy Loss

In therapy for pregnancy loss, there are often not one but two individuals with a reproductive story that has somehow been violated, "stolen," and fundamentally changed (Jaffe, 2014). Many therapists who are attracted to pregnancy loss and infertility work have struggled through similar experiences as those of their clients. One survey of nurses and mental health professionals working in reproductive medicine found that 52 percent had a history of infertility and 71 percent started this work after their infertility experience (Covington & Marosek, 1999). This suggests that to varying degrees, mental health professionals in this field likely have conscious and unconscious reasons for choosing to focus on the very kind of traumatic losses that most people in our society go to great lengths to minimize or avoid (Markin & Zilcha-Mano, 2018).

Some therapists may decide to specialize in pregnancy loss or infertility to try and make sense of and process their own chaotic experience of reproductive trauma and loss, while others are searching for that feeling of control and mastery that they could not find throughout their personal reproductive journey. Some of these therapists may seek to give their clients the support that they yearned for, yet lacked, during their own pregnancy loss experience, walking a fine line between meeting the client's need for empathy and validation and the therapist's need to nurture in her clients what was left uncared for in herself. Of course, not all therapists working with reproductive loss issues will have prior personal experiences with this kind of unique loss. Yet, some of these clinicians might be intimately familiar with other kinds of "silent" and "invisible" losses; for example, the traumatic loss of a family member by suicide that was never talked about or acknowledged by close others. For these individuals, the pain of being alone in the anguish of loss and of losing someone prematurely is both identifiable and fresh. Perhaps another therapist has never known what it is like to lose a pregnancy or to experience infertility per se, but she knows what it's like to feel betrayed by her

Psychotherapy for Pregnancy Loss. Rayna D. Markin, Oxford University Press. © Oxford University Press 2024.
DOI: 10.1093/oso/9780197693353.003.0007

body after a diagnosis of breast cancer. Alternatively, another therapist, as a child, may have helplessly watched his mother bury her stillborn baby and unsuccessfully tried to save her from the tidal wave of depression that followed. He may find some form of healing through helping women in similar situations yet struggle to contain the urge within him to "save" his clients, unintentionally confirming for these women that there is indeed something wrong with them in need of saving. Because of these shared experiences between reproductive loss clients and their therapists, *countertransference*, in one form or another, will always be present, whether it be in the background or the foreground of therapy. Thus, it is important not to deny countertransference, but to acknowledge, understand, use, and manage it for the benefit of the client, so that it does not unconsciously leak out through therapist nonverbal and verbal behaviors to the detriment of the treatment (Gelso & Hayes, 1998).

This chapter begins with a brief theoretical and empirical review of various aspects of countertransference, particularly *countertransference management* and its relation to psychotherapy outcome. Evidence-based relationship principles derived from research on countertransference in psychotherapy are then applied to the treatment of clients who have suffered a pregnancy loss specifically. Pregnancy loss with and without infertility are examined in this chapter because both represent reproductive traumas that can have a significant impact on an individual's sense of self and other, which, in turn, can cause powerful transference–countertransference dynamics in the therapy relationship. Based on theory and research, possible signs of internal countertransference reactions and overt behaviors are explored, including inappropriate therapist self-disclosure. Common transference–countertransference themes when working with pregnancy loss and infertility are discussed, including when either the therapist or client becomes pregnant. Detailed case examples demonstrate the application of these ideas. First-person language is used in these clinical vignettes and elsewhere, unlike in other chapters, due to the highly personal nature of countertransference. Clinical challenges to managing countertransference and clinical implications are offered.

CASE VIGNETTE: COUNTERTRANSFERENCE MANAGEMENT

Hana[1] was a 33-year-old second-generation Korean American married cisgender female who entered treatment with me after a diagnosis of primary infertility and repeated pregnancy losses. She was currently pregnant again and, as is typical during pregnancies after loss, struggled with a great deal of anxiety over another potential loss. She was troubled by fantasies of throwing herself in front of a moving car to rid herself of the pregnancy, despite stating

---

1. The events and client descriptives in this case have been substantially altered and merged with other similar cases to protect client confidentiality.

that she wanted this baby and sacrificed much to "get here." I understood her fantasies as an attempt to take control of the possibility of yet another loss before it once again could take control of her. She was also a practicing therapist at the beginning of her career. Hana lamented that she got "a late start in life." She felt behind in comparison to her peers in terms of her career advancement and family planning. Her parents had wanted Hana to go into medicine, but 3 years into medical school she suddenly dropped out, which caused much tension with her family. She subsequently enrolled in graduate school to obtain her master's in social work (a field she stated her parents did not understand), where she met her now husband. Hana reported feeling a great deal of pressure from her parents to continue the family lineage and often felt blamed by them for her fertility struggles, particularly because Hana married later in life than her parents had wanted and was normative in traditional Korean culture. Hana's mother would often chastise her that the stress of starting her practice was causing her to miscarry and, instead, she should focus on her husband and on starting a family. Hana stated that her parents have always had high expectations of her that she could never live up to, and, as a result, has always felt like a disappointment to them.[2] Failing to produce grandchildren represented a major area in which Hana felt like a disappointment to not only her parents but also her husband and his parents and family. This all led to feelings of shame and inadequacy for Hana and chronic pressure to "catch up" to prove her worth. It should be noted that some of the conflicts described by Hana in her relationship with her parents may, in part, be explained by differences in level of acculturation, as Hana came to identify more with Western values than her parents.

From the very start of therapy, there was an undercurrent of competition and envy that was sometimes difficult to put one's finger on, but always there. Hana would often push the therapist–client boundaries by asking personal questions of me that would take the focus off her and onto me. She would try to steer the conversation in a direction more consistent with that of two friends or colleagues chatting. In effect, Hana would often compare herself to me (setting up a competition or comparison), while simultaneously pushing the boundaries of our relationship. For example, she would ask about my career trajectory, what age I was when I started a practice, and how long it took me to build a client base. She lamented that my office was nicer than her own and that I was more "established." One time she stated that I would not understand what it feels like to be behind in life, as compared to others, because I seemed "like a pretty

2. Hana's description of her mother was consistent with the "tiger mom" stereotype (Chua, 2011; Lui & Rollock, 2013), wherein children are taught to value hard work, educational achievement, and perfection, and children's failures are seen as reflecting poorly on the family. However, empirical studies have not confirmed that there is one parenting style in East Asian cultures (Kim et al., 2017). In one study of Chinese American families, multiple parenting profiles emerged (supportive, tiger, easygoing, and harsh) (Kim et al., 2013), and the tiger parenting profile was associated with greater academic pressure, more depressive symptoms, and alienation.

put-together person." This comment and ones like it, on one level, were meant as a compliment but were always dripping with hostility and envy, leaving me unsure of how to respond. It did not help the situation that, at the time, I was also in the early stage of pregnancy. I decided to disclose this to her in our first session because I felt she had the right to know in order to decide for herself whether, in the long term, having a pregnant therapist would interfere with her ability to do the work of therapy (as, on some level, I must have suspected it would). She would continually bring the focus back to me and my pregnancy with comments like, "We don't have to meet today if you aren't feeling well" or "How much weight have you gained? I can't imagine you gained a pound! How far along are you? You look smaller than me! I'm sure you're nauseous, so it must be hard to see so many patients." Again, while these comments, on the surface, were meant to be "nice," they were always wrapped in unspoken hostility and competition. I felt put on the spot and pressured to disclose more about myself than I typically would. Already feeling vulnerable after disclosing my own precarious pregnancy, additional self-disclosures, as innocuous as they might seem on the surface, left me feeling extra-vulnerable and "off my game."

At the time, I was aware that Hana's efforts to compare herself to me were a sign of just how inadequate she felt and that I represented yet another person who reminded her of all that she felt she lacked. I wanted to help her with this, but I felt irritated that she continually pushed me away by putting the focus on me. This made it hard for me to do my job, leaving me feeling inadequate. Being "put on the spot" also made me feel vulnerable, right when I was already feeling vulnerable in my pregnancy. I also felt irritated that she assumed, and made a point of letting me know, that everything had come easily to me, from my career accomplishments to my pregnancy. Her constant comparisons between the two of us (in which I always came out "on top," while feeling chastised for it) felt like both a reminder of my fears, anxieties, and insecurities regarding my current pregnancy, and, at the same time, a dismissal of them. In short, I came to dread my sessions with her, which alerted me to the fact that I needed to better understand my countertransference. Upon reflecting on my internal countertransference reactions to her, I realized that Hana was unconsciously making me feel as vulnerable, flawed, criticized, and exposed as she felt in our relationship (a projective identification that was successful because I was indeed already feeling vulnerable and exposed). I came to understand that my discomfort in the role of her therapist mirrored Hana's discomfort in the role of my client, and I needed to better understand the terror that was motivating Hana to avoid this role so ardently, much to her own detriment. I was then able to use my feelings to better empathize with Hana's experience and explore it. I reflected to Hana,

I find myself in a bind. I could continue to answer your questions and keep the focus on me, but I have a hunch that that would not really help you, and that there is something very terrifying for you about allowing us to really focus on you? There is almost a real terror of being seen in here. And I think it's important we understand that terror, and how I can help you feel safe in here.

This led to a productive exploration of how, for Hana, accepting that she was the client in this relationship meant that she had failed once again, and was indeed as inadequate and flawed as she felt inside (and as she perceived her family, and particularly her mother, to see her). Moreover, Hana feared that if the true extent of her inadequacies were exposed, then her parents would permanently reject her, meaning that she was indeed as unlovable as she feared. Similarly, Hana explained that she worked hard in therapy to put the focus on me so I would not see just how inadequate and flawed she truly was, which would reinforce her inner self-critic and confirm her worst fears about herself, and possibly lead to me rejecting her and withdrawing my support.

Interestingly, Hana never asked me about my history of pregnancy loss and/or infertility because she assumed that she was the "defective" one in the room, and I was the "perfect" one. One week, Hana commented that she could not make a subsequent appointment due to a doctor's visit, and that I was "*so lucky*" that I did not have a high-risk pregnancy and had to make "all these additional appointments." "Otherwise, I would have time to dress nice like you," she explained. I reflected back to her,

> I have a reaction when you say that, so maybe it's worth stopping and thinking about it together. I think I immediately felt like I had done something wrong and maybe a little wary of your anger and not wanting to make you angrier. While some of that may be coming from me, it does make me stop and think, "Wow, you are really angry, and feel really cheated," and maybe that's worth directly looking at together.

This felt different than previous disclosures because it was on my terms, I did not feel pressured to disclose it, and it was for the benefit of the work. This led to a productive and more direct conversation about Hana's anger at an unjust world, envy of other women who seem to have it all, including me as the therapist, and, most of all, anger at herself for her own perceived failures and inadequacies. I asked Hana why she chose to see me and other women as more accomplished, more fertile, and all around better than her, when, after all, she lacked the facts to really know this in most cases and doing so only seemed to make her feel worse about herself. In response, Hana described attempting to take control by criticizing and belittling herself before others could do so. I never disclosed to Hana whether I had a history of infertility or loss, or not, because it would not have helped Hana or me to do so; what was important was understanding why she went to so much effort to idealize others only to devalue herself.

In summary, this case demonstrates how countertransference can either hinder or help the client and treatment, depending on the therapist's ability to manage it and the therapist's and client's capacity to negotiate their relationship and tolerate difficult feelings. Hana's competition and envy elicited from me a more *chronic countertransference* reaction of feeling guilty about my own successes or accomplishments, as if reproduction was some sort of skill or test that one passed or failed, which led me to feel both guilty and resentful in our relationship. My own countertransference and guilty feelings motivated me to disclose more than I typically would (and Hana also "pulled" this from me). While I never disclosed too much personal information and these disclosures may have seemed minimal and insignificant to others, for me, they represented a deviation from my baseline and were offered within the context of feeling pressured to do so, as if I needed to make up for the "successes" Hana perceived me to have "over her." However, once I was able to understand and work through my own countertransference reactions, I could hold Hana's anger and envy, making room for us to explore these feelings safely and more directly. At the same time, this specific client and situation elicited an *acute countertransference* reaction within me that was specific to this client, relationship, and time in my life. Hana had a way of pushing boundaries in relationships and of putting other people down within a comment that was framed as a compliment. This would lead anyone to feel "disarmed" (which I did), and to absorb some of the vulnerability, anger, and inadequacy that Hana experienced but did not want to own. In addition, for me, it touched upon a soft spot in the sense that her constant comparisons between the two of us set up an identification between us that I did not want to have at the time (I did not want to feel vulnerable and uncertain in my current pregnancy as she did), and, simultaneously, dismissed my own experience, as she assumed everything had come easily for me. This made it hard for me to emotionally join with her, as I was working hard to keep some self/other differentiation between the two of us. Yet, once I understood and processed my reactions, I was able to join Hana on a more emotional level around the fear of confronting one's own vulnerabilities and perceived inadequacies. Lastly, the anger and aggression I felt from Hana, and the subsequent uneasiness I felt getting emotionally close to her, were, in part, rooted in Hana's attachment insecurities and conflict over dependency. Specifically, Hana feared that I would reject and criticize her as she perceived her own mother to do, so, in a self-protective and preemptive move, she became critical of and angry with me before I could do so with her. Her attempts to push me away with distracting comments and disparaging remarks were all attempts to protect herself from becoming dependent on me, and then, as she feared, disappointing me and eliciting my criticism. At the same time, Hana deeply craved acceptance and closeness in the therapy relationship, as she did in her relationship with her mother and family. This left her chronically unsatisfied in her relationship with me because while pushing me away made her feel safer, it also left her feeling alone and unlovable. Yet, she could not tell me this in words initially, and examining my own countertransference feelings gave me a window into understanding Hana on a deeper level.

Lastly, there were several emotional indicators of my *internal countertransference*, including anxiety, guilt, and irritation or anger. My overt *countertransference behaviors* included disclosing more about myself than typical for me. Importantly, while not a behavior per se, my way of being with Hana deviated from how I typically am with clients. I felt more on guard and defensive, irritated toward and critical of Hana, and less emotionally available—which, by no coincidence, is how Hana perceived her own mother to be in their relationship. While these countertransference and transference dynamics made therapy with Hana challenging, examining them proved to be the best way of truly understanding those experiences that Hana could not yet put into words. The case of Hana is revisited under the section "Common Countertransference Themes in Psychotherapy for Pregnancy Loss" later in the chapter.

COUNTERTRANSFERENCE MANAGEMENT: AN EVIDENCE-BASED RELATIONSHIP PRINCIPLE

Over time, countertransference has evolved from something almost shameful or taboo that was believed to be located solely within the therapist to something co-created by the therapist and client, which could either help or hinder the therapeutic work (Hayes et al., 2019). From a more contemporary perspective, whether countertransference is ultimately a detriment or an aid to therapy depends largely on how the therapist manages it and how the dyad negotiates transference–countertransference dynamics. If adequately understood and managed by the therapist, countertransference could potentially increase the therapist's empathy of the client and the client's self-understanding (Hayes et al., 2019). Though clients may contribute to therapists' countertransference, the onus is still on therapists to know themselves and to consistently exercise the skill needed to understand and manage their countertransference reactions, as to not harm the client (Hayes et al., 2019; Jaffe, 2015).

Definitions

Freud (1910) first proposed what is now often termed the *classical definition* of countertransference, which he believed was the therapist's unconscious conflict-based reaction to the client's transference. The client's transference was believed to trigger unresolved childhood issues within the therapist and to interfere with treatment. Contrary to this, the *totalistic* conception of countertransference (Heimann, 1950; Kernberg, 1965; Little, 1951) later emerged to encapsulate all of the therapist's reactions to the client, which could and should be used to advance the therapist's understanding of the client and the client's impact on others, including the therapist, for the benefit of the work. A third idea of countertransference was developed in interpersonal relations and object relations theory (e.g., Anchin & Kiesler, 1982; Butler et al., 1993; Levenson, 1995), wherein the client's style pulls for a certain style in others. For example, the client who has an oppositional style tends to generate oppositional (or hostile) thoughts and feelings in the therapist. As in the totalistic viewpoint of countertransference, therapists are encouraged to use their reactions to a particular client to better understand the client and, specifically, the client's interpersonal problems (see Hayes et al., 2019, for a detailed review).

Integrating aspects from each of these definitions of countertransference, Gelso and Hayes (1998, 2007) define it as "the therapist's internal and external reactions, in which unresolved conflicts of the therapist, usually but not always unconscious, are impacted" (Hayes et al., 2019, p. 525). As Hayes et al. (2019) explain, in this conception of countertransference, like the classical perspective, the therapist's unresolved conflicts are seen as the source of countertransference. However, this definition differs from the classical one in that countertransference is seen as a potentially useful phenomenon if the therapist successfully understands personal reactions and uses them to better understand the client. It also differs from the classical viewpoint in that countertransference is believed to be the therapist's reaction not only to the client's transference, but also to many other factors both internal and external. Countertransference is believed to be inevitable because all therapists have unresolved conflicts and unconscious vulnerabilities that are touched upon with clients (Hayes et al., 2019). This integrated definition allows for the conceptualization of countertransference within a variety of theoretical orientations, and not just in psychoanalysis where it first began (Hayes et al., 2019). In the field of psychotherapy for pregnancy loss and infertility, Jaffe and colleagues have also argued that countertransference is an ongoing phenomenon across theoretical perspectives that can either aid or hinder therapeutic progress depending on the therapist's self-awareness and ability to manage it (Jaffe, 2015; Jaffe & Diamond, 2011). *Countertransference management* typically refers to the therapist's ability to identify and understand internal countertransference reactions so that they do not manifest in harmful overt behaviors (Gelso & Hayes, 1998).

Countertransference and Outcome

In a recent meta-analysis, Hayes et al. (2019) examined whether different dimensions of countertransference significantly predicted psychotherapy outcome. In a meta-analysis of 14 studies, the correlation between countertransference reactions and psychotherapy outcome was significant ($r = -.16$), indicating that more frequent countertransference reactions were associated with poorer outcomes. Studies were included in this meta-analysis that defined countertransference reactions as therapist behaviors or emotional reactions that were specific to therapist unresolved issues, perhaps pulled for or influenced by the client, but excluded studies that defined countertransference reactions as therapist reactions in general. Furthermore, studies included in this meta-analysis defined psychotherapy outcome as the quality of a given session and the client's well-being or functioning at termination (Hayes et al., 2019). However, once publication bias was considered, the relation was no longer significant. On the other hand, in a separate meta-analysis of nine studies, the correlation between countertransference management and outcome was significant ($r = .39$). When taking publication bias into account, the correlation changed but remained significant ($r = .51$), suggesting a medium to medium-large effect

size. This finding indicates that better countertransference management is associated with larger gains in outcome. Lastly, in a third meta-analysis of 13 studies,
the correlation between countertransference management and countertransference
reactions was also significant ($r = -.27$), indicating that better countertransference
management was associated with fewer countertransference reactions (Hayes et al.,
2019). While these meta-analyses did not include therapies for reproductive loss
specifically, their results may be tentatively applied to such cases. The results suggest that while it is not necessarily detrimental to treatment for therapists working
with pregnancy loss and infertility clients to have had similar experiences, countertransference reactions that arise from similar experiences, but are not understood
or managed, can negatively impact outcome. Additionally, the more "raw," or unresolved, the therapist's personal experiences are, the harder it will likely be for that
therapist to manage internal countertransference reactions. Therapists should process their own experiences of reproductive trauma and loss before working with
this client population, although therapists must continually work on themselves and
monitor their internal reactions (Jaffe, 2015).

Acute versus Chronic Countertransference

Gelso and Hayes (1998) differentiate between acute and chronic countertransference. Hayes et al. (2019) define *acute countertransference* as therapist responses that
occur "under specific circumstances with specific clients" (Reich, 1951, p. 26). For
example, a therapist who is typically very attentive and attuned to her clients may
stop listening to the details of a client's stillbirth, dissociate in the moment, and have
difficulty later recalling the events of the session, because the experience "hits" too
close to home to her own experience of loss. In contrast, *chronic countertransference*
reflects a habitual and pervasive need of the therapist, such that it has become part
of the therapist's personality structure (Hayes et al., 2019). For example, a therapist
may emotionally withdraw from a client's experience of giving birth to a stillborn
baby, and then offer advice in order to prevent this from happening again in a subsequent pregnancy (e.g., "Have you tried acupuncture, meditation, genetic testing?"),
because this therapist has a chronic need to fix emotional pain and suffering across
clients due to childhood experiences of failing to rescue an emotionally fragile caregiver. In the case of Hana above, the therapist's chronic countertransference to Hana
involved feeling guilty about success (something specific to the therapist across
clients, although pulled for by Hana's issues related to competition and envy), and
her acute countertransference included feelings of vulnerability, anger, and inadequacy that were specific to this client and period of the therapist's life.

Internal Countertransference

Gelso and Hayes (1998) differentiate between countertransference as an internal state or an overt expression (see Tables 7.1 and 7.2). As an *internal state*,

countertransference may be manifested emotionally, cognitively, or somatically (Hayes et al., 2019). On a cognitive level, countertransference may take the form of daydreams or fantasies, or failure to accurately recall therapy-related events (Hayes et al., 2019). For example, Rachel, a therapist who is in the middle of a very arduous adoption process, after a long and traumatic infertility journey that involved multiple pregnancy losses and failed IVF attempts, is troubled by fantasies of "snatching" her pregnant client's baby and carrying it in her uterus. Because she is preoccupied by her own fantasies and the anxiety that they engender, Rachel has difficulty concentrating on the client and remembering what the client talked about in session. Emotionally, anxiety is probably the most common affective cue or signal that a therapist is having a countertransference reaction, as it indicates that the therapist perceives some form of internal threat (Gelso & Hayes, 1998; Hayes et al., 2019). Shame and guilt may also be emotional signals that some countertransference reaction is being stirred within the therapist, as these are inhibiting emotions that signal the presence of other unacceptable feelings or experiences (McCullough et al., 2003). Looking at the example of Rachel once more, when her client suddenly experiences a pregnancy loss at 16 weeks gestation, Rachel is overcome with guilt. She worries that her fantasies, and feelings of anger and envy of the client's capacity to carry a viable pregnancy and have a genetically linked child, somehow caused the miscarriage. She feels ashamed and anxious that somehow the client will discover her thoughts and feelings and blame her for the loss. Lastly, on a somatic level, researchers have found that common visceral countertransference reactions include therapist sleepiness, muscular tension, and headaches (Booth et al., 2010). For instance, Rachel experiences unexplained headaches after sessions with this particular client.

Selective Inattention

One type of internal countertransference reaction that can be classified as a cognitive process is *selective inattention*, which refers to any thoughts, feelings, or dynamics occurring in the therapy that are not known or consciously attended to by the therapist (Essig, 2005). Selective inattention is considered to be a sign of countertransference, as therapists are believed to fail to consciously acknowledge some thought, feeling, or experience because it generates unacceptable levels of anxiety in them (Essig, 2005). Selective inattention can be harmful to the therapeutic process because it keeps the therapist and the client in the dark, unable to see important processes and experiences occurring within the therapist and/ or client (Essig, 2005). Further, as Essig (2005) argues, what is not consciously known or attended to cannot be worked through and resolved. For this reason, Essig (2005) suggests that therapists routinely ask, "What is *not* going on in the therapy relationship or process?"

The case of Sofia[3] provides an example of how countertransference reactions can lead to therapist selective inattention, and how selective inattention can be used to aid the therapy if recognized and managed. Sofia came to see me in a state of crisis after experiencing several early-term miscarriages over the past year and a half. These losses led her and her husband to seek an evaluation at the fertility clinic, where she was eventually told that the repeated miscarriages were likely due to uterine abnormalities and fibroids. Upon entering treatment, she could not eat, sleep, or think clearly, and was overcome by anxieties and obsessions. However, it was not the diagnosis of infertility that was causing Sofia stress but rather the fear that starting fertility treatments would have the result of producing a live baby with some sort of "defect," which would ruin her life "forever." Interestingly, every session Sofia would somehow work into the conversation that she really thought CBT was "great," which, as Sofia knew, was not the kind of therapy I practiced. Despite the frequency of these kinds of statements, for some reason, I never attended to them or explored their meaning. I finally asked myself, "Why not?"

As I got to know Sofia better, it became apparent that she experienced a great deal of guilt and anxiety over separating from her mother, which having a baby and becoming a mother represented. She feared making her own decisions and ardently needed her mother's approval for even minor choices. On an unconscious level, Sofia feared that her autonomy and healthy self-assertion would incite her mother's anger and disapproval and result in the loss of their relationship. Sofia sacrificed much of her separateness to maintain this connection, yet, on another level, resented her mother for it. For example, Sofia's mother would frequently give her advice that did not feel empathic or attuned to Sofia's needs and wants. Yet, Sofia would religiously follow her mother's instructions without ever acknowledging her dissatisfaction. I believe that because Sofia did not feel safe to directly express, or even acknowledge (or attend to), her anger toward her mother, it manifested consciously as anxiety. These dynamics were recreated within the therapeutic relationship. Specifically, by not attending to and exploring Sofia's "CBT-related" statements, I was failing to attend to her unspoken dissatisfaction in our relationship, and with the ways in which my "help" differed from how she wanted to be helped, much like in her relationship with her mother. On an unconscious level, I was afraid that if I acknowledged our differences and her dissatisfaction Sofia would leave therapy, just as Sofia feared that her separateness would destroy her relationship with her mother. This new understanding began with me asking myself what I was *not* attending to and ended with me changing the focus of treatment to help Sofia feel safe to disagree with me and assert herself.

3. The details of this case and client descriptives have been substantially altered and combined with other similar cases so no one client can be identified.

Table 7.1. Internal Countertransference Reactions
and Possible Cues/Signals

Type of Internal Countertransference Reaction	Emotion/Affective	Somatic	Cognitive
Cue or signal of internal countertransference (any deviations from the therapist's typical reactions to clients in affective, somatic, or cognitive experience should be explored as possible signals of countertransference reactions)	Anxiety, guilt, shame, irritation, or anger	Headaches, muscle tension, fatigue	Selective inattention, difficulty with recall of session, daydreams

Overt Countertransference Behaviors

Overt countertransference behavior has been studied in terms of therapist withdrawal, underinvolvement, or avoidance to the client's material, or as overactivity and overinvolvement (Gelso & Hayes, 2007; Hayes et al., 2019). As Hayes et al. (2019) describe, therapist avoidant reactions are those that inhibit, discourage, or divert session content, such as ignoring or mislabeling affects, changing topics, or allowing prolonged silences (Bandura et al., 1960). As opposed to therapist underinvolvement or avoidance, Jaffe and Diamond (2011) discuss how therapists with a history of pregnancy loss or infertility can become overinvested or overinvolved in their client's reproductive decisions, as the boundaries between their own experiences and needs and those of the client may merge, particularly when experiences from the therapist's reproductive past are not resolved or resurface. For example, Kerry, a reproductive therapist, carries much unresolved guilt and loss over her decision to terminate a much-wanted pregnancy due to the diagnosis of a genetic anomaly. When her client is confronted with the same awful decision, Kerry may either steer her client in the direction of choosing termination as she once did, because, unconsciously, she cannot tolerate contemplating other options, or, alternatively, steer the client away from termination in an attempt to "save" her from the pain Kerri cannot save herself from. From a therapeutic standpoint, the issue in either scenario is not whether terminating the pregnancy is the "right" decision for this particular client or not, but that Kerry's unresolved feelings are getting in the way of the client exploring her own thoughts, feelings, needs, and wants. As seen here, countertransference behavior can be harmful to the therapy process because it involves the therapist acting in accordance with the therapist's needs and not in terms of the best interest of the client (Hayes et al., 2019).

Sometimes, however, countertransference behavior may be beneficial; for example, when it alerts the therapist that something is awry and requires attention (Hayes et al., 2019). Deviations from the therapist's baseline activity level, especially, may be an indicator of underlying conflictual countertransference feelings and can be considered a behavioral signal or cue of countertransference (Keisler, 2001). In the above example, Kerry recognizes that she is being more directive (and even intrusive) than usual because of unresolved feelings related to her own pregnancy termination. Moreover, when Kerry catches herself pushing the client toward terminating the pregnancy, she realizes that her countertransference left the door wide open for the client to project onto her that part of the client that wants to terminate the pregnancy, but that the client feels too ashamed to acknowledge. Kerry then uses this understanding to help the client hold conflicting feelings around terminating a much-wanted pregnancy, and to empathize with how hard such a decision is for any parent. In the case of Hana above, the therapist's internal countertransference involved feelings of anxiety, guilt, and irritation/anger and her countertransference behaviors involved more than typical self-disclosure.

Table 7.2. OVERT COUNTERTRANSFERENCE BEHAVIORS AND POSSIBLE CUES/SIGNALS

Type of Overt Countertransference Behaviors	Withdrawal/ Underinvolvement/ Avoidance	Overactivity/ Overinvolvement
Cue or signal of overt countertransference (any deviations in therapist's baseline behavior should be explored as possible signals of countertransference)	Therapist changes topic, or inhibits, discourages, or diverts client content or affect, mislabels affect, prolonged silences	Overinvolvement or overinvestment in client's reproductive decisions and outcomes, overly directive, too much or inappropriate use of self-disclosure

THERAPIST SELF-DISCLOSURE: HELPFUL INTERVENTION OR COUNTERTRANSFERENCE BEHAVIOR?

Therapeutic self-disclosure can be defined as "therapist statements that reveal something personal about the therapist" (Hill & Knox, 2002, p. 256). Hill et al. (2019) further narrowed this definition to involve a verbal revelation about the therapist's life or person outside of therapy. Disclosures can be about feelings, similarities, insights, or strategies (Hill et al., 2019). Whether the therapist should disclose personal experiences with pregnancy loss and infertility is a much-debated and "hot" topic within the field of infertility counseling and reproductive psychology (Jaffe, 2015; Jaffe & Diamond, 2011). Within this context, a careful examination of when therapist self-disclosure is a helpful intervention, and when it is a type of countertransference behavior that reflects the therapist's overinvolvement and hinders the treatment, is needed. While the amount and type of self-disclosure that therapists make likely varies by theoretical orientation (Jaffe & Diamond, 2011), it is almost a universal phenomenon that therapy for pregnancy loss and infertility serves as a lightning bolt for issues around therapist self-disclosure. Arguably, this is because many mental health professionals drawn to this work have experienced some form of reproductive trauma and loss themselves (Covington & Marosek, 1999; Marrero, 2013).

These therapists are challenged to use their similar experiences of pain and loss to empathize with the client for the benefit of the therapy, without overidentifying with the client and blurring the boundaries between self and other (Jaffe & Diamond, 2011; Leon, 2015). Self-disclosures that assume sameness in experience between the therapist and client, although often well intentioned, are offered in the service of what the therapist needs and not what the client ultimately needs (Jaffe & Diamond, 2011). Thus, a possible "con" of therapist self-disclosure is that it has the unintended side effect of building a relationship with the client that is based on a false sense of sameness (Essig, 2005). As Essig (2005) describes, defining a relationship based on common experiences can give the illusion of empathy and understanding but, in reality, confuses where the therapist begins and the client ends. In this situation, the client often does not feel safe to disclose and, rather, denies parts of her experience that differ from the therapist's because the connection is built on sameness (Essig, 2005). Such a relationship does not leave room for the client's separateness and autonomy in the therapy relationship.

It is not uncommon for reproductive therapists to use this work to find meaning and purpose from the trauma of loss that they have experienced in their personal life. Making meaning from trauma and loss is in fact a hallmark of post-traumatic growth (Gillies & Neimeyer, 2006; Tian & Solomon, 2020). In doing so, however, these therapists are faced with the complex task of using the work to make meaning from their personal trauma, while keeping the focus of the treatment on the needs of the client (Jaffe, 2015). As Jaffe (2015) writes, being wounded does not in itself make one an expert. Therapists must understand and process these wounds in order to use their experiences to the benefit of the client. Otherwise, the therapist's own healing may interfere with that of the client (Jaffe, 2015). Therapist self-disclosures often serve as an "easy" mechanism through which unresolved issues and open wounds can "slip out" into the treatment, shifting the therapeutic focus from the client to the therapist. In fact, therapist self-disclosure has been found to be much riskier if the therapist is in the midst of unresolved problems (Knox & Hill, 2003). In essence, therapist self-disclosure is intricately tied to countertransference and countertransference management because decisions to self-disclose or not are made within the context of the therapist's reactions to the client, including the therapist's countertransference reactions (Jaffe & Diamond, 2011).

Although there are certainly potential perils of therapist self-disclosure, there are also potential advantages or benefits of it to the treatment, particularly with this client population (Jaffe, 2015). The therapist disclosing personal experiences of reproductive trauma and loss could help to normalize clients' feelings, help them to feel understood and less alone, promote an atmosphere of safety and emotional "holding," and encourage clients' self-disclosure in turn (Essig, 2005). Studies have found that therapists use disclosures to establish a bond, to help clients feel normal or understood, and to encourage more client disclosure (Hill, 2014; Knox et al., 1997). In a qualitative meta-analysis, Hill et al. (2019) looked at the clinical consequences of therapeutic self-disclosures and found that the most frequently occurring clinical consequences were enhanced therapy relationship, client gained insight, client mental health functioning improved, and overall helpful for the client. Consistent with this, therapist self-disclosures of past experiences with pregnancy loss, or other reproductive traumas, may be particularly meaningful and impactful for reproductive loss clients, who often enter treatment feeling ashamed, misunderstood, defective, different, and alone (Jaffe, 2015). Importantly, Hill et al. (2019) point out that, though their meta-analytic results suggest that therapeutic self-disclosure has, overall, a positive impact on clients, previous research has shown these strategies are relatively infrequent in psychotherapy (Hill et al., 1988, 2014). Furthermore, meta-analytic findings and clinical experience suggest negative clinical consequences from therapists using self-disclosure for self-gratification (Hill et al., 2019). From this, Hill et al. (2019) stress the need to use self-disclosures sparingly, for appropriate reasons, and to meet the client's needs.

Lastly, therapists may choose to self-disclose not necessarily because of the benefit of disclosure itself, but because of the potential harm in refraining from self-disclosure. For instance, especially when the therapist is a woman of reproductive age, clients will always wonder about the reproductive story of the therapist (Jaffe & Diamond, 2011). They will often ask if the therapist has children and if she has experienced pregnancy loss or infertility (Jaffe & Diamond, 2011). Sometimes clients will ask this because they are searching for a competent figure to identify with, or someone who can finally understand what they are going through and help them to feel less alone, while others will ask out of a sense of competition and envy. Regardless, these are not innocuous questions for the client or for the therapist and, instead, are loaded with personal meaning (Jaffe & Diamond, 2011). Refusing to answer the client's question outright may feel like a rejection or criticism, reinforcing her sense of feeling different and defective (Jaffe, 2015). On the other hand, a disclosure such as, "Yes, I have personal experience with this kind of devastating loss so I know how difficult this can be, but I never want to assume that my experience is the same as yours," may help to normalize and validate the client's experience without putting too much focus on the therapist, while sending the message that the client need not have the same experience as the therapist. On the other hand, therapists who have not had personal experience with pregnancy loss or infertility often feel in a bind because disclosing this, especially early in the treatment when the alliance has not yet been established, may alienate the client and reinforce her sense of feeling different and alone. Yet, refusing to answer the question outright may be perceived as defensive or withholding to the client (Jaffe, 2015). One way of dealing with this dilemma is to disclose something like, "While I can't know exactly what you are going through, I have had personal experiences of feeling like I've lost someone prematurely, but I'm here to listen to you and learn about your unique experience."

IMMEDIACY

As opposed to therapeutic self-disclosure, Hill et al. (2019) define *immediacy* as "a discussion of the therapeutic relationship by both the therapist and client in

the here and now involving more than social chitchat" (Hill et al., 2014, p. 299).
Immediacy can include interventions asking the client about immediate feelings
and thoughts, statements of immediate therapist feelings, drawing parallels with
other relationships, or acknowledgment of an alliance rupture and attempts to repair. Hill et al. (2019) conducted a qualitative meta-analysis on the most frequent
clinical consequences of immediacy, which were found to be enhanced therapy
relationship, client opened up, and overall not helpful. Their results suggest that
immediacy may be a helpful intervention but should be well thought out, as it
may have the potential to be unhelpful as well. Importantly, these researchers
found that therapists frequently use immediacy when there are problems in the
therapeutic relationship in the hope of working through them (Hill et al., 2019).
Similarly, immediacy may be used to address transference–countertransference
dynamics in the relationship, and a mechanism for both managing the therapist's
countertransference and using it to the benefit of the therapy. For instance, the
following intervention, from the above case example of Hana, is an example of
immediacy:

> I have a reaction when you say that, so maybe it's worth stopping and thinking
> about together. I think I immediately felt like I had done something wrong
> and maybe a little wary of your anger and not wanting to make you angrier.
> While some of that may be coming from me, it does make me stop and think,
> "Wow, you are really angry, and feel really cheated," and maybe that's worth
> directly looking at together.

This intervention gave the therapist a productive outlet for her countertransference feelings, so they did not leak out into her behavior, while putting the focus
back on the client's unresolved anger and envy.

THE CLIENT ROLE

Countertransference is best understood in terms of an interaction between the
therapist's unresolved conflicts and aspects of the client that touch upon or stir up
the therapist's conflicts (Gelso & Hayes, 2007). Hayes et al. (2019) argue that research does not support the view that there are common client characteristics that
universally provoke the same countertransference reactions from all therapists
(Hayes & Gelso, 1991; 1993; Robbins & Jolkovski, 1987; Yulis & Kiesler, 1968).
Instead, these authors suggest that the same client will elicit a different reaction
from different therapists, depending on the therapist's own issues and personality
structure. In the context of pregnancy loss, one therapist may respond to a client's
grief after miscarriage by withdrawing and changing the topic, for this therapist
learned in early attachment relationships that "loss happens" and you "just have
to move on." Another therapist, however, may respond to that same client's grief
by becoming overly involved, recounting to the client numerous stories of other
people who experienced miscarriages and went on to have viable pregnancies,

not letting the client get a word in. This therapist, early on, learned to help her family cope with and deny the loss of her baby brother by filling in the space with manic-like monologues. At the same time, clients will have different ways of coping with loss, which will interact with their therapists' way of coping with and defending against loss. For instance, a client who copes with loss by focusing on facts and figures will likely frustrate a therapist who copes with loss by focusing on her sadness.

COMMON COUNTERTRANSFERENCE THEMES IN PSYCHOTHERAPY FOR PREGNANCY LOSS: APPLICATION TO THE CASE OF HANA

Although each client and therapist–client dyad are unique, based on clinical experience and theory, there are proposed to be common transference–countertransference themes in psychotherapy for pregnancy loss, sometimes in the context of infertility and other reproductive traumas. These themes are delineated below and exemplified in the case of Hana.

Therapist Unresolved Reproductive Trauma and Loss

A critical element of therapy for reproductive trauma and loss is the client telling and retelling her story of loss, repeatedly, with as much detail as possible (Jaffe, 2015; Leon, 2015). She must feel free to disclose to you, as her therapist, the gory details of her miscarriage, the shocking pain of an ectopic pregnancy, the physical trauma of being poked and prodded during IVF, or to show you pictures of her cherished stillborn baby (Jaffe, 2015). In turn, as therapists, we are challenged to remain open to listening to the details of the client's story without becoming overwhelmed or dysregulated ourselves. If, as the therapist, we are unresolved regarding our own reproductive trauma and loss, then it will be difficult to stay empathically attuned to the client's experience and to act as safe base for the client to process trauma and loss.

Supporting this, Rosenberger and Hayes (2002) found that therapists may become anxious, have distorted perceptions of their clients, and exhibit avoidance behaviors when unresolved issues have been aggravated. Another study found that, in grief therapy, therapists with unresolved grief were seen by their clients as having less empathy, whereas therapists who had worked through their grief were perceived to better empathize, make better treatment decisions, and offer hope to their clients (Hayes et al., 2007). Perhaps, therapists with unresolved grief were more focused on themselves and their own grief than that of their clients (Hayes et al., 2007; Jaffe, 2015). The implication of these studies for therapy for pregnancy loss and infertility is clear: Therapists' own experiences can either hinder or help the client, depending on the degree to which therapists are resolved in respect to their reproductive trauma and loss (Jaffe, 2015). It is important to note that infertility and pregnancy loss often leave behind scars that even once healed can be aggravated and reopened (Jaffe, 2015). Consequently, therapists with a history of reproductive trauma and loss must always be aware of their vulnerabilities and work to manage them (Jaffe, 2015). Related to this, therapists should examine their personal history, vulnerabilities, and unresolved feelings related to other types of prior losses, and how grief and loss were dealt with in their family of origin and culture. In the case of Hana, the therapist's anxiety over a potential pregnancy loss kept her from identifying and empathizing with Hana's terror and fear over another potential loss on a deeper and more emotional level. This was of course complicated by the fact that Hana attempted to identify with the therapist as another pregnant woman through passive-aggressive comments such as, "How much weight have you gained? I can't imagine you gained a pound! How far along are you? You look smaller than me!" However, the therapist's inability to initially look past this passive-aggressiveness and identify with the fear of loss that lay beneath it was in part due to her own unresolved issues.

Self/Other Integration and Boundaries

Particularly when the therapist is unresolved with respect to reproductive trauma and loss, the therapist may be in danger of overempathizing or overidentifying with the client, blurring the boundaries between self and other. This is important because self/other integration is considered to be an important facilitator of countertransference management (Gelso & Hayes, 2001). For instance, a therapist who chose to pursue multiple trials of IVF should not allow her choice to interfere with the decision-making of a client who may not want to pursue multiple trials (Kronen, 1995). Without firm self-other boundaries, the therapist is at risk of merging with the client's pregnancy or infertility successes and failures (Kronen, 1995), making it impossible for the therapist to remain neutral and focused on the client and the client's needs (Jaffe & Diamond, 2011). Clinical experience suggests that therapist difficulties with self/other integration or boundaries most often are expressed through the therapist becoming overly active, friendly, invested, or directive with the client; for example, making inappropriate or excessive self-disclosures. However, a therapist may also withdraw from the client in a self-protective maneuver to preserve their sense of self and separateness. In the case of Hana, the therapist both disclosed more than was typical of her with other clients and emotionally withdrew to preserve self/other boundaries between herself and the client.

Therapist Reactions to Idealization and Devaluation

As with other clients and types of therapies, in therapy for pregnancy loss and infertility, clients may, at altering moments, have a need to idealize and/or devalue the therapist, which can pull for powerful countertransference reactions. Client idealization and devaluation can range in intensity, from overt and very strong to subtle and covert. There are several reasons specific to pregnancy loss and infertility why clients may devalue, or have negative feelings toward and projections of, the therapist. One, pregnancy loss and infertility are often experienced as massive assaults on a woman's self-esteem and identity, leaving her with intense feelings of shame and inadequacy (Diamond & Diamond, 2017). From this, the client may project her strong self-critical voice onto the therapist and interpret even benign comments by the therapist as critical or attacking. Second, the experience of pregnancy loss and of not having important others available for support and comfort, during an intense moment of distress, can raise early attachment experiences of similar instances of trauma and loss wherein attachment figures were emotionally unavailable or unresponsive (Markin, 2018). In this case, clients may transfer onto the therapist early attachment experiences with unsupportive and unattuned caregivers that have been resurrected by the loss of a pregnancy (Markin, 2018). Third, pregnancy loss clients, perhaps for the first time, feel a fundamental lack of control over their own bodies. When infertility is involved, clients may feel at the mercy of reproductive medicine doctors who seem to have all the resources and power (Raphael-Leff, 2012). This degree of dependency and lack of control can breed anger and resentment, and the therapist may come to be seen as yet another person who has control or power over the client. In the case of Hana, the client transferred onto the therapist past experiences with early attachment figures of feeling criticized and rejected during moments of intense distress. Further, Hana came to see the therapist through the lens of her own self-critical voice, as a potentially attacking or critical figure, which reinforced Hana's damaged sense of self as fundamentally flawed and unlovable. This negative sense of self likely started in early attachment relationships and was reinforced by experiences of infertility and loss. Lastly, Hana came to resent her need for the therapist's support and understanding, as this gave the therapist the power to reject and hurt her, as she experienced in past relationships. Hana attempted to take back that control by pushing the therapist away before she could be rejected.

Regardless of the exact reason for client negative feelings toward the therapist, these are powerful client reactions that can stimulate equally powerful countertransference reactions in the therapist. Most commonly, for therapists who have a chronic need to be seen as "nice," perhaps to ward off hostility, criticisms, or perceived attacks from others, it will be difficult to remain neutral and to hold and explore clients' negative feelings toward them. Often, therapists will need to "catch" subtle and fleeting "flashes" of the client's negative feelings toward them and help the client to feel safe enough to directly express these feelings. If the therapist cannot tolerate the client's anger, or other negative feelings toward him or her, then it will be difficult for the therapist to acknowledge and hold these client reactions. In the case of Hana, once the therapist better understood her countertransference reactions, she was better able to tolerate Hana's hostility and envy and help Hana to explore these feelings.

Contrary to devaluation and negative feelings toward the therapist, pregnancy loss and infertility clients most often come into therapy hungry for the therapist's support and understanding, overwhelmed by their intense distress with few or no support persons to turn to. For this reason, they often move toward the therapist, and the support, comfort, and understanding you provide them (Diamond & Diamond, 2017). Some clients may see the therapist as the supportive mother-figure that they both wished they had as a child and urgently need in the present, as they struggle to mourn the loss of their baby and hopes and dreams for the future. Relatedly, idealization of the therapist may help some clients to feel safe enough to approach feelings of trauma and loss previously too terrifying to give voice to or acknowledge.

Positive feelings toward the therapist can elicit strong countertransference reactions, just as negative ones can. Some therapists, because of their own discomfort with client positive feelings of them, may dismiss, deny, interpret away, or minimize the client's idealization too quickly, leaving the client feeling unsafe once again. Alternatively, other therapists, who have a chronic need to be admired, may not appreciate the cost that the client must pay for her excessive admiration—for, often, the more the client idealizes the therapist as the perfect, all- nurturing and fertile woman, the more she devalues herself. Hana idealized the therapist as having everything she lacked, and resented her for it, as she always felt "less than" in comparison. Hana's idealization and subsequent resentment touched upon a soft spot within the therapist, related to feeling guilty over accomplishments and successes.

WHEN ONE OF US IS NOT LIKE THE OTHER: TRANSFERENCE AND COUNTERTRANSFERENCE ISSUES WHEN THE THERAPIST OR CLIENT BECOMES PREGNANT

One of the dangers of building a therapist–client relationship based on sameness (i.e., therapist and client common experiences with pregnancy loss and/or infertility) is this: What happens to the relationship and the treatment when one person is no longer the "same," or like the other, and becomes pregnant? A therapist's pregnancy may leave the client filled with a multitude of intense emotions toward the therapist. She may feel abandoned, angry and resentful, envious, or jealous. Where there was once a sense of safety and connection from a false sense of sameness, now, for the client, there may feel like a divide between, or separation from, the therapist. She may feel emotionally abandoned by the therapist, as she had felt that they were "in this" together.

Sensing the client's anger or aggression, the pregnant therapist may feel vulnerable and not want to invite the client's negative or hostile feelings (Jaffe & Diamond, 2011). She may feel protective of her unborn baby and want to shield it from the client's hostility. In reaction, therapists may withdraw from the client as a self-protective mechanism, or, alternatively, they may become overinvested and overly "nice," attempting to ward off the client's hostility. Either way, as a result, the client's negative feelings toward the therapist are never processed. In fact, clients may prematurely drop out of therapy because of difficulty expressing negative feelings toward the pregnant therapist (Jaffe & Diamond, 2011). Lastly, because of the envy and rage that clients often feel upon learning of their therapist's pregnancy, if the therapist has a miscarriage, then the client may fear that her envy and rage caused it (Jaffe & Diamond, 2011). At the same time, loss of the therapist's pregnancy can feel like a relief to the client, who now no longer must worry about competition or abandonment (Jaffe & Diamond, 2011). Both these factors can lead to clients' guilty feelings that interfere with their ability to speak freely.

As exemplified above, Hana experienced anger and envy toward the therapist related to her pregnancy. At first, these negative feelings were expressed indirectly through passive-aggressive comments. In turn, the therapist felt on guard, attacked, and vulnerable, and emotionally withdrew from Hana out of a need for self-protection. At the same time, the therapist overly self-disclosed to placate Hana and her hostility. Once the therapist was able to step outside her countertransference, she could tolerate and emotionally "hold" Hana's anger and envy, which afforded Hana the space to process these feelings. In general, the more the therapist can tolerate clients' negative projections, the more the client will be able to own and process negative feelings. Sometimes, a client's negative transference toward her pregnant therapist is just too intense and a referral to another therapist may be in the best interest of both individuals. The pregnant therapist is vulnerable herself, and staying in a therapeutic relationship with unmanaged primal rage and envy can be harmful to the therapist and the client.

Likewise, a therapist who has experienced pregnancy loss, and perhaps infertility, may have intense reactions to a client's pregnancy during treatment. The client's pregnancy may be experienced by the therapist as yet another thing that does not feel fair in the world, leading to feelings of resentment toward the client. The therapist may feel jealous, angry, and competitive with the client. As Jaffe and Diamond (2011) point out, it may be difficult for the therapist to celebrate the client's hard-won battle when finally achieving a viable pregnancy and/or to maintain neutrality. If the client is aware that the therapist is trying to conceive, the client may feel guilty about her own pregnancy success and may feel the need to take care of the therapist (Jaffe & Diamond, 2011). Professional consultation or personal therapy may be needed for the therapist to manage her countertransference reactions to the client in such situations.

COUNTERTRANSFERENCE REACTIONS TO TRAUMA

Physical trauma is inherent to many experiences of pregnancy loss and infertility (Watson, 2005). Often, therapists can personally relate to their clients' trauma of being poked and prodded during IVF; of obsessively checking for blood and finding it; of bleeding out one's baby and seeing the remains; or of a room full of seemingly detached medical providers who watch as her insides are put on full display. Clients going through pregnancy loss and infertility often share an experience fundamentally similar to that of clients who report other kinds of physical trauma, of feeling violated and out of control and unsafe in their own bodies. Because of this, listening to these experiences can stir therapists' own experiences not only of reproductive trauma, but also of other kinds of past physical traumas, including sexual trauma (Watson, 2005). Once past experiences of physical and/or sexual trauma are triggered within the therapist by the client's content, the therapist may feel flooded emotionally. In this dysregulated state, the traumatized therapist may dissociate with clients. Dissociation is a common defense in cases of trauma that is used to protect the self from fragmentation of self-states (Bromberg, 1998). It projects the illusion of a coherent self, but in actuality leaves the therapist dysregulated and cut off from important parts of self (Freeman, 2005). Once removed from important feelings and parts of self, the therapist cannot be present to help the client integrate aspects of the trauma that the client is dissociating, nor can the therapist help to regulate the client's intense distress.

Vicarious Trauma

Vicarious trauma describes the therapist's negative transformation after being exposed to a client's trauma (Jaffe, 2015). Listening to the details of a client's traumatic experience can affect us deeply, and, as sensitive and attuned therapists, we can often absorb the client's trauma, sometimes even before it is directly voiced or acknowledged. Jaffe (2015) differentiates between vicarious trauma and countertransference in that vicarious trauma is a direct reaction to traumatic client material and is not a reaction to past personal life experiences. However, as Jaffe (2015) argues, vicarious trauma can evoke countertransference issues when the traumatic experiences that are shared are similar to those of the therapist. A common reaction to vicarious trauma is the therapist feeling helpless and wanting to fix the client's problem. However, most often there is nothing a therapist can do to fix the wounds inflicted upon clients by pregnancy loss and infertility, and the therapist can only be there with them and open to hearing their story.

CLINICAL CHALLENGES TO COUNTERTRANSFERENCE MANAGEMENT

Countertransference management in cases of pregnancy loss with or without infertility is inherently difficult because reproduction and parenthood are deeply personal to both client and therapist. Research, theory, and practice all suggest that good countertransference management starts with therapists working through their own reproductive trauma and loss. That being said, there are some wounds that never fully heal and some scars that will always leave their mark. While some therapists may never fully be "resolved" in terms of personal trauma and loss, these experiences do not always need to feel raw, fresh, and new, but can become integrated into one's experience and life story. Clinicians walk a thin line between being in touch with just enough pain to empathize with the client, but not too much pain as to overidentify. This, in a nutshell, is the challenge of the work that we do.

A common area of difficulty concerning countertransference management has to do with what happens when the therapist and client hold different perspectives on anything from reproductive choices to morals, ethics, and spiritual issues (Jaffe & Diamond, 2011). There are endless decisions that often need to be made when it comes to fertility, and the choices of the client will not always line up with those of the therapist. For example, a therapist may disagree with her client's decision to decide the sex of the baby during IVF, or with a couple's decision to selectively reduce one or more fetuses in a multiple pregnancy after IVF, especially if the therapist is struggling to become pregnant and have a baby at the same time. What may be the right course for the client may not be right for the therapist, and vice versa. Often therapists are called to put aside their own personal moral, ethical, or religious choices to focus on the needs of the client and remain impartial and supportive (Jaffe & Diamond, 2011). Therapists putting aside their own personal beliefs to remain neutral and supportive to the client seems particularly relevant to cases in which clients are deciding whether or not to terminate a wanted pregnancy, perhaps because the fetus has been diagnosed with a genetic anomaly or because the pregnancy poses a significant health risk to the mother, as sometimes is the case with ectopic pregnancies, for example. Such situations may be especially difficult for therapists and clients to navigate in states that have restricted abortion access.

CLINICAL IMPLICATIONS

The following clinical implications are adapted from Hill et al. (2019) and Hayes et al. (2019) but are applied to therapy for pregnancy loss specifically below.

- Self-insight and reflection are key to identifying and managing one's countertransference. Understanding oneself helps us to recognize when and why we are having strong internal reactions to clients or acting in ways that deviate from our typical behavior. Self-insight also helps us to separate our own experiences from those of the client. Particularly when the therapist has also experienced reproductive trauma and loss, it is imperative to process these experiences to avoid overidentifying with the client.
- Therapists should work on their own psychological health, including healthy self/other boundaries with clients. This is particularly relevant to infertility and pregnancy loss therapists, who often personally identify with client experiences. The therapist processing one's own history of trauma and loss is critical to being able to separate self and other, pointing to the importance of therapy for the therapist (Geller et al., 2005).

- Therapists can benefit from therapy, supervision, and self-care. Is this work depleting you, or filling you up? When therapists feel depleted from this work it is likely due to unmanaged vicarious trauma and/or countertransference reactions.
- Understanding what a client pulls from you and why is the first step in being able to use countertransference to help the client and the therapy along. In the context of pregnancy loss, understanding what a client pulls from you may reveal what aspects of the grief and loss experience the client is defending against.
- Be cautious, thoughtful, and strategic about using self-disclosure; make sure self-disclosures are focused on the client's needs and not the therapist's; keep self-disclosures brief and with few details.

8

Client Attachment in Therapy for Recurrent Pregnancy Loss and Infertility

Theory, Research, and Clinical Guidelines

The experience of separation from an attachment figure is an incredibly painful and anxiety-ridden one. From an evolutionary perspective, infants come into the world biologically pre-programmed to experience stress and anxiety upon separation so that they feel motivated to reestablish proximity to a caregiver, who can then help the infant to physically and psychologically survive when a threat is experienced as coming from either outside or within the self. In ideal circumstances, when an infant experiences separation distress and naturally seeks out an available and sensitive caregiver, the caregiver will consistently provide a reunification that is emotionally soothing, organizing, and supportive. However, in less-than-ideal attachment circumstances, an infant seeks out an attachment figure for comfort and reconnection, but, whether the attachment figure is somehow unavailable, rejecting, preoccupied, or intrusive, reunification either does not happen at all or is tainted by negative emotion and confusion. These types of recurrent inadequate or traumatic attachment experiences become internalized as guiding expectations of the self and others in relationships throughout the lifespan.

In this sense, early attachment experiences set our expectations regarding how available and capable others are of providing the support and comfort we need in times of separation distress, and how effective we are at eliciting care and comfort from others (Bowlby, 1969,1982). Later in life, when a woman dreams of becoming a mother herself, but a pregnancy or unborn baby is tragically lost, past attachment experiences related to eliciting and receiving support

Psychotherapy for Pregnancy Loss. Rayna D. Markin, Oxford University Press. © Oxford University Press 2024.
DOI: 10.1093/oso/9780197693353.003.0008

and comfort from others in times of separation distress are often evoked, as she once again finds herself in the painful and anxiety-ridden state of separation and in search of support and comfort from a trusted other. Women who experience recurrent pregnancy loss (RPL) in particular are constantly in a state of separation distress and often experience heightened attachment needs as a result. The therapist establishing himself, herself, or themself as a secure attachment figure who can be trusted to sensitively respond to the client's distress, providing support, understanding, and comfort, helps the client feel safe enough to approach and process feelings of grief and loss, perhaps contrary to past attachment experiences.

CHAPTER OVERVIEW

This chapter begins by reviewing attachment theory and research and how attachment theory can be used as a clinical guide in psychotherapy for pregnancy loss with individuals and couples. Research on client (and therapist) attachment style and the process and outcome of therapy is subsequently discussed. From this research, it is argued that client attachment plays an important role in treatment, especially with clients affected by pregnancy loss, and thus therapists should adjust their approach and relational style to meet the attachment needs of the client (Levy et al., 2019). More generally, therapists adjusting their approach or style depending on client factors has been termed *therapist responsiveness* (Norcross & Wampold, 2019). Lastly, the final section of this chapter addresses how attachment theory can help us understand the various ways in which individuals and couples cope with feelings of separation and grief or loss following RPL. Finally, treatment implications and next steps are discussed. Chapter 9 builds upon the present chapter and offers specific guidance on how therapists should adjust their approach and relational style to fit client attachment style.

Below, we are introduced to a client named Marni, who has experienced multiple devastating setbacks to her dream of becoming a parent. She initially seeks individual therapy as a single woman trying to conceive through assisted reproductive technology. This case provides an in-depth illustration of therapist responsiveness to a client with a more anxious attachment. The vignette also portrays how attachment style can impact a client's experience of RPL and ability to cope with the resulting distress, and, moreover, how clients learn to better cope with feelings of separation and grief/loss within a secure attachment relationship with the therapist. We later return to the case of Marni in Chapter 9 within the context of couples therapy to demonstrate therapist responsiveness to an anxious and avoidant partner.

Case Vignette: Client Attachment and Therapist Responsiveness

Marni[1] is a 37-year-old cisgender single woman who entered therapy after experiencing recurrent miscarriages of pregnancies achieved through intrauterine insemination and sperm donation. She reported being diagnosed with polycystic ovary syndrome when she was 19 years old and has since known that she would likely experience infertility. Marni described a pattern of unstable romantic relationships, all of which would become intensely close very quickly and in which Marni would initially believe she had found the perfect man for her and to father her children. However, just as quickly as they began, these relationships would fall apart in dramatic ways that left Marni feeling rejected and abandoned. Marni longed for the unconditional love and closeness of a child and at 34 decided she would no longer wait to find a husband to father her children, whom, she reasoned, would only inevitably reject or abandon her anyway. Since then, for the past 3 years, Marni has undergone IUI after IUI, in the hope of achieving a viable pregnancy. However, each round has either failed to achieve a pregnancy or resulted in a pregnancy that has miscarried. Marni feels dependent on her doctors, yet angry at them for not providing her with more care and support. She has switched fertility clinics multiple times, each time at first feeling like she has found the perfect doctor, only to eventually feel disappointed and neglected by yet another doctor and the clinic staff.

Marni was raised by a single mother and never knew her father. Her mother's "career," according to Marni, was finding, marrying, and divorcing rich men. As a result, Marni's mother was in and out of relationships and Marni had to move around a lot. When her mother was "in between men," Marni reports basking in her mother's full attention and always doing fun and crazy things together. However, when Marni's mother would get remarried, according to Marni, she would turn her attention to her new husband and become largely absent in Marni's life. When Marni was 13 years old, her then stepfather wanted to send her away to boarding school. Marni pleaded with her mother not to send her, and, in response, her mother scolded Marni, telling Marni not to ruin "this" for her. At boarding school, Marni would call her mother daily, hysterically crying, begging to come back home, until her mother stopped taking her calls. Then, Marni started experiencing extreme depression, and turned to alcohol and drugs, sexual acting out, and self-cutting as drastic attempts to signal her mother to her intense distress and to elicit her proximity and care. However, Marni's efforts were to no avail, and she remained at boarding school for the next 3 years. As a result of her early inconsistent caregiving experiences, Marni can be described as having a more anxious or preoccupied attachment style, seeing herself as unlovable, unworthy, and helpless, and others as rejecting, unavailable, and inconsistent or preoccupied.

---

1. This case is an amalgamation of several cases so no one patient can be identified.

Marni starts every therapy session sobbing, inconsolable, and in intense distress. While weeping, she often attacks herself and is intensely self-critical, blaming herself and her "defective" body for the infertility and losses. She sees herself as fundamentally unlovable and attacks herself for not being able to find a father for her future child. "Who would want to spend their life with me? No one wants to stick around and love me, not a man, not even a baby!" she laments. At first, the therapist was "pulled in" to Marni's attachment style and emotionality, and, like Marni, felt emotionally flooded, confused, and overwhelmed. She felt sorry for Marni, empathized with her pain, and made interventions to deepen Marni's already intense emotions. However, eventually the therapist came to feel frustrated with Marni and her relentless escalation of distress, combined with her refusal to accept the therapist's help, empathy, and support. At the same time, Marni was, in passive ways, voicing frustration with the therapist and her perceived lack of availability, although the therapist felt she was jumping through hoops to be available to Marni and to demonstrate her support and care. In response, the therapist felt frustrated and angry and withdrew from the relationship and was less emotionally present and validating with the client. The therapist's inconsistent provision of sensitive care most likely mirrored, or reenacted, Marni's mother's inconsistent care and attention, and was further emotionally injurious to Marni.

The therapeutic process started to change for the better when the therapist realized what was being reenacted within the therapist–client relationship and adjusted her relational style accordingly. The therapist adopted the stance of a reliable and consistent presence, who calmly listened to Marni when in distress, but did not react reflexively to it with more emotional distress. The therapist showed up each session and did not reject Marni, contrary to Marni's expectations. With increased awareness into what was being evoked in the therapy process, the therapist was now better able to withstand the emotional chaos that Marni experienced and evoked within her, which allowed her to be more consistent, reliable, and understanding. The therapist's stance was primarily reflective and curious, helping Marni to put her intense feelings into words and reflect upon them, rather than getting carried away by them. During one session toward the middle of therapy, Marni entered the therapy room in tears, stating that she had another miscarriage and was so devastated that she reached out to her mother, asking if she could please just come over and be there with her, to which her mother stated that she had a prior commitment at the country club. When Marni protested, her mother stated, "You always have to ruin everything for me with your problems."

Upon recounting this story to the therapist, Marni immediately started attacking herself, stating that she was "stupid" for reaching out to her mother. "What did I expect from her? Of course, no baby would want to stay in my womb, my own mother can't even find something to love about me!" she cried. As Marni became more emotionally escalated, the therapist stayed empathic, yet consistent and calm, but not aloof, gently listening without reacting. She then attempted to help Marni make sense of her overwhelming feelings and to regulate them, unlike her early attachment figures. The therapist stated:

You are so angry with yourself right now, but I imagine at the time, even if just for a moment, you were angry at your mother for failing to be there for you in your time of need, and worse, for blaming you for it. Of course, you would reach out to your mother for comfort, that's what children of any age naturally do when upset and in distress.

In response, Marni seemed to slow down and cry genuine tears of grief and sorrow, rather than defensive weepiness. The therapist continued, "You are stuck in this awful position of not only having to grieve the loss of your baby and hopes and dreams for the future, but also of not having your mother's support and comfort when you need it once again." Marni responded, "I was already feeling so alone after I miscarried and when she wouldn't come over, I felt even more alone and unwanted." The therapist reflected how quickly Marni's sorrow and anger turns into self-criticism and asked Marni if they could, together, look past this self-criticism to her valid feelings of grief and anger. It is important to note that Marni had to first grieve the loss of an available and supportive attachment figure in times of distress before she could grieve the loss of her unborn babies and reproductive capacities.

Marni was eventually able to explore her longstanding difficulty directly expressing anger to her mother, particularly over her mother's lack of consistent and sensitive care and support in times of loss, whether that be the temporary loss of her mother after being sent away to boarding school, or the permanent loss of her unborn babies after miscarrying. The therapist reflected,

If you were to directly express your anger to your mother, then you fear you might lose whatever crumbs of understanding she gives you, and then you would really feel alone, and that would be too painful to bear, especially now when you are feeling the loss of your babies so acutely. Your pain and need for her right now are so great that you are willing to stuff your anger, or turn it against yourself, if that means saving the relationship.

The therapist went on to wonder,

Can this be a place, in this relationship with me, where you can come to feel safe to show your genuine feelings when in distress and trust that I will be here to offer my understanding and support without in some way punishing or criticizing you?

Over time, the establishment of a safe, emotionally containing, and consistent therapeutic relationship helped Marni to internalize the therapist's empathy as self-soothing and self-compassion, and to use the therapist as a safe base from which to explore feelings of trauma and loss. This helped Marni to grieve not only her recurrent pregnancy losses, but also the lack of a consistent attachment figure who provides support and comfort in times of separation and loss. Through the process of grieving, Marni's internal working models shifted to more secure, as she experienced the therapist as someone who would reliably and sensitively respond to her distress, and, subsequently, Marni felt more valuable and worthy.

WHAT IS ATTACHMENT THEORY AND HOW CAN IT BE USED AS A CLINICAL GUIDE IN INDIVIDUAL AND COUPLES THERAPY FOR PREGNANCY LOSS?

John Bowlby's (1969) ideas on attachment theory were first conceived from his observations of children who were separated from their caregivers during World War II. His theory provided a novel way of understanding both relational closeness and human bonding, as well as separation and loss in relationships with close others. Bowlby, and his student Mary Ainsworth, observed differences in how children cope with separation from a caregiver and in how they experience comfort or soothing upon the caregiver's return, which gave rise to the concept of attachment styles, also sometimes referred to as attachment patterns, organizations, types, or categories. Attachment style refers to a person's characteristic way of relating to an intimate caregiver and to other important persons (called *attachment figures* or *objects*), particularly one's parents, children, and romantic partners (Levy et al., 2019). Although unborn babies or fetuses are not typically thought of as attachment objects in Western society, research shows that mothers often attach to their unborn baby relatively early in the pregnancy (Siddiqui & Hägglöf, 2000). Further, a mother's characteristic attachment style influences how she thinks about, imagines, and mentally represents her unborn baby (Benoit et al., 1997), and how she copes with separation upon the loss of a pregnancy/unborn baby (Scheidt et al., 2012).

Attachment Definitions and Important Concepts

As Levy et al. (2019) explain, attachment style involves one's level of confidence in the consistent availability of close others to act as a *secure base* from which one can freely explore the world when not in distress, and one's capacity to use others as a *safe haven* to which one can turn to for support, protection, and comfort in times of distress (Bowlby, 1988). Exploration of "the world" includes not only the physical world, but also the examination of one's relational and intrapsychic world, including one's own thoughts and feelings and the thoughts and feelings of others (Levy et al., 2019). In the context of therapy for pregnancy loss, the client's capacity to use the therapist as a safe haven from distressing and overwhelming feelings related to reproductive trauma and loss allows the therapeutic relationship to function as a source of emotional soothing and regulation for the client. Once more emotionally regulated, the client can then use the therapist as a secure base from which to explore new feelings and experiences associated with the loss(es) that were previously believed to be too painful or overwhelming to approach or acknowledge, which facilitates the processing of trauma and loss (Leon, 2015). For instance, 9 months into treatment, Naz felt safe enough with her therapist to finally process the traumatic experience of being in the Neonatal Intensive Care Unit (NICU) for the 15 days leading up to her son's death, 11 years earlier, an experience that Naz previously felt was too painful to even think about.

In couples therapy, the therapist similarly functions as a secure base from which partners feel safe to (a) explore their own thoughts and feelings as well as those of their partner's, and (b) try new ways of being and behaving in the relationship that meet one another's attachment needs for support and understanding when in distress (Johnson & Sims, 2000). In couples therapy for pregnancy loss, it can be helpful to make explicit that while we cannot irradicate grief, partners can learn to rely on each other for support, understanding, and comfort when in distress, so they do not feel alone in their grief and sorrow. After Naz processed the trauma of the NICU experience with her therapist, she was able to, for the first time in 11 years, talk about these experiences with her partner in a joint session. For Naz, finally talking to her husband about her memories of the NICU and of their infant son, of her deep regret that she never got to breastfeed him, and of her private fear that she caused his death by going into labor early helped her to feel less alone in her feelings of grief and loss and a sense of relief. Essentially, Naz came to experience her partner as a safe haven from unbearable feelings of trauma and loss, or as someone she could go to when in intense distress for comfort and support.

Relative differences in one's capacity to use others as a secure base and/or safe haven are reflected in Bowlby's (1969) three attachment patterns: secure, anxious ambivalent, and avoidant. Ainsworth eventually renamed the anxious ambivalent pattern as anxious resistant, and identified a fourth pattern called disorganized. Later, other researchers have referred to these basic patterns using similar but slightly different names; for example, dismissing for avoidant and preoccupied for anxious ambivalent. Regardless, the caregiver's "reliable and sensitive provision of loving care is believed to result in what Bowlby called a *secure bond* between the infant and the caregiver" (Levy et al., 2019, p. 17). Attachment patterns or styles are believed to derive from repeated interactions with primary caregivers, through which the infant is believed to form *internal working models* (IWMs) of self and other. These internal working models include expectations, beliefs, and emotional appraisals and rules for processing and excluding information (Bowlby, 1969, 1973, 1980). In turn, infants' IWMs predict individual differences in the degree to which relationships are characterized by security (Levy et al., 2019).

Because of varied early experiences with caregivers, some adult clients enter treatment with a history of feeling abandoned in relationships, focus on others to manage their emotions, experience overwhelming anxiety when alone, and fear rejection and abandonment. These clients fall on the more anxious adult attachment spectrum, and they tend to have internal representations of themselves as not worthy and of others as abandoning or rejecting (Bowlby, 1988; Holmes, 2001; Wallin, 2007). Other adult clients avoid dependency, are fearful of intimacy, suppress their feelings, and minimize their distress. These clients fall on the avoidant spectrum and tend to have internal representations of themselves as self-sufficient and of others as unavailable (Bowlby, 1988; Holmes, 2001; Wallin, 2007). Research supports the notion of attachment styles as dimensional, from low to high attachment anxiety and from low to high attachment avoidance. Secure individuals would score low on both these dimensions, whereas fearful avoidant individuals would score high on both these dimensions (Brennan et al., 1998).

Attachment as a Clinical Guide

Bowlby believed, and empirical research has supported (e.g., Fraley, 2002; Mallinckrodt et al., 1995; Sroufe et al., 2005), that the attachment system operates throughout the lifespan, from "cradle to grave," and across a variety of relationships, including the therapy relationship (Bowlby, 1977, 1988). Clients look to their therapist to provide many of the same functions that their primary caregiver(s) once did, including support, understanding, and comfort. Bowlby (1975) assumed that clients relate to their therapist much like they once related to attachment figures in childhood. Clients with an insecure attachment benefit from therapy by developing a secure attachment to the therapist, as they learn to rely on the therapist during times of duress in order to explore current issues, better tolerate painful or new emotions, and ultimately revise internal working models and develop new ways of coping (see Daniel, 2006, for a review). Pregnancy loss represents one such time of duress when insecure clients can benefit from therapy by developing a secure attachment to the therapist, as they learn to rely on the therapist for the support, understanding, and emotional containment needed to process feelings of sadness and loss. To reach this goal, Bowlby (1988) suggested five main psychotherapy tasks, which are outlined and applied to individual and couples therapy for pregnancy loss in Table 8.1.

HOW DOES ATTACHMENT RELATE TO THE PROCESS AND OUTCOME OF THERAPY: ATTACHMENT AS AN EVIDENCE-BASED THERAPIST RESPONSIVENESS PRINCIPLE

Below, research is reviewed that highlights the important role that client attachment plays in the process and outcome of therapy. Client attachment may play a particularly important role in therapy for pregnancy loss when the client's attachment needs for comfort and support are heightened. With the client's attachment system activated, it is important that the client come to experience the therapist (and the partner in couples therapy) as a secure attachment figure from which distressing feelings of trauma and grief and loss can be safely approached and processed.

Table 8.1. BOWLBY'S (1988) FIVE PSYCHOTHERAPY TASKS AS APPLIED TO THERAPY
FOR PREGNANCY LOSS

Attachment Task(s)	Application to Individual Therapy for Pregnancy Loss	Application to Couples Therapy for Pregnancy Loss
Task 1: Establish a secure base, which involves providing clients with a strong internal felt sense of trust, care, and support, in which clients feel free to more fully and safely explore the world; the physical world, but also the internal subjective world of self and other (see Levy et al., 2019).	As the client develops an internal felt sense of the therapist as sensitive, caring, and trustworthy, she generally feels safer to approach and process traumatic affects associated with the loss(es) and/or other adverse reproductive events, for she knows she is no longer alone in her feelings (Leon, 2015).	The therapist acts as a secure base from which partners feel safe to explore their own thoughts and feelings as well as those of their partner, which helps each partner to make sense of and process their own experience of reproductive trauma and loss and that of their partner. From this, the couple can grieve and process reproductive trauma and loss together, giving and receiving support, understanding, and comfort.
Task 2: Explore past attachment experiences and past and present relationships. Task 3: Explore the therapeutic relationship, which involves how it may relate to relationships or experiences outside of therapy. Task 4: Link past experiences to present ones.	Past inadequate or traumatic attachment experiences in which the client turned to her early attachment figures for support and comfort in times of distress, particularly distress due to separation and loss, are likely to be evoked after the loss of a pregnancy and reenacted within the therapy relationship and need to be worked through and grieved (Markin, 2018).	Past inadequate or traumatic attachment experiences in which partners turned to their early attachment figures for support and comfort in times of distress, particularly due to separation and loss, are likely to be evoked after the loss of a pregnancy and reenacted within romantic relationships, leading individuals with an insecure attachment to overestimate their partner's negative intentions and underestimate their availability, support, and care. Therapists should help partners identify how past attachment experiences are being reenacted in the context of current marital/ partner distress, and work toward facilitating more secure attachment experiences within the couple (Johnson & Sims, 2000).

(continued)

Table 8.1. CONTINUED

Attachment Task(s)	Application to Individual Therapy for Pregnancy Loss	Application to Couples Therapy for Pregnancy Loss
Task 5: Revise IWMs.	IWMs are revised as clients have a different, more secure, attachment experience with the therapist in which painful and overwhelming feelings related to the experience of pregnancy loss(es) are sensitively and reliably responded to by the therapist, contrary to the client's expectations. Clients learn that others are available for support, emotional soothing, comfort, and understanding in times of distress and that the self is capable and worthy of eliciting such support.	IWMs are revised as partners have a different, more secure, attachment experience with their romantic partner (see Johnson & Sims, 2000), in which painful and overwhelming feelings related to the experience of pregnancy loss(es) are sensitively and reliably responded to, contrary to expectation. Partners come to experience each other in a new light and as someone who can give the support, emotional holding, and understanding that their early attachment figures could not when needed.

EMPIRICAL FINDINGS: CLIENT ATTACHMENT AND THERAPY OUTCOME

Early studies yielded conflicting results as to whether securely attached clients benefit more from therapy than insecurely attached clients (Berant & Obegi, 2009; Fonagy et al., 1996). In a recent meta-analysis of 36 studies (Levy et al., 2019), the effect size for the association between attachment security, regardless of attachment style, and psychotherapy outcome was in the small to moderate range ($r = .17$, $d = .35$). Moreover, in-treatment improvement in attachment security was related to improvement in treatment outcomes ($r = .16, d = .32$) such that larger improvements in attachment security predicted larger improvements in outcome. The results of this meta-analysis suggest that client attachment is important to the outcome of therapy, and it appears particularly important to help insecure clients become more secure over the course of treatment. Lastly, interpersonal therapies were found to be less hindered by attachment insecurity ($r = .15$, $d = .30$) than non-interpersonal therapies ($r = .33$, $d = .70$) (Levy et al., 2019), suggesting that it is important for therapists to focus on the here-and-now of the therapy relationship when working with insecure clients. For instance, Marni's therapist could have reflected,

I see how much pain you are in right now and how devastated this loss has left you feeling. Yet, I sense you are trapped in between wanting my comfort to ease the pain and not feeling safe to really let my empathy and care "in," so you are always left feeling unsatisfied in here with me.

EMPIRICAL FINDINGS: CLIENT ATTACHMENT AND THE THERAPY PROCESS

Client Attachment and the Working Alliance

The relationship between client attachment and the therapeutic alliance has been the focus of a robust body of literature (e.g., Diener & Monroe, 2011; Eames & Roth, 2000; Kanninen & Punamaki, 2000; Kivlighan et al., 1998; Marmarosh et al., 2014). A meta-analysis of 17 studies suggested that clients' comfort with intimacy and dependency and their attachment security had a positive relationship with alliance, whereas insecure attachment had a negative relationship with alliance (Diener & Monroe, 2011). Because the alliance predicts therapy outcome (Flückiger et al., 2019), it is important to identify how clinicians can adjust their relational style to foster positive alliances with insecure clients. Further, it is difficult to imagine a client experiencing the therapist as a secure base when there are significant problems in the alliance. Therapists need to pay attention to carefully calibrating their relational stance to a client's attachment needs to facilitate a positive alliance and secure attachment experience.

Therapist Attachment Style and Early Working Alliance

The client is not the only person in the room with an attachment style that can impact the therapist–client relationship. As such, researchers have examined the association between therapist attachment style and the working alliance. Black et al. (2005) found that therapist attachment security correlated with therapists' positive perceptions of early alliance, whereas therapist attachment anxiety correlated with therapists' negative perceptions of the alliance. Sauer et al. (2003) examined the relation between therapist attachment style and client-reported alliance. They found that therapist attachment anxiety was positively related to client-reported alliance early in treatment, but over the course of treatment it had a negative effect on alliance. The authors proposed that the positive relationship between therapist attachment anxiety and early alliance was due to more anxiously attached therapists focusing on forming and maintaining a positive relationship with the client and avoiding conflict. Therapist attachment has been associated with other aspects of the therapy relationship. Prior research has found that therapist attachment avoidance is related to less empathy (Rubino et al., 2000; Westmaas & Silver, 2001), more emotional distancing (Mikulincer & Shaver, 2005), hostile countertransference in dyads with anxious clients (Mohr et al., 2005), and rejecting interpersonal behaviors (Bartholomew & Horowitz, 1991), whereas therapist attachment anxiety is related to less empathy in response to therapeutic ruptures (Rubino et al., 2000). This research suggests that therapist attachment style is activated within the therapy dyad and impacts the quality of the relationship in multiple ways. To form effective relationships with clients of different attachment styles, therapists must be aware of their own attachment insecurities (Marmarosh et al., 2014).

Therapist Attachment, Client Attachment, and Alliance

Though most studies have focused on either client or therapist attachment style, a few have examined the interaction between client and therapist attachment on the alliance and have yielded inconsistent results. Some evidence suggests that therapist and client complementary insecure attachment styles negatively impact the alliance, perhaps because insecurely attached therapists get pulled into acting out in complementary ways to clients who are similarly insecurely attached (Dozier et al., 1994; Tyrrell et al., 1999). Secure therapists may be better at meeting the needs of different clients without getting pulled into any one response (Mallinckrodt, 2010). However, not all studies support the theory of noncomplementary attachment styles yielding better outcomes (Sauer et al., 2003; Romano et al., 2008; Rubino et al., 2000).

Marmarosh et al. (2014) examined the impact of complementary attachment styles on early working alliance in therapist–client dyads, using an advanced statistical procedure called the Actor–Partner Interdependence Model (APIM; Kenny & Cook, 1999). Contrary to prior research, these researchers did not find any direct effects of client or therapist attachment on client early alliance ratings. However, they did find one significant interaction, indicating that client-perceived early alliance was higher when more anxious therapists worked with clients with decreasing anxiety, and less anxious therapists worked with clients with increasing anxiety. As Marmarosh et al. (2014) suggest, high-anxiety clients may not want to work with high-anxiety therapists, who are most likely not as adept at providing the emotional soothing and containment that these clients need when in distress. On the other hand, clients with less anxiety may benefit from a more anxious therapist's emphasis on closeness and support. While it remains unclear when exactly complementary attachment styles are helpful or harmful to the therapy process, research and clinical experience suggest that therapists should refrain from getting pulled into or reflexively reacting to the client's insecure attachment style (Levy et al., 2019).

COPING WITH RPL AND INFERTILITY THROUGH AN ATTACHMENT THEORY LENS

Attachment theory can provide us with a framework for understanding how different clients cope with the extreme distress that typically follows various types of traumatic and/or compounded losses, such as RPL and infertility, which relates to what these clients need out of therapy to learn new and more adaptive ways of coping with loss.

Attachment and Mourning: Implications for Grieving Parents

Bowlby (1980) made important parallels between separation anxiety and mourning. He observed that adults who are mourning typically go through the same stages as infants do following moments of separation from a caregiver, including sadness, anxiety, protest (anger), and grief. Bowlby believed that the experience of permanent separation from a close other through death conjures past experiences of temporary separation from attachment figures in early life and, perhaps more importantly, how early attachment figures responded to the infant's separation distress (see Fraley & Shaver, 2016). This is exemplified in the case of Marni, who felt similarly scolded, rejected, unlovable, and alone after reaching out to her mother for support and comfort following the loss of yet another pregnancy, as she once did when attempting to elicit her mother's closeness and understanding as a child after being sent to boarding school. As seen here, the experience of not having a sensitive and reliable attachment figure following the devastating loss of a wanted pregnancy creates new emotional injuries, while also reopening old attachment wounds related to the perceived lack of a supportive and understanding caregiver in earlier times of separation and loss (Markin, 2018). These clients need to grieve past attachment experiences before they can grieve current losses (Leon, 2015).

Early separation experiences with attachment figures are believed to ultimately organize an individual's attachment system and predict one's characteristic way of responding to various types of losses, including pregnancy loss, and the degree to which these various characteristic grief responses are adaptive (Fraley & Shaver, 2016). For instance, Marni responded to feelings of separation and loss in her relationship with her mother similarly to how she responded to feelings of grief and loss after multiple miscarriages, with excessive self-criticism and chronic hypervigilance to signs of potential future loss, keeping her chronically depressed and anxious. In essence, because pregnancy loss grief can be understood as a natural reaction to the loss of an attachment object (Condon, 2000), such losses may activate a grieving parent's attachment system and the same attachment behaviors as once employed in early life when in distress over feeling separated, abandoned, or disconnected from attachment figures (Bowlby, 1980). Unfortunately, for more avoidant or anxious individuals, attachment behaviors that first developed in early life to help cope with the experience of feeling alone in one's distress are no longer adaptive in the present and interfere with the grieving process (Fraley & Shaver, 2016).

Mourning and Attachment Anxiety

Research suggests that individuals who are high in attachment-related anxiety are more likely than those who are low in anxiety to have complicated or disordered grief reactions (see Fraley & Shaver, 2016, for a review). These individuals are at risk for experiencing what Bowlby (1980) called *chronic mourning*, as they find themselves overly preoccupied with thoughts of their deceased loved one and unable to return to normal functioning for months or even years after a loss. They may experience prolonged symptoms of depression, anxiety, and aspects of PTSD (see Fraley & Shaver, 2016, for a review). This pattern of bereavement is similar to what some clinicians and attachment researchers have called *unresolved grief* (e.g., Ainsworth & Eichberg, 1991; Main & Hesse, 1990; Zisook & DeVaul, 1985), which has been found to predict not only a woman's own mental health outcomes following pregnancy loss, but also a subsequent infant's attachment status (Engelhard et al., 2003; Hughes et al., 2001; Main & Hesse, 1990, 1992). Consistent with these findings, in a rare study that looked at pregnancy loss grief specifically, maternal anxious attachment predicted somatization and post-traumatic stress symptoms 9 months after a pregnancy loss (Scheidt et al., 2012). Anxious individuals, as infants, never knew when their unreliable caregiver(s) would become physically and/or emotionally unavailable, so they learned to anticipate separation and loss before it even occurred in an attempt to try and prevent it through drastic or excessive measures. Thus, these individuals are chronically "stuck" in the distress of loss, sensing that abandonment lies around every corner. Marni, for example, had a difficult time processing valid feelings of perinatal grief because she remained chronically anxious about experiencing future losses and of not having others available to comfort and support her after such losses.

Mourning and Attachment Avoidance

In contrast to anxious individuals, Bowlby (1980) believed that others may express relatively little distress following loss, continue in their daily activities without any noticeable disruption, and seek little support or comfort from others. These individuals, as infants, displayed similar "mini-grief" responses upon separation from a caregiver, exhibiting a cold, detached-like response when the caregiver left the room and when the caregiver returned. These infants learned to suppress feelings of sadness and loss over separation, rather than feel alone or humiliated in their distress. This bereavement response is associated with an avoidant attachment and has been described as *delayed* or *absent grieving* (Fraley & Shaver, 2016). Bowlby believed that this manner of reacting to loss is a defensive reaction, one that has the potential to break down and give rise to intense feelings of grief and sorrow down the road and even to adverse effects on physical health (Fraley & Shaver, 2016). Consistent with Bowlby's (1980) prediction, research suggests that while attachment-related anxiety is associated with prolonged grief symptoms, more avoidance is associated with long-term difficulties adjusting to loss (Jerga et al., 2011). Bowlby acknowledged that some avoidant individuals are not necessarily avoiding grief; rather, they never attached in the first place to feel grief upon loss. He believed that these individuals pay a high price for sparing themselves feelings of grief and loss, as they never get to experience the joy of bonding

(Fraley & Shaver, 2016). This is consistent with the observation that avoidant mothersreport less strong prenatal attachments and worse mental health during the first and third trimesters of pregnancy and rely on more distance coping during the entire pregnancy (Mikulincer & Florian, 1999).

There is disagreement among bereavement scholars as to whether delayed or absent grieving is in fact a "disordered" form of grief, as Bowlby predicted (e.g., Bonanno, 2009). Some research suggests that it is important to take into consideration the type of avoidant attachment when predicting whether delayed grieving is adaptive or not, and that while fearful avoidant individuals are at risk for depression, anxiety, and PTSD following loss, the delayed grieving pattern is not necessarily problematic for dismissing-avoidant individuals (see Fraley & Shaver, 2016, for a review). Despite this, this book focuses on dismissing-avoidant individuals. Several studies suggest that dismissing-avoidant individuals suffer more general health problems (Meier et al., 2013) and experience elevated levels of PTSD and depressive symptoms (Fraley et al., 2006) after different kinds of traumatic losses. This suggests that stressful or traumatic events might undermine the utility of avoidant strategies that in other circumstances might function relatively effectively (see Mikulincer & Shaver, 2008, for an in-depth discussion of this point). Pregnancy loss, especially RPL, which is often associated with a felt sense of powerlessness to conceive a biological child, is a type of traumatic loss in which dismissing-avoidant strategies may similarly break down and lead to maladaptive outcomes. Though avoidant individuals might rationalize their wish to become a parent as "just something people my age do," the experience of RPL confronts these clients with previously disowned attachment needs and fears in a new way that can be utilized in therapy.

EMPIRICAL FINDINGS ON RPL AND INFERTILITY STRESS: AN ATTACHMENT TRIGGER

The attachment system is activated during times of stress when the need for an emotionally soothing, understanding, and supportive other is heightened. Unfortunately, individuals with an insecure attachment tend to have characteristic ways of coping with separation and loss that are maladaptive and are likely intensified in situations of ongoing and chronic loss, such as RPL and infertility. Both these experiences, uniquely and in combination with one another, represent a series of adverse and stressful life events that trigger the attachment system and the affected woman's need for comfort and support (Donarelli et al., 2016). RPL, defined as the loss of two or more clinical pregnancies (American Society for Reproductive Medicine, 2012), has a tremendous impact on a woman's emotional well-being, as well as that of her partner's well-being (Voss et al., 2020). Affected women are at risk for developing chronic grief, depression, anxiety, stress, lower quality of life, obsessive-compulsive disorder, and PTSD (Chen et al., 2020; Tavoli et al., 2018; Voss et al., 2020). While most studies have examined the experience of women suffering from RPL, Voss et al. (2020) looked at heterosexual couples experiencing RPL and found that both men and women were at significant risk for high levels of anxiety, depression, and poor social support. Women were at somewhat higher risk for depression and anxiety and men for poor social support. Many men feel the burden of responsibility to support their partner, causing them to suppress their own feelings and needs and to delay grieving. Further, it is less socially acceptable for men to show feelings of sadness and loss, especially within the context of paternal grief (Voss et al., 2020).

One explanation as to why affected men and women experience these profound emotional consequences is that RPL exposes them to ongoing and chronic *traumatic loss* (Markin, 2023), defined as an abrupt or unexpected loss that is so devastating that it overwhelms the mind's usual ways of coping with distress and of making sense of the world (Neria & Litz, 2004). Parents are challenged to cope with the shock and devastation of multiple consecutive losses and to make sense of a world in which such bad things can repeatedly happen. In a continued state of shock and devastation, it is difficult for these parents to process their feelings at the time of each loss and to make sense of events and of their reactions. Unprocessed feelings of grief and loss therefore compound after each miscarriage, infertility setback, and/or invasive medical procedure, the sum of which can overwhelm a parent's typical way of coping (Markin, 2023). On top of this, subsequent pregnancies can trigger post-traumatic stress reactions (Turton et al., 2001), including chronic hypervigilance, anxiety, and emotional avoidance. In fact, pregnancies after loss are most often characterized by (a) *pregnancy-related anxiety*, or fears related to the health of the baby and pregnancy outcomes, (b) *chronic hypervigilance* to signs of another potential loss, and (c) *emotional cushioning*, wherein women fear another loss, and thus, to varying degrees, protect their emotions by avoiding prenatal bonding (see Diamond & Diamond, 2016, for a review). These clients vacillate between grieving the traumatic loss of yet another pregnancy and struggling with post-traumatic stress symptoms when pregnant again.

RPL often occurs within the context of infertility, defined as the inability to conceive a child after 12 months of regular unprotected sexual intercourse because of an impairment in a person's capacity to reproduce as an individual or with his/her partner (Zegers et al., 2017). Infertility affects 9 percent of couples worldwide, and about 56 percent of these couples will seek medical assistance to conceive (Boivin et al., 2007). The risk of miscarriage in women with infertility has been reported to range widely, from 7 to 70 percent (Hakim et al., 1995; Molo et al., 1993). Both research and clinical experience suggest that the powerlessness to conceive a child leads individuals and couples to suffer from elevated and multifaceted stress (Cousineau & Domar, 2007; Matthiesen et al., 2011). In turn, the stress of infertility itself, and in combination with RPL, likely activates attachment-seeking behavior with primary attachment figures (Lowyck et al., 2009). In romantic relationships, the primary attachment figure is the partner (Mikulincer & Shaver, 2007). Thus, partners' attachment insecurities are often heightened during stressful experiences with RPL and infertility, causing conflict in relationships and often leading couples to seek therapy.

Couple Attachment and Infertility Stress

Couples experiencing infertility and RPL are constantly bombarded with devastating news and difficult choices that leave them with mounting anxiety, overwhelming stress, and unbearable emotional pain, triggering the need for support and comfort from one another. Yet, giving and receiving support and comfort when in distress is relatively more or less difficult depending on a partner's attachment history and style. Supporting this, recent studies have found that men and women with an anxious attachment style tend to experience more infertility stress (Bayley et al., 2009), and that men and women with a secure attachment report more well-being during ART treatments (Lowyck et al., 2009). When controlling statistically for the nesting of partners between couples, Donarelli et al. (2016) found that wives with more attachment avoidance experienced more infertility distress, perhaps because they could no longer rely on their usual self-reliant coping mechanisms to cope with the overwhelming stress of infertility and were instead confronted with their previously denied need for support and comfort from others.

More statistically advanced studies on how a partner's attachment influences the other partner's distress due to infertility suggest partners of securely attached individuals experience less infertility distress than partners of insecurely attached individuals, perhaps because securely attached individuals have a greater capacity to regulate their own distress and provide support and comfort to others (Donarelli et al., 2012; Mikulincer et al., 1998). Donarelli et al. (2016) found that husbands tended to feel more infertility distress when their wives had more attachment anxiety, whereas wives felt more infertility-related distress when their husbands had more attachment avoidance. These researchers suggest that this may have to do with the fact that while men typically use distancing coping strategies to deal with infertility stress, women typically rely on emotion-focused coping strategies (Peterson et al., 2006). In this way, the partner patterns observed in their study may reflect the pursuit–distance and demand–withdrawal patterns (Betchen, 2005) described by couple researchers, in which one partner typically pursues or "demands" emotional closeness from the other, which triggers the withdrawal and avoidance of the other partner, and so forth. From an attachment perspective, such patterns emanate from the separation distress that one partner experiences when perceiving the other as inaccessible or unresponsive (Johnson & Sims, 2000). Such negative cycles of conflict emerge in relationships when more anxious clients attempt to deal with their separation distress by pursuing excessive closeness to their partner and avoidant clients cope by preemptively withdrawing from the relationship altogether before they can feel rejected or humiliated.

Attachment-Informed Couples Therapy for RPL and Infertility: Treatment Implications

As Johnson and Sims (2000) write, attachment theory can be viewed as a theory of trauma, wherein the absence of or break in a secure connection to others is a source of anxiety and traumatic stress (Atkinson, 1997). From this perspective, it is the absence of, or break in, a secure connection to one's partner or spouse that creates considerable distress (Johnson & Sims, 2000). This is evident among couples affected by RPL and infertility, who often experience increased relationship conflict and decreased marital satisfaction (Peterson et al., 2006; see Samadaee-Gelehkolaee et al., 2016, for a review). Typically, these couples are traumatized not only by the loss of multiple pregnancies and by the powerlessness to conceive a much-wanted child, but also by the break in or absence of connection to one another during a time of intense distress. The separation distress that results from feeling disconnected from one's romantic partner (or current attachment object), just as one is feeling emotionally vulnerable and overwhelmed and in need of comfort and support, tends to activate earlier attachment experiences of feeling alone in one's separation distress. In fact, researchers have documented how marital distress resembles separation distress in early attachment relationships. In particular, lack of emotional engagement with an attachment figure during times of stress appears to be a key aspect of separation distress in both early caregiving and marital relationships (see Johnson & Sims, 2000, for a review). From this, reestablishing emotional engagement and closeness in couples may help to not only repair the relationship, but also to help the couple cope with the trauma and loss of RPL and infertility, through giving each partner an experience of not feeling alone in overwhelming feelings of distress.

SUMMARY AND NEXT STEPS

- *Summary:* Therapists should strive to facilitate a secure-base experience in which the client develops a sense of the therapist as a trustworthy and reliable source of support and comfort. Knowing that one is not alone in one's distress helps the client feel safe to approach and process feelings of separation and grief/loss, particularly in situations of ongoing, chronic, and compounded losses like RPL. In this process, IWMs shift to more secure as the client learns to rely on others for support and comfort in times of distress.
  - *Next Steps:* The subsequent chapter identifies ways in which therapists should adjust their relational style to meet the client's attachment needs and facilitate a secure-base experience, with the dual goal of shifting IWMs to more secure and processing feelings of grief and loss associated with RPL.

- *Summary:* Client and therapist attachment style impacts the process (particularly the working alliance) and outcome of therapy. Importantly, research suggests that therapist and client attachment style interact in complicated ways to predict the quality of the therapy relationship, which in turn predicts outcome.
  - *Next Steps:* Since client insecure attachment negatively impacts the alliance and treatment outcome, the subsequent chapter addresses how therapists should adjust their relational style depending on client attachment to facilitate a positive alliance and secure-base experience. Moreover, the subsequent chapter explores specific ways in which therapist and client insecure attachment styles may interact to negatively impact the therapy relationship and process within the context of therapy for RPL.
- *Summary:* Research suggests that attachment style predicts an individual's characteristic way of coping with grief and loss and the relative adaptiveness of these responses.
  - *Next Steps:* The next chapter will explore how a client's attachment style impacts her response and ability to cope with pregnancy loss and with pregnancies after loss, and, moreover, the kind of relationship clients of different attachment styles need to learn new and more adaptive ways of coping with grief and loss.
- *Summary:* Couples affected by the stress of RPL and infertility often experience negative cycles of conflict that activate negative internal working models and perpetuate a traumatic break in connection, precisely when each partner needs the other's support and comfort to cope.
  - *Next Steps:* The subsequent chapter addresses how therapists can facilitate a secure-base experience within the couple in order to stop negative cycles of communication so that both partners feel safe to process reproductive trauma and loss and, in the process, develop a more secure romantic partner attachment.

9

Relational Guidance on Therapist Responsiveness to Client Attachment in Individual and Couples Therapy for Recurrent Pregnancy Loss and Infertility

Theory, practice, and research all suggest that attachment theory has important implications for the therapy process and outcome (see Chapter 8 in this book for a review). As Levy et al. (2019) conclude, it seems particularly important for therapists to adapt their approach, interventions, and relational style to the unique attachment needs of the client. Yet, *how* exactly should therapists adapt their approach and relational style to "fit" a client's attachment needs? While, from an attachment perspective, the effectiveness of individual therapy rests upon the client coming to experience the therapist as a secure base, or temporary attachment figure (Bowlby, 1988), little clinical guidance exists for therapists on what they should actually do, or how they should *be* in the relationship, to facilitate a secure-base experience with clients of different attachment styles. The kind of relational experience that contributes to a client's internal sense of the therapist as a sensitive and trustworthy attachment figure likely differs for clients with different attachment styles, and therapists need to know how to adjust accordingly. Similarly, from an attachment perspective, in couples therapy, the primary task is to help each partner develop an internal sense of the other as a sensitive and trustworthy secure base from which feelings and distress can be explored and co-regulated (Johnson, 2019). This chapter offers guidance on how therapists should adjust their relational style depending on client attachment to facilitate a secure-base experience with individuals and couples affected by RPL and infertility, who need a secure base from which to process feelings of reproductive trauma and loss (Leon, 2015; Markin, 2023).

Psychotherapy for Pregnancy Loss. Rayna D. Markin, Oxford University Press. © Oxford University Press 2024.
DOI: 10.1093/oso/9780197693353.003.0009

OVERVIEW

This chapter applies the attachment theory, research, and clinical guidance reviewed in Chapter 8 to a specific clinical context. Marni, a client with a more anxious attachment who was introduced in Chapter 8, is again referred to throughout this chapter as a clinical illustration. Below, markers for identifying more anxious or avoidant clients affected by RPL and infertility are suggested as an aid to help clinicians form an initial diagnostic impression of a client's attachment style (see Box 9.1). Then, based on theory and research, guidance on how therapists should adjust their relational style and approach to facilitate a secure-base experience with avoidant and anxious clients is discussed and demonstrated within a hypothetical couple session vignette. The relational guidance offered below is believed to be relevant to therapy for pregnancy loss in general but is explored within the context of RPL and infertility specifically. These adverse reproductive events represent a series of ongoing stressful life experiences that often overwhelm a client's typical way of coping, triggering the attachment system to seek support and comfort from others (Donarelli et al., 2012, 2016). In turn, the triggering of IWMs provides an opportunity to rewire the attachment system. This chapter concludes by exploring challenges to therapist responsiveness to client attachment and clinical implications.

IDENTIFYING THE MORE ANXIOUS CLIENT IN THERAPY FOR RPL AND INFERTILITY

IWMs of Self and Other

More anxious clients often present to treatment with perceptions of others as preoccupied, distant, and inconsistent and the self as unlovable, helpless, and fragile (Marmarosh et al., 2013). This IWM of others is exemplified in the case of Marni, who, after an initial "honeymoon" period, would ultimately come to perceive the doctors and staff of multiple fertility clinics as uncaring and unavailable, a theme that was also evident in her romantic relationships and later on with her therapist. Concerning the more anxious client's IWM of self, although infertility and pregnancy loss are typically experienced as assaults on one's self-esteem and identity (Leon, 2015), for more anxious clients, these events confirm a pre-existing sense of self as unlovable and unworthy and are experienced as deeply injurious to an already fragile sense of self. Marni experienced her miscarriages and fertility struggles as confirmation of her lack of worth and destiny to be abandoned and alone because of her perceived inadequacies. More anxious clients fear rejection and abandonment (Simpson & Rholes, 2017) and often experience RPL as a series of abandonments, or as a rejection of their very self and body. This is demonstrated in Marni's cry, "Who would want to spend their life with me? No one wants to stick around and love me, not a man, not even a baby!"

Box 9.1.

CHECKLIST FOR IDENTIFYING ANXIOUS CLIENTS AFFECTED BY RPL
AND/OR INFERTILITY

☐ Client possesses negative internal working models of self as unlovable
   and helpless and of others as preoccupied and rejecting. When seeking
   support after yet another miscarriage, they often feel that others are too
   busy to care and have abandoned and disappointed them yet again in
   their time of distress. Infertility is experienced as confirmation of their
   basic inadequacy and unlovability.

☐ Client's experience of pregnancies after loss is dominated by pervasive
   and severe pregnancy-related anxiety, and each loss is experienced as
   another abandonment or rejection. Anxiety, in this context, can be
   understood as both an understandable reaction to the trauma of repeated
   losses and as an attachment cue to alert others to their overwhelming
   distress.

☐ Client uses hyperactivating strategies to elicit support and comfort from
   others to cope with feelings of distress, typically overwhelming and
   pushing away support persons with excessive demands for closeness and
   reassurance. Fervent efforts to maintain proximity and avoid rejection
   in relationships to cope with the trauma of RPL and infertility seem to
   interfere with the client's capacity to reflect on the actual experience of
   reproductive trauma and loss.

☐ Client quickly becomes overwhelmed and disorganized when asked about
   her reproductive story. She cannot reflect on her experience of RPL and/
   or infertility and instead gets swept away by intense emotions.

☐ Client expresses overwhelming distress when talking about her
   experience of RPL and/or infertility but cannot seem to take in the
   therapist's empathy and support and seems to hardly recognize the
   therapist is there at all sometimes.

☐ Client quickly becomes flushed in the face, sweaty, and tense, especially
   when discussing experiences of loss and of turning to attachment figures
   for support and comfort.

☐ Client expresses much ambivalence toward attachment figures. While she
   longs for them to support and understand her and frequently demands it,
   she also harbors a long list of grudges and feels chronically disappointed
   in their lack of availability.

☐ In couples, the anxious partner typically pursues or demands support
   and reassurance by using hyperactivating strategies, which tends to
   overwhelm, frustrate, and push away the other partner, creating a self-
   fulfilling prophecy wherein the anxious partner feels abandoned and
   alone in one's feelings of grief and loss.

In couples, because of their negative IWM of others, anxious partners may overestimate how preoccupied or rejecting their partner is and underestimate their partner's availability and care. Simultaneously, because of their negative IWM of self, anxious partners may underestimate their ability to elicit support and care from others and hyperactivate their distress in an effort to get their attachment needs met, overwhelming and pushing away their partner (Simpson & Rholes, 2017). In the context of RPL, anxious individuals often perceive their partner as unavailable, rejecting, and unsupportive when grieving after each miscarriage and similarly inattentive to their anxiety over another potential loss when pregnant again. Partners of anxious individuals often feel overwhelmed by the intensity of their anxious partner's distress, on top of their own feelings of distress, and withdraw in response.

Characteristics of Pregnancies After Loss: Grieving a Pregnancy Loss and Becoming Pregnant Again

Women affected by RPL vacillate between grieving the loss of a much-wanted pregnancy and fearing yet another imminent loss when pregnant again (Markin, 2023). While it is understandably difficult to grieve miscarriage after miscarriage irrespective of attachment style, anxious individuals, who are more likely to experience unresolved grief following other types of losses (Fraley & Shaver, 2016), may experience even more difficulty processing this kind of compounded grief. It is important for clinicians to understand that RPL represents an anxious client's worst attachment fear: that one will be abandoned, at any moment, unexpectedly, and repeatedly. Because each lost pregnancy is experienced as a part of self, these clients are left feeling as if they cannot even trust their own body not to reject or abandon them. There is essentially no safe haven, not even within oneself or one's womb. As a result, anxious clients may appear preoccupied with thoughts of past lost pregnancies/babies and with becoming pregnant again (and the fear of yet another potential loss), to such an extent that it is difficult for them to return to normal functioning. They may experience prolonged grief, as they continue to yearn for that which was lost and may continue to "seek out" the babies they have lost through engaging in frantic attempts to get pregnant again with what has been termed a *replacement child* (Cain & Cain, 1964). This grief response was first developed in early life, as the preoccupied infant continued to yearn for and seek out an absent attachment figure.

When pregnant again, anxious individuals likely remain chronically fearful of another potential loss, for wired into their attachment system is an expectation that felt security or closeness cannot be trusted because one could lose it any time. While *pregnancy-related anxiety*, or the fear of yet another loss, typically characterizes pregnancy after loss (Côte-Arsenault & Mahlangu, 1999), it tends to be more overwhelming, preoccupying, and dysregulating for women with more attachment anxiety (Markin, 2018). These anxious clients find themselves in a precarious position because finally obtaining what they want (i.e., a viable pregnancy) is experienced not as the answer to their intense distress, but rather as a source of further distress, for they immediately begin fearing an additional potential loss. This is consistent with research suggesting that when highly anxious individuals face stressful events (like RPL), they tend to use hyperactivating/emotion-focused coping strategies, which direct their attention to the source of distress and cause them to ruminate over "worst-case" scenarios, making it difficult to solve the problem at hand (Simpson & Rholes, 2017). In therapy, it is often difficult to explore genuine feelings of grief and loss related to miscarriage after miscarriage with anxious clients because they tend to ruminate over the inevitability of "worst-case" scenarios in the future. It is important for clinicians to keep in mind that pregnancy-related anxiety is typical of pregnancies after loss and not necessarily pathological or indicative of an anxious attachment. A key difference is that whereas more secure clients can typically identify their fear of another potential loss as a feeling and reflect upon the meaning of their fears and anxieties, more anxious clients typically cannot identify their fears and anxieties as subjective experiences.

Hyperactivating Strategies

Individuals with a more anxious attachment engage in hyperactivating strategies, or frantic efforts to find support and relief in interpersonal relationships that typically involve demanding, clinging, and possessive behaviors. Anxious clients use these strategies to help control their anxiety over abandonment by minimizing emotional distance and soliciting displays of affection from others (Bartholomew & Horowitz, 1991; Feeney & Noller, 1990). Such strategies were learned in early attachment relationships, where they were necessary to get the attention of an inconsistent and preoccupied caregiver (Dozier et al., 1999; Main, 1995; Wallin, 2007). The desperation, loss, and sense of abandonment that anxious clients feel upon miscarriage after miscarriage tend to exacerbate pre-existing hyperactivating strategies in close relationships. This is because wired into the attachment system of anxious clients is a "rule" that to get their attachment needs met for emotional containment, support, and understanding during times of distress, they must cling to others and amplify their emotionality and helplessness (Simpson & Rholes, 2017). Consequently, more anxious clients often enter therapy after overwhelming fertility clinic staff and doctors with their excessive demands for support and attention, and after pushing away and overwhelming romantic partners and other support persons. Despite anxious clients' frantic efforts to elicit closeness, they typically feel helpless to actually obtain the closeness they so desire and actively pursue (Cassidy & Kobak, 1988). For instance, the helplessness that Marni experienced in her efforts to have a healthy child reaffirmed and magnified her engrained sense of powerlessness to secure the love she so desperately craved. After all, she could not even do the "one thing" that she was "born" to do and birth a child who would love and never leave her.

Ambivalence in Relationships

Anxious clients express ambivalence toward attachment figures, such as caregivers, spouses/partners, friends, and even temporary attachment figures like fertility doctors, nurses, and staff. They appear preoccupied with past wrongs in relationships and unable to "let it go" (Marmarosh et al., 2013). For example, while Marni was perpetually angry with her fertility doctor for not giving her enough attention and support, she fervently pursued closeness to him and seemed convinced that he would be the one to "get me pregnant." Similarly, while Marni seemed preoccupied with lamenting the ways in which her mother continually wronged her throughout her life, she was also desperate for her mother's support and understanding and would often seek her out when in distress—for example, after her most recent miscarriage. Internally, Marni experienced much ambivalence over her own attachment needs, for while she longed for closeness to her mother, she also held a great deal of unprocessed rage toward her, which she would often turn inward as a relentless self-attack.

RELATIONAL GUIDANCE FOR ANXIOUS CLIENTS STRUGGLING WITH RPL AND INFERTILITY

Research suggests that anxious clients are more likely to report infertility stress and to experience long-lasting negative mental health outcomes, such as post-traumatic stress and somatization, after a pregnancy loss (Bayley et al., 2009; Scheidt et al., 2012). Despite their apparent need for psychological services and support, these clients tend to have a difficult time forming a trusting relationship with their therapist and collaborating on the tasks and goals of therapy (Diener & Monroe, 2011). Fortunately, irrespective of these obstacles to treatment, anxious clients are more likely to benefit from therapy when they make greater gains in attachment security over the course of treatment (Levy et al., 2019). Thus, it is important for clinicians to identify these clients early on in treatment and to adjust their relational style to meet the client's attachment needs. Specifically, when working with anxious clients, based on recommendations made by Levy et al. (2019) and Pando-Mars (2016), it is suggested that therapists adjust their relational style to (a) avoid reacting reflexively, going too far in acting in contrast or in a complementary fashion to a client's more anxious attachment, (b) act as a calm, non-reactive, focused, reflective, and emotionally soothing container that can withstand the client's emotional chaos, and (c) encourage genuine relatedness instead of defensive clinginess.

Avoid Reacting Reflexively to a Client's Anxious Attachment

As Levy et al. (2019) suggest, therapists should avoid reacting reflexively to a client's attachment anxiety by either acting in contrast or in a complementary fashion to it. This is evident in the case of Marni, wherein her therapist initially

responded to Marni's attachment anxiety in a complementary manner with further emotional intensity, before then reacting in contrast to it, growing aloof and
withdrawn in the relationship out of a sense of frustration with Marni's relentless
escalation of distress, yet inability to accept the therapist's empathy and care. As
seen here, therapists are often initially pulled into the overwhelming emotional
distress of the anxious client, and then mirror the client's emotional intensity and
dysregulation by becoming affectively overwhelmed and dysregulated themselves.
The therapist may unknowingly collude with the client's defenses through, for example, asking questions to deepen the client's already dysregulated emotionality
(Levy et al., 2019). Therapists may use various interventions to deepen, or further intensify and explore, the already overwhelming and chaotic emotionality
of anxious clients because, in the moment, it feels as if doing so communicates
empathy while helping the client to work through distressing feelings. However,
as Marni's therapist experienced, such attempts usually end in further emotional
dysregulation for anxious clients, and confusion and frustration for therapists,
who do not understand why their fervent attempts to empathize with, join, and
deepen the client's distress seem to consistently backfire.

  This dynamic typically occurs when the therapist has mistaken the anxious
client's *emotionality*, or defensive and maladaptive affects that are attention-
seeking, for the *genuine expression of primary emotions* (Marmarosh et al., 2013;
Pando-Mars, 2016; see Chapter 5 in this book). For instance, in the context of
RPL, anxious clients are more likely to express defensive "weepiness" that escalates
the client's sense of helplessness than primary feelings of grief/sadness and loss.
Differentiating defensive sadness from genuine feelings of grief and loss can be
particularly difficult in the context of RPL, where one would expect intense feelings
of sadness and loss associated with the experience of compounded grief. However,
while mirroring and deepening a client's primary feelings of sadness and loss usually lead to the client feeling "better," less alone, and more regulated and understood,
deepening the client's defensive emotionality usually leads to further defensiveness
and emotional dysregulation. In response, the frustrated, overwhelmed, confused,
and demoralized therapist often withdraws from the relationship, acting in contrast to the client's anxious attachment and confirming what the anxious client
feared all along, that she will be left alone in her distress with no one to turn to.

  While this dynamic in the therapy relationship is not uncommon with anxious clients, it is important for therapists to be able to identify and "step outside"
of it. Secure therapists appear better at identifying this unfolding dynamic in the
therapy relationship and then responding in a more flexible and less reactive manner
(Mallinkcrodt, 2010). Marni's therapist, for example, observed this dynamic unfold in
the therapy relationship and used her new awareness to better empathize with Marni.

The Interaction of Client Anxiety and Therapist Attachment

Therapists' specific response to anxious clients likely depends on the therapist's
own attachment style. Anxious therapists may be more likely to react in a

complementary fashion to the excessive emotionality of anxious clients, which, in turn, further escalates the client's distress and emotional dysregulation (Levy et al., 2019). How the therapist feels inside, including the neurophysiological state of emotional dysregulation, is likely communicated to the client through relational and affective pathways. These forms of communication involve right hemispheric processes in the brain that are highly relational and nonverbal, and expressed through such things as facial expression, tone of voice, vocal quality, and eye contact (Schore, 2003). In essence, in dyads where both participants are more anxious, the emotional dysregulation of one participant likely activates a similar reaction in the other on a nonverbal and automatic level. Once activated, the anxious therapist may simply be too dysregulated to just *be* with the client in the client's emotional pain and distress (Schore, 2012). Yet, often, the only thing that a therapist *can* do to help clients process the loss of multiple pregnancies is to just *be* with their feelings of grief and loss, devastation, powerlessness, and anger. The experience of the therapist affectively joining and holding the client's distress is emotionally regulating in itself (Greenberg, 2014).

Clients affected by RPL and infertility with an anxious attachment tend to experience the "typical" internal disorganization that comes from the devastating experience of losing pregnancy upon pregnancy, on top of their characteristic level of hyperarousal and emotional dysregulation. Therefore, especially at this time, these clients need a secure attachment object who can just be with them in their distress, providing emotional organization and soothing. As such, therapists working with anxious clients should remain non-reactive, simply listening to the client's reproductive story with care and concern. This may be difficult for more anxious therapists who are similarly dysregulated. Consistent with this, one study found that more anxious clients form better relationships with less anxious therapists (Marmarosh et al., 2014). On the contrary, an avoidant therapist may feel overwhelmed by an anxious client's emotional intensity and neediness and quickly disengage from the relationship. In turn, the therapist's withdrawal tends to reinforce the client's expectation of rejection and abandonment in relationships and stymies the grieving process. As Levy et al. (2019) suggest, when working with anxious clients, therapists should titrate their interpersonal style as to not appear too disengaged, or uninterested, as consistent with avoidant therapists, while also refraining from escalating the client's emotional distress with their own emotional chaos, as consistent with anxious therapists.

Act as an Empathic yet Focused, Non-reactive and Reflective, Emotionally Soothing Container That Can Withstand the Client's Emotional Chaos

More anxious clients need the therapist to be empathic and nurturing yet focused, especially when they become overwhelmed by their emotions and unable to slow down and reflect upon them (Pando-Mars, 2016). The more the anxious client displays escalated and defensive emotionality and becomes increasingly

disorganized, the more the therapist needs to remain nonreactive and stay focused on helping the client make sense of her chaotic and overwhelming emotional experience (Pando-Mars, 2016). The therapist's empathic and soothing
yet focused approach provides these clients with emotional organization and
containment, so that they can then stop and reflect upon the meaning of their
thoughts, feelings, and behaviors (Marmarosh & Tasca, 2013; Pando-Mars, 2016).
Often, more anxious clients will vehemently attack the self for the recurrent losses
they have suffered, which tends to interfere with the grieving process. Sometimes
it is helpful to reframe the client's belief that her losses were her fault as a feeling
(rather than a fact) that can be reflected upon and understood. Anxious clients
typically need to understand that their tendency to attack the self in times of
separation and loss first started in early attachment relationships. After all, if the
reason one's caregiver is unreliable is one's fault, then at least one potentially has
the power to do something about it in the future. This false sense of control over
preventing further separation and loss comes at the price of the anxious client's
self-esteem and autonomy.

While reflecting on thoughts and feelings to gain some emotional distance is
typically most helpful for anxious clients (Levy et al., 2019; Marmarosh et al.,
2013; Pando-Mars, 2016), actually doing so within the therapy relationship is
complicated by the fact that reflecting on internal experience has not historically
felt like a safe endeavor to anxious clients. Early caregivers of these clients were
often too preoccupied, anxious, and inconsistent to be depended upon to help the
child make sense of overwhelming distress. Contrary to these past attachment
experiences, the therapist's consistent, non-reactive, and focused curiosity into
the thoughts and feelings of the anxious client sends a message that the client is
not alone in her distress and that her intense feelings are capable of being understood. For example, the therapist may need to consistently and empathically point
out the client's tendency to attack the self when approaching genuine feelings of
grief and loss after a miscarriage and inquire what feelings may come up for the
client if such self-criticism were temporarily put to the side.

Similarly, the therapist's non-reactive and consistent presence sends the message that, despite the intensity of the client's emotions and attachment needs, the
therapist can provide emotional soothing and comfort (Levy et al., 2019). In cases
of RPL, anxious clients need to come to trust on an implicit level that their intense
need for support and comfort from a trustworthy and sensitive other during such
times of intense distress will neither destroy them nor drive the therapist away, in
order to feel safe enough to access genuine feelings of grief and loss. Contrary to
past attachment figures, these clients need to experience the therapist as someone
who is capable of helping them to make order out of the emotional chaos they
feel inside, through offering consistent support, comfort, and understanding. One
client described this experience as organizing a disheveled closet with one massive heaping pile of undifferentiated clothes, hanging up each item of clothing one
by one.

In the vignette from Chapter 8, Marni's attachment anxiety was especially triggered after she reached out to her mother for support and comfort following a

recent miscarriage, and, in response, felt rejected and criticized, rather than cared for and comforted as she had hoped. Marni came into the following therapy session spiraling out of control affectively, hardly able to get out a complete sentence before sobbing or yelling uncontrollably, was consumed by resentment and self-criticism, and had little capacity to reflect on her experience. As seen in the case write-up in Chapter 8, in response, the therapist acted as an emotional container for Marni's intense affect by (a) clarifying and focusing on Marni's primary emotions and attachment needs (i.e., anger toward her mother for emotionally abandoning her in moments of profound distress and the attachment need for support and comfort when in distress), (b) bringing Marni's attention back to her immediate experience (i.e., redirecting her attention away from excessive resentment and self-criticism and toward her primary feelings and reactions in the moment), and (c) reflecting on the client's experience and trying to understand it within her attachment context, rather than reacting with emotional intensity and dysregulation. In essence, contrary to past attachment figures, the therapist demonstrated to Marni that she was capable of holding and helping Marni to make order out of the intense and chaotic emotions Marni felt inside. This helped Marni to develop a sense of herself as someone who is capable of withstanding difficult experiences and feelings and as others as available for support and comfort when needed, eventually helping Marni to feel safe enough to approach and process genuine feelings of grief and loss.

Encourage Genuine Contact and Not Defensive Clinginess

No person, insecurely attached or not, can mourn and process the overwhelming number of traumatic losses associated with RPL and infertility alone. Rather, we all need an empathic and supportive relationship in which to mourn and process trauma and loss (Markin & Zilcha-Mano, 2018). Yet, counterintuitively, despite anxious clients' preoccupation with closeness, they have massive resistance to genuine relatedness that makes it difficult for them to take in the care and concern of others. As Pando-Mars (2016) explains, they tend to use words and excessive emotionality as a shield against genuine contact. Their intense desire for closeness, on one hand, and their overwhelming fear of abandonment, on the other, often lead them to pull for the care and concern of others, while failing to recognize and take in empathic support when offered (Pando-Mars, 2016). This is why it is so difficult for anxious clients to process their experience of RPL even when they find an empathic and caring therapist, for the therapist's attention and care is both what they want and what they fear. In this case, clients need to first rewire their attachment IWMs to more secure before they can process pregnancy loss grief within the therapy relationship (Leon, 2015). Without the ability to take in the therapist's empathy, support, and emotional soothing, talking about their devastating and even traumatic RPL experiences to the therapist is only likely to lead to further emotional dysregulation for anxious clients.

The therapist can expand the client's capacity for genuine contact in relationships with interventions that make explicit the therapist's implicit presence, as different from the presence of early attachment figures (Pandora-Mars, 2016). For instance, after Marni came into therapy feeling devastated by her mother's lack of responsiveness to her feelings over her latest miscarriage, the therapist genuinely felt sorrow for Marni's adult and child self, both of whom were so often left alone in their feelings of separation and loss. The therapist could have stopped and said to Marni, "I feel very connected to your sadness right now and your sense of aloneness. I'm wondering if you sense that? Can we pause and really let that in right now and see what that's like for you?" Interventions like this facilitate genuine contact in the therapy relationship through helping the client to experience the therapist as someone who is capable of providing empathy and soothing, contrary to past attachment figures. Anxious clients have been historically deprived of such genuine contact and relatedness because of their caregiver's own preoccupation or narcissistic absorption and have thus internalized a sense of others as preoccupied and emotionally unavailable. To help these clients take in the presence of the therapist as separate from that of early attachment figures, the therapist needs to make explicit how the therapeutic relationship is different and new (Pando-Mars, 2016). This is a fundamental principle in experiential and attachment-based treatments, such as Accelerated Experiential Dynamic Psychotherapy (Fosha, 2000; Pando-Mars, 2016).

Relational Guidance as Applied to Couples Therapy with an Anxious Partner

When working with couples with an anxious partner, the therapist's emotionally soothing and focused relational style helps to contain and deescalate conflict and negative cycles of interaction within the couple. One common negative cycle of interaction that has been observed among heterosexual couples experiencing infertility distress is the pursuit–distance or demand–withdrawal pattern (Donarelli et al., 2016; Peterson, 2015; see Chapter 8 in this book). This pattern may be understood, in extreme cases, as an interaction between one partner's more anxious attachment and the other partner's more avoidant attachment style (Johnson & Sims, 2000). For example, Mary angerly demands that her partner Bill immediately reassure her that the new fertility drug they just started will "work," and becomes enraged when Bill shows the slightest hesitancy in his reassurance, calling him unsupportive and uncaring. In response, Bill tries to assuage Mary's anxiety with facts and figures, denial, and persuasion, rather than emotionally engage her, which Mary experiences as an emotional abandonment, perpetuating the cycle. In this chapter, couples with one more anxious and one more avoidant partner are focused on for two reasons. The first reason is that the demand–withdrawal cycle that is commonly observed among couples experiencing infertility distress can be understood as the interaction of one partner's more anxious attachment and the other partner's more avoidant attachment (Johnson & Sims, 2000). Second, a literature review on self-reported adult attachment and romantic partner preference found evidence to support the hypothesis that adults of complementary (i.e., avoidant and anxious), not similar, attachment styles are more likely to prefer one another in long-term relationships (Holmes & Johnson, 2009).

Unfortunately, anxious partners often possess little understanding of what thoughts and feelings motivate their behaviors and those of their partner (Johnson & Sims, 2000). For example, Mary lacked conscious understanding that her excessive demands for reassurance from Bill reflected an attempt to manage her long-engrained attachment fear of being abandoned when in distress and difficulty with self-soothing. Anxious partners start to feel safe enough to gradually explore the thoughts and feelings that motivate their excessive pursuit of reassurance and closeness from others, particular when in distress, and to similarly understand what internal experiences motivate their partner's withdrawal in response, when the therapist functions as a secure base. As anxious partners come to feel as if they can depend on the therapist to help contain and make sense of their chaotic emotional experiences, and to provide support and comfort when needed, they typically begin to turn inward and reflect upon thoughts and feelings, which no longer seem as scary and overwhelming. The therapist's genuine curiosity into the anxious partner's internal experience may similarly spark the client's curiosity into thoughts and feelings, within oneself and one's partner. Anxious partners are then more likely to slow down and think about their internal experience, instead of looking to their partner to provide relief from the overwhelming anxiety and loneliness they feel inside. They may start to wonder why they are so quick to blame their partner for their own infertility distress and why their partner's efforts to support them never seem to stick. As anxious partners get in touch with their unmet attachment need for closeness and intimacy (which is often brought to the forefront and amplified in cases of RPL and infertility), and their feelings of desperation and loneliness, they can locate the source of their distress as coming from their own attachment fears, insecurities, and needs, rather than blaming their partner (Johnson & Sims, 2000), which challenges the demand–withdrawal pattern. This process is exemplified in the session dialogue below with Marni and her now husband Joe, as the therapist works with Marni to identify the attachment needs and fears that motivate her demands of, and disappointments in, Joe.

Sometimes, before couples can try new attachment behaviors with one another in the present, they first need to contend with certain attachment "ghosts" from the past. Anxious partners may not be able to stop demanding excessive closeness, support, and reassurance from their partner until they grieve early attachment experiences in which such hyperactivating strategies were needed to gain the attention of a preoccupied caregiver. In this case, the therapist should make explicit how past attachment experiences are impacting the couple's relationship and work toward differentiating past and present attachment experiences (Bowlby, 1988). Marni, in the session vignette below, must first grieve the loss of a supportive and understanding maternal figure during earlier times of separation and loss before she can fully put her hyperactivating behaviors to rest and form a more secure attachment relationship with Joe, which is more important now than ever because of the immense duress that both partners are currently experiencing due to struggles with RPL and infertility.

IDENTIFYING MORE AVOIDANT CLIENTS STRUGGLING WITH RPL AND INFERTILITY

IWMs of Self and Others

Avoidant clients tend to have internal representations of themselves as self-sufficient and of others as unavailable, disappointing, and rejecting (Bowlby, 1988; Holmes, 2001; Wallin, 2007). These individuals learned in early attachment relationships that their distress, as well as their need for closeness and support when in distress, will be ignored, discouraged, and/or shamed by primary attachment figures, while being "strong" and self-reliant will be rewarded (Ainsworth et al., 1978). Consistent with this, avoidant adults may be less likely to seek out support and comfort from others to help cope with the distress of RPL and infertility, potentially leading to higher levels of infertility distress (Donarelli et al., 2016). For example, one client who suffered her third miscarriage of a wanted pregnancy checked into a hotel room while miscarrying, stating that she preferred to deal with it on her own. She blamed her partner for not being more available during the miscarriage but stated she preferred it that way anyway. These desperate attempts to prove one's excessive self-reliance during times of extreme adversity occur alongside mounting distress and the growing need for comfort and support, as well as increased reliance on outside intervention to achieve a viable pregnancy. Avoidant patients affected by infertility are often forced to rely on fertility doctors, clinics, and ARTs to do what one "should" be able to do on one's own. This can bring about intense feelings of shame/humiliation and neediness within the avoidant individual, who prizes self-reliance.

In the session dialogue below, Joe, who has a more avoidant attachment, ardently resists his doctor's diagnosis of male-factor infertility and the doctor's recommendation for sperm donation. Instead, as is typical of avoidant individuals, Joe engages in defensive self-enhancement, suppressing negative aspects of self and focusing on personal strengths (Mikulincer & Shaver, 2007), stating that there is nothing wrong with his "swimmers" and that the doctor is just jealous of him. This defensive self-enhancement maintains Joe's internal working model of self as strong and self-reliant by projecting his sense of shame and inadequacy onto an envious doctor. Yet, underneath Joe's denial and narcissistic self-enhancement lie intense feelings of shame and humiliation around needing help to do something as primal as fathering a child, which contradicts his internal representation of self as virile, strong, and self-reliant. As seen in the session below, Joe's IWM of others as unavailable and rejecting is apparent in his fear that if he were to disclose to Marni his feelings and distress, she would humiliate or reject him rather than comfort him.

Characteristics of Pregnancies After Loss: Grieving a Pregnancy Loss and Becoming Pregnant Again

Avoidant adults, as children, learned to suppress feelings of sadness and loss upon separation from a caregiver because these feelings were experienced as shameful and weak (Bowlby, 1969), and have been shown to similarly display absent or delayed grieving after the death of a close other (Fraley & Shaver, 2016). From this, women with a more avoidant attachment may deny feelings of grief and loss after even recurrent miscarriages (Markin, 2018), perhaps stating that they were "chemical pregnancies anyway." Yet, they may report somatic symptoms, irritability, or panic attacks (Kotler et al., 1994), as consistent with Bowlby's (1969) belief that while individuals with an avoidant attachment defensively exclude feelings of grief and loss, these feelings still come out in other ways through, for example, problems with physical health. When pregnant again, avoidant individuals may take extra measure to deny feelings of closeness to the fetus/unborn baby, conceptualizing the fetus as an "it" rather than assigning it personhood and talking about the pregnancy in a cool and detached manner. When asked to describe how she imagines the personhood of her unborn baby, the pregnant mother with an avoidant attachment may reply, "What do you mean? I don't know. That's a strange question" (Markin, 2018). This exemplifies how avoidant individuals may engage in extreme forms of *emotional cushioning* (see Chapter 8 in this book), mentally and emotionally distancing themselves from the fetus/unborn baby in an effort to avoid feelings of grief and loss upon another potential miscarriage (Bowlby, 1969; Markin, 2018).

Deactivating Strategies

More avoidant individuals simultaneously deactivate their attachment need for closeness and relatedness and their affective experience. These deactivating strategies were first learned within early attachment relationships (Schore, 1994, 2002). These infants were often left alone in overwhelming and distressing situations for too long, crying for a long period of time before being picked up (Beebe & Lachmann, 2002). Even when trying to comfort their infants, these caregivers may have expressed disgust, frustration, or annoyance with physical touch and proximity (Main & Weston, 1982). These infants thus learned that proximity seeking does not facilitate soothing or modulate distress, but rather leads to further emotional hurt (Schore, 1994). Having one's attachment needs for closeness and comfort repeatedly rejected leads to a defensive process in which the infant turns off proximity-seeking behaviors and shifts attention away from attachment figures during distress, therefore reducing emotional rejection and shame (Marmarosh et al., 2013). These infants learn to be defensively independent and self-reliant (Sroufe et al., 1983) as a way of avoiding the painful experience of suffering alone in distress with no comfort. Consistent with this, as adults, avoidant clients are likely to be quite adept at dealing with the practical and medical aspects of RPL and infertility but struggle to cope with the associated feelings. For example, in the session vignette below, Joe would rather suffer in silence than disclose his feelings of vulnerability and distress to Marni and risk feeling alone, ashamed, and inadequate, as he once did as a child.

Because of their deactivating strategies, avoidant clients generally express a restricted range of affect in session and appear cut off from their emotional experience of RPL and infertility. They typically fail to show emotion, particularly sadness, where one would generally expect to find it. For example, they may talk about the details of their recurrent miscarriages in a detached and medical manner and deny mourning their recurrent losses, but show their feelings indirectly through their nonverbal behaviors, such as crossing arms, avoiding eye contact, or leaning away from the therapist. Avoidant clients are likely to answer the therapist's questions with brief, superficial, and idealized answers, avoiding real answers, experiences, and emotions (Marmarosh et al., 2013). In couples, avoidant individuals will often project feelings of distress onto their partner, and then devalue in their partner what they cannot own in the self. When the other partner has a more anxious attachment, the projections of the more avoidant partner have somewhere "to land," as anxious individuals function as a receptacle for distress. When Joe and Marni first entered treatment, Joe appeared unaffected by the couple's infertility struggles and instead asserted that Marni's emotionality was the problem that needed to be fixed. Yet, Marni was essentially "carrying" both her own and Joe's anxiety and feelings of sadness and loss. As Marni started to get better, Joe actually started to feel worse, because he was now forced to hold his fears, sense of shame, and feelings of grief.

Defenses

The deactivation that is typical of more avoidant individuals is maintained through defenses against both emotional experience and relatedness (Pando-Mars, 2016). *Defenses against emotion*, such as shutting down or disconnecting from oneself and others, help avoidant individuals to manage feeling affectively overwhelmed and serve to protect them from having to feel alone in their distress since they did not consciously experience their distress in the first place (Pando-Mars, 2016). Avoidant individuals often use defenses such as intellectualization and detachment to distance themselves and others from their emotional experience and often, for the same reason, use second-person language (Marmarosh et al., 2013). For example, when Joe was asked about his reaction to the diagnosis of male-factor infertility, he stated, "You can't take it too seriously. You just have to stay focused on the goal and keep trying." While Joe denied having an emotional reaction to the diagnosis of male-factor infertility, upon receiving the news, he escaped to his woodworking shed for days, not speaking to anyone. As seen here, avoidants' defenses against emotional experience make it difficult for them to work through feelings of grief and loss, for their feelings are avoided at all costs. Similarly, avoidant individuals rely on *defenses against relatedness* to protect themselves from feeling rejected, humiliated, disappointed, or intruded upon by close others (Fosha, 2000; Pando-Mars, 2016). They simultaneously defend against their attachment need for closeness as well as their emotional experience through dismissing their feelings and their need for comfort and support from others (Pando-Mars, 2016). Joe's escape to his woodworking shed served to distance himself and Marni from his feelings of distress, which, on one hand, protected him from feeling vulnerable and potentially humiliated or rejected, but, on the other hand, averted any chance of experiencing genuine relatedness or comfort and working through his feelings.

Box 9.2.

CHECKLIST FOR IDENTIFYING AVOIDANT CLIENTS AFFECTED BY RPL AND/OR INFERTILITY

☐ Client possesses IWMs of self as self-reliant and strong and of others as unavailable, rejecting, shaming, and disappointing. These clients may engage in defensive self-enhancement to cope with the shame brought about by pregnancy loss and infertility. They deny being affected by RPL and/or infertility and prefer to handle things on their own.
☐ Client's experience of pregnancies after loss is dominated by pervasive and severe emotional cushioning.
☐ Client uses deactivating strategies, or defenses against relatedness and emotional experience, to cope with feelings of grief and loss and with infertility distress. The client denies having any feelings related to past losses or to infertility and similarly denies needing the comfort and support of others. The client is quite adept at dealing with the practical, concrete, and medical aspects of infertility but cannot deal with the emotional aspects.
☐ Client appears cut off from her emotions when asked about adverse reproductive events. For example, the client tells her therapist about getting her tubes removed as if she were reciting a math equation.
☐ Client gives vague, brief, and superficial responses to questions about her experience of recurrent miscarriage and infertility.
☐ Client may deny feelings of sadness and loss but express feelings nonverbally by crossing arms, avoiding eye contact, or leaning away from the therapist.
☐ Client relies on intellectualization and detachment as primary defenses so talks about experiences with loss and/or infertility in a detached, vague, and o19al manner.

RELATIONAL GUIDANCE FOR AVOIDANT CLIENTS STRUGGLING WITH RPL AND INFERTILITY

Avoidant clients are likely to experience problems in the alliance (Diener & Monroe, 2011) and yet, from an attachment perspective, need the therapy

relationship to work through current sources of distress and gain greater attachment security, which has been linked to better treatment outcomes (Levy et al.,
2019). Thus, it is important for clinicians to identify these clients early on in treatment and to adjust their relational style to meet the client's attachment needs,
helping avoidant clients feel safer to tolerate and express vulnerable feelings of
distress in the presence of another. In particular, avoidant clients affected by RPL
and infertility often experience distress (Donerelli et al., 2016) on such an intense
level that their avoidant defenses can no longer keep feelings at bay. Although
this results in more distress in the short term, this breakdown in the avoidant's
defenses provides an ideal therapeutic opportunity to shift IWMs to more secure,
as the client has an experience in the therapy relationship in which the client does
not feel alone or humiliated when vulnerable as expected, but rather accepted
and comforted. To this aim, based on recommendations made by Pando-Mars
(2016) and Levy et al. (2019), when working with more avoidant clients, therapists
should adjust their relational style to (a) strike a balance, as to not overwhelm the
client, (b) be validating and accepting without intrusive, exploring the benefits
and the costs of the client's self-reliance, and (c) build affective and relational
capacities. Table 9.1 summarizes the relational guidance on therapist responsiveness to clients with more attachment anxiety or avoidance.

Table 9.1. SUMMARY OF GUIDELINES FOR THERAPIST RESPONSIVENESS
TO CLIENT ATTACHMENT

	Anxious	Avoidant
How should therapists adjust their relational style depending on client attachment?	• Avoid going too far in acting in contrast or in a complementary fashion to a client's more anxious attachment. • Act as a calm/non-reactive, focused, reflective, and emotionally soothing container that can withstand the client's emotional chaos. • Encourage genuine relatedness, not defensive clinginess.	• Strike a balance between being active but not too active. • Be validating and accepting without being intrusive. • Build affective and relational capacities through accepting and validating whatever feelings the client offers.
What kind of relational experience does the client need to come to experience the other (i.e., therapist and/or pattern/spouse) as a secure base?	• Client experiences the other as consistently available for support and understanding, and as someone who can help organize and soothe the client's distress, particularly chaotic and unprocessed affective experiences.	• Client has an experience in which it feels safe to share feelings and distress, and, once vulnerable, feels supported and understood, but not intruded upon.

Striking a Balance as to Not Overwhelm the Client

Practice and research suggest that therapists should titrate their interpersonal style as to not overwhelm more avoidant clients. These clients require the therapist to walk a thin line between being active but not too active, engaged but not too engaged, giving them space to feel in control, autonomous, and safe (Levy et al., 2019; Marmarosh et al., 2013). Levy et al. (2019) suggest that therapists should resist the understandable pull to play out a chase-and-dodge dynamic with avoidant clients, a sequence first observed among mothers and infants (Beebe & Lachman, 1988). In this, the avoidant client attempts to evade the therapist's questions about personal emotional experiences, and, in response, the therapist tries even harder to chase after and extract the client's emotions. In turn, this is experienced as intrusive by the avoidant client and causes the client to dodge the therapist even more. The chase-and-dodge dynamic often occurs when avoidant clients discuss their experiences of recurrent miscarriage with little expressed emotion, and, in response, the therapist chases after the client's grief and sadness. This often leads the client to dig in the client's heels and essentially say, "No, I am *not* sad about this" while the therapist covertly or overtly demands, "Yes, you are!" As the therapist becomes increasingly active and tries to extract the client's feelings of loss, the avoidant client feels intruded upon and becomes more withdrawn and dismissive. In the vignette below, Joe and Marni enact their own chase-and-dodge dynamic, as Marni "chases" after Joe to share her feelings of sadness and loss in an effort to bring them closer together and mitigate her attachment anxiety; in response, Joe feels overwhelmed and withdraws. Initially, the therapist unintentionally enacts the same dynamic with Joe by pursuing his feelings of grief and loss, despite nonverbal signals that he is feeling overwhelmed and embarrassed in the moment.

The Interaction of Client Avoidance and Therapist Attachment

The avoidant attachment style of the client is likely to interact with the attachment style of the therapist, with some therapists responding to client avoidance by becoming too active and others becoming too disengaged. Because avoidant clients act excessively self-reliant and tend to reject or belittle any support or genuine contact the therapist offers, more avoidant therapists might feel intimidated, humiliated, or rejected and then disengage and under-function (Pando-Mars, 2016). On the contrary, a more anxious therapist is more likely to hyperactivate, actively pursue, try to please, and become generally intrusive with avoidant clients to minimize emotional distance (Pando-Mars, 2016). Secure therapists may, on the other hand, respond to client avoidance with curiosity, despite their internal emotional reactions (Marmarosh et al., 2013). Regardless of therapist attachment style, most therapists, to varying degrees, feel as if their comments are dismissed, ignored, or belittled by avoidant clients and feel frustrated and ineffective as a result (Pando-Mars, 2016), causing some therapists to either disengage or under-function, as consistent with a more avoidant therapist, or actively pursue and over-function, as consistent with a more anxious therapist (Pando-Mars, 2016).

Be Validating and Accepting

When working with avoidant clients, the therapist must walk a thin line between being validating and accepting but not intrusive. Pando-Mars (2016) suggests that it is important for the therapist to accept what is given by the avoidant client without pushing for more. What seems like an insignificant self-disclosure to the therapist likely feels both exposing and risky to the avoidant client. In this spirit, therapists should remain open to processing feelings of trauma and loss associated with RPL and infertility, without demanding it. Instead of trying to break down the client's avoidant defenses to get to underlying feelings and vulnerabilities, the therapist should validate and respect the client's self-reliance, and all the successes and accomplishments that have come from the client's ability to be self-reliant and strong, while also exploring the costs (Levy et al., 2019; Marmarosh et al., 2013; Pando-Mars, 2016). Take, for example, a more avoidant client who dismisses any hint of sadness or loss associated with her multiple miscarriages of wanted pregnancies and instead focuses on the medical aspects of RPL. A therapist may respond,

> When you lost your mother as a child, you were the one who held your family together with your strength and resilience. You couldn't afford to break down because where would that have left you and your family? Now, through all these devastating miscarriages, gosh, if it wasn't for your strength, you and your partner would not have been able to make it through blow after blow trying to have a baby. Your self-reliance and strength have always been something you can count on to get you and others through tough times, and yet, I also wonder if it ever gets lonely or tiring always having to be so strong?

Build Affective and Relational Capacities

Although clients affected by RPL and infertility often enter therapy in a state of distress, those with an avoidant attachment are likely to have difficulty accepting the help that they need, and with acknowledging that they need help in the first place. Avoidant clients may instead express their distress as frustration or irritability with fertility doctors and with the medical field or science in general, perhaps calling the field of reproductive medicine "voodoo science" and describing fertility doctors as charlatans. They often see their "overly emotional" partner as the problem and deny having any feelings of distress themselves, except perhaps for anxiety and panic, which they possess little insight into and tend to attribute to some organic cause. Because they locate the source of their distress in external sources or people, it is difficult for the therapist to know how to help them or in what ways they need or want help, which often makes the therapist feel ineffective (Pando-Mars, 2016).

Underneath their defensiveness lies an attachment fear that if they were to let the therapist see how much they are struggling inside, then the therapist would see them as someone who needs help, which would make them feel weak and needy (Pando-Mars, 2016). While these kinds of avoidant strategies may typically "work" in other situations, the powerlessness to conceive a child engenders a unique kind of intense distress that triggers an individual's attachment need for support and comfort. Being in such intense distress, wherein one *needs* the support and comfort of others, touches upon the avoidant's core conflict, "If I let you see me, for sure you will later reject me and I would attack myself for being a fool and bringing on that pain. . . . In fact, I won't be vulnerable at all, for that is dangerous. . . . Better to hide behind my wall and suffer in silence" (Pando-Mars, 2016, pp. 41– 42). However, hiding behind one's walls and suffering in silence is not an effective long-term strategy because, once ignored, dismissed, or devalued, feelings of reproductive trauma and loss compound after each miscarriage, invasive medical procedure, and devastating setback to one's dream of becoming a parent.

To help avoidant clients feel safe enough to step out from behind their defensive wall and expose their vulnerability and distress, the therapist must help them notice what is *different* in the here and now of the therapeutic relationship as opposed to past attachment relationships (Fosha, 2000; Pando-Mars, 2016). Therapists must use extreme sensitivity to titrate their responses as to not overwhelm the client, giving the client the space to approach the therapist on the client's own terms. A therapy relationship in which the client's vulnerabilities are appreciated and accepted on the client's terms and in which the client's distress is validated and soothed, instead of shamed or dismissed, can provide a corrective attachment experience for avoidant clients. Through this kind of relationship, the avoidant client may learn that *having needs* need not be associated with *being needy* and weak (Pando-Mars, 2016). Avoidants build their affective and relational capacities as they learn through corrective attachment experiences with the therapist that it is safe to show their emotions to close others and to rely on them in times of distress, like RPL and infertility.

In couples therapy, avoidant partners similarly build their affective and relational capacities through daring to expose increasing amounts of vulnerability to their partner and feeling validated and accepted in return. This process is exemplified through an event that occurred *after* the couples session in the vignette below with Joe and Marni. Upon hearing the news from the fertility doctor that the couple is now officially out of options and will likely never conceive a biological child together, Joe withdrew to his woodshed as usual. Yet, Marni did not respond in her typical manner, pursuing and demanding Joe's vulnerability and closeness and criticizing his lack of availability and emotional expression. Instead, she joined him in the shed and sat next to him in silence, holding his hand but not looking at him, so as to not overwhelm or shame him. The space, kindness, and acceptance that Marni showed Joe in that moment began to crack his wall of self-reliance, as tears quietly rolled down his cheek. In the following session, the therapist used interventions to make explicit what felt different to Joe about this experience with Marni, as opposed to past attachment experiences. She asked, "What was it like for you for Marni to know your grief and to share your sadness? What allowed you to be vulnerable with her? How did this experience differ from past experiences?" Joe's attachment narrative began to change from a story in which seeking support and comfort from others leads to further emotional pain to one in which relying on others can feel comforting and healing.

Relational Guidance as Applied to Couples Therapy with an Avoidant Partner

The overarching therapeutic goal of couples therapy for RPL and infertility is to help both partners feel safe enough to share their feelings and distress with one another, and for them to have an experience in which, once shared, feelings and distress are understood, supported, and co-regulated, leading to a joint sense that the couple is in this difficult process together. Promoting a sense of safety and trust in the couple's relationship starts with the therapist establishing himself or herself as a reliable and trustworthy figure who can sensitively respond to the unique attachment needs of each partner. In couples with one anxious and another avoidant partner, the therapist is confronted with the challenge of responding to the more anxious partner with one relational style, while responding to the more avoidant partner with a completely different relational stance. Whereas the anxious partner requires the therapist's consistent support and understanding, emotional regulation, and soothing, the avoidant partner needs the therapist to be validating but not effusive, and to gently encourage affective expression without demanding it. What feels like support and care to the anxious partner will likely feel engulfing and intrusive to the avoidant partner, and the therapist must constantly adjust accordingly.

What does this process look like specifically for avoidant individuals who have an anxious partner? First, as the avoidant partner comes to internalize the therapist as a trustworthy and reliable figure who is sensitive to underlying attachment needs and fears, the client eventually feels safe enough to use the therapist as a secure base from which to try new ways of being and behaving in romantic relationships. From the secure base of the therapist, the avoidant client may risk, in tolerable doses, acknowledging and exposing personal distress and the need for support and comfort to the avoidant's partner. When the more anxious partner subsequently follows the therapist's example of validating whatever crumbs of vulnerability the more avoidant partner shares with patience and understanding, instead of further demands and criticisms, then the avoidant's attachment fears and expectations are challenged, leading to even greater relational safety and emotional risk-taking. While the anxious partner's every impulse is to give less space, not more, the anxious partner has now seen firsthand that when the therapist is patient and respects the avoidant partner's attachment need for autonomy, then the avoidant partner actually approaches rather than retreats. The combination of the anxious partner demanding or pursuing less, and the avoidant partner engaging more, automatically alters the demand–withdrawal pattern that these couples frequently find themselves stuck in. Altering this negative pattern of interaction puts the couple in a better position for processing grief and loss and infertility stress, together, for one partner is no longer demanding emotional support and engagement while the other avoids the experience of it altogether.

Lastly, like Marni, to truly change his attachment behaviors and expectations in current relationships, Joe had to first contend with his attachment "ghosts" from the past. Despite his overt defensive self-reliance, covertly, Joe found the experience of disconnection from Marni to be emotionally painful. On some level, he was terrified of exposing his needs and weaknesses to Marni and having her feel disgusted with and reject him the way his parents once did when he was a child. He withdrew in their relationship to prevent Marni from seeing how "defective" he really was and then rejecting him, just as his parents once rejected him for being a "defective" and "inadequate" child. Being diagnosed with male-factor infertility evoked experiences from Joe's childhood of feeling like something was fundamentally wrong with him that drives others away. Early on, he learned that it was best to hide his struggles, and perceived "deficiencies" and vulnerabilities, and to act strong to elicit closeness. In couples therapy, Joe had to grieve for his child-self, who was left alone, ashamed, and confused, in a state of extreme distress, before he could allow himself to experience Marni as someone who would be willing to support and comfort him, and himself as someone who was worthy of such love and care.

THERAPIST–COUPLE VIGNETTE

The vignette below is from the fourth session of couples counseling with Joe and Marni, who sought counseling with the goal of learning how to better communicate and cope with the stress of infertility. The couple has been in a constant state of conflict while trying to conceive for the past 3 years. Marni previously knew she would need ART to conceive due to a medical condition and experienced RPL before meeting Joe (see vignette in Chapter 8). However, they had both assumed Joe was fertile. Joe (47 years old) said he never had any intention of marrying or having children until he met Marni, who, he explained, drew him out of his "shell" with her outgoing personality. Marni (43 years old) had "given up" on romantic love when she first met Joe and, at the time, was focused on satisfying her need for closeness through becoming a mother. For both Joe and Marni, the other was an unexpected life surprise. Though Marni can be classified as having a more anxious attachment, she "earned" more attachment security through her work in an earlier individual therapy, as described in Chapter 8. Though she regresses when under stress toward greater attachment anxiety, she is also capable of insight, of emotion regulation, and of depicting the thoughts and feelings underlying her own behaviors and those of others, especially when these capacities are supported by the therapist. Joe, on the contrary, possesses a more avoidant attachment and has never undergone prior therapy. Below, the relational guidance offered in this chapter (see Table 9.1) is demonstrated throughout the hypothetical session dialogue that is based on an amalgamation of clinical experiences.

MARNI: I didn't think it was possible to get more bad news! Just when I think every single bad thing that could possibly happen to someone trying to have a baby has already happened to me, another one comes out of nowhere and smacks me in the face! What are we going to do? Tell me, Joe, tell me! He refuses to talk about this with me, and we need to decide what we are going to do next. I just can't believe this is happening. I can't eat, sleep, or work. This is all my fault; why didn't I insist we do these tests earlier? *[Marni's arms and legs start shaking and she is sobbing uncontrollably with her head in her hands, rocking back and forth.]*

THERAPIST: I can see how much distress you are in, Marni. Let's try and slow down together and look at these feelings. You are not alone in this. Start from the beginning. *[Therapist's non-reactive and soothing tone of voice helps focus and contain Marni's overwhelming and dysregulated emotions. "You are not alone in this" is an example of an intervention that likely feels comforting to an anxious client (satisfying her need for connection) but intrusive to an avoidant client. Here, the therapist sends the message that she will affectively join the client and can withstand her chaotic emotionality.]*

MARNI: *[In a relatively more calm and coherent voice]* This week our doctor told us that Joe is basically shooting blanks. That, combined with all my fertility issues, I feel like we are doomed. *[Marni's face turns red and she turns toward Joe and points her finger at him.]* I told you something like this was going to happen, but you wouldn't listen to me! If you had just listened to me and gotten these tests sooner, then we wouldn't have wasted all this time trying to get pregnant with your bad sperm! We could have started looking into sperm donation months ago! I told you I had a feeling something wasn't right, and you just dismissed me and made me feel crazy! *[Marni escalates her distress in an attempt to garner Joe's support and attention, yet she expresses her needs by demanding and criticizing Joe, which perpetuates his withdrawal.]*

THERAPIST: Marni, I wonder what you were feeling just now? It seemed as if a strong feeling came up for you right before you pointed your finger at Joe. *[Therapist encourages Marni to reflect on the feelings underlying her behaviors, with the goal of slowing her down and accessing more primary emotions.]*

MARNI: Angry, I'm so angry. He never listens to me. He's so dismissive.

THERAPIST: Right, right. So, this is really very important to you, that he listens to you and takes your feelings seriously *[Marni nods in agreement]*. I get the sense that you also had a feeling come up right before the anger, when you said, "I feel like we are doomed." *[The therapist tries to make order out of Marni's chaotic emotional experience by teasing apart emotions and better understanding them. The therapist is validating and empathic but stays focused on Marni's underlying feelings and attachment needs. The therapist emotionally containing and organizing Marni's emotional experience helps establish her as a secure base from which Marni can explore thoughts and feelings.]*

MARNI: I guess sad, just very sad. *[Tears well up and Marni seems to slow down.]*

THERAPIST: There is a lot of sadness there that has built up over time, layer on top of layer. *[Therapist holds and soothes the primary emotion of sadness and loss underneath the anger.]*

MARNI: Yes, exactly, so much. I've been through so many losses. I've lost so many babies. This just can't be how it ends. I finally meet someone and get married and I'm still alone with no baby to show for everything I've been through. It's like no matter what I do, everyone leaves me. This might sound strange, but when the doctor told us the results of the semen analysis, it felt like another miscarriage to me, and I started to fixate in my mind on every miscarriage I've ever had.

THERAPIST: It doesn't sound strange at all. Every loss adds another layer of grief, and there are so many layers now that you probably can't even tell them apart anymore, and you are left with an overwhelming amount of sadness. *[Therapist validates healthy feelings of grief.]* And, maybe to take it a step further, as you are grieving the loss of your babies, you are also feeling the loss of something in your relationship with Joe.

MARNI: Yes, yes, exactly. I feel like we aren't as close as we used to be. I try to talk to him about what he wants to do next, what's the plan, but he just tells me I need to relax, and I'm like, "I thought we were in this together, why are you pulling away?"

THERAPIST: These are really important and valid feelings of loss that we are talking about now. Why, I wonder, do these feelings of sadness and loss come out so quickly as anger toward Joe? *[Therapist encourages more genuine relatedness through the expression of core feelings of sadness and loss instead of defensive anger and criticism.]*

MARNI: I mean, Joe doesn't really do sadness, so maybe I'm afraid that if I show him those feelings, he will reject me and then I'll feel even more abandoned and alone than I already do. So I get kind of panicked and angry and I'm just trying to get his attention. He can be so distant. It's hard for me to know if he wants a baby as much as I do, if he wants a baby with *me*?

THERAPIST: What is your anger so afraid of?

MARNI: I just can't give up on having a baby, and I guess my anger is afraid Joe is going to give up on having a baby . . . and on me, like I'm just too much for him . . . *[Marni is now reflecting on her attachment needs and fears and on the feelings underlying her behaviors.]*

THERAPIST: What's your reaction to all this, Joe? I'm aware of how quiet you have been.

JOE: *[In a stoic tone of voice]* We are not considering sperm donation, there is nothing wrong with my swimmers. That doctor has always been jealous of me. He's a jerk. Marni, we are going to be fine. We just need to keep trying. Getting emotional is not going to change anything.

MARNI: *[Sighs and rolls eyes]* What is wrong with you? After everything I just said and shared, that is your response! You still aren't listening to me! Don't you care about me?

[A few moments of silence ensue as Marni anxiously awaits a response and Joe withdraws, looking down and away, avoiding eye contact.]

THERAPIST: Joe, I imagine you have some complicated feelings about the doctor's diagnosis and about the feedback Marni is giving you right now. You do appear unaffected on the outside, but I imagine you are really hurting on the inside. *[Like Marni, the therapist misses Joe's intense shame and subtly "chases" after his emotional expression.]*

JOE: Nope, I'm fine. She's the one that loses control of her emotions. *[Joe further withdraws in response to feeling intruded upon, criticized, and overwhelmed.]*

MARNI: I'm not a child, Joe.

THERAPIST: I'm wondering if what is happening in here right now (which maybe I just contributed to in a way) is what happens at home? Marni, when you feel Joe withdrawing, you seem to pursue him even more, mostly with anger that covers up all the sadness and loss you are holding inside. But I think you are just trying to get some sort of emotional reaction out of him, so you feel less alone. Joe, the more she pursues you, the more you seem to withdraw, which only makes Marni pursue you more intensely, and so forth. So, you both are trapped in this cycle that probably doesn't feel good to either of you. *[Therapist makes the negative cycle of interaction explicit.]*

MARNI: Definitely. Like after we got home from the clinic when the doctor told us about your test results, Joe, I wanted to cry with you, but you escaped out back to your woodshed, and I felt so abandoned. You left me all alone with all these feelings. *[Turning toward therapist]* I probably should have given Joe more space, but I followed him out back, and I know I was angry and yelling. I couldn't help it in the moment. I couldn't be alone with all this disappointment.

THERAPIST: So, there is something about feeling disconnected from Joe that is painful to you, but that kind of gets lost in your anger and pursuit of him.

MARNI: Yes, I'd say that's accurate, yes. I so badly want us to be close like we used to be before we started trying. Joe has never been the most affectionate guy, but we had fun together and I always knew he cared in his own way. I miss that.

THERAPIST: I hear a real pleading in there, a yearning, to pull him back toward you. Does that feel familiar? *[Exploring the connection between past and present attachment relationships]*

MARNI: When I was little, I was so lonely. It was just me and my mom, and I have memories of begging my mother to pick me up from boarding school, but she abandoned me there for yet another husband, who she ended up tossing aside when she got bored. As a child, I couldn't wrap my mind around how she could be so loving and attentive one minute and so cold and distant the next, so I would plead even harder to try and get her attention. Even though I'm 43 now, when it comes to my mother, I'm still that desperate and anxious kid. When I was trying to have a baby on my own, before I met Joe, I had repeated miscarriages. I was so devastated after each one. Even then, knowing that never in my entire life has she once shown up when *I* needed her, I sought her out for comfort. I was just so lonely and devastated and I needed my mother. I thought as a woman, as a mother, she could relate to me, but no, comforting me was too much of an imposition on her. And I became that kid again, anxious and desperate.

THERAPIST: That sounds so painful and like those experiences left behind this very tender unmet need for closeness and to feel like you can depend on someone to be there for you no matter what. So, I imagine when you feel Joe disappearing or withdrawing, it really strikes a nerve, because you don't know the next time he will "be back," so to speak. *[Therapist begins to identify how past attachment experiences are impacting the present romantic/attachment relationship and remains soothing, organizing, and reflective.]*

MARNI: Definitely. Through all the stress and the failures trying to get pregnant, I feel him slipping away from me, and it just makes me feel afraid and desperate. But whenever I try to talk to him about how I feel, he runs away to the woodshed, and I feel like that kid at boarding school all over again, begging him to come back to me. But he doesn't respond, and it drives me crazy.

THERAPIST: In some ways, you keep demanding of Joe what you have always wanted from your mother *[tears well up in Marni's eyes and she nods in agreement]*. On some level, you must have hope that he can respond to you in a different way than your mother and meet your needs.

MARNI: I have hope, but I just don't know why he shuts me out. What did I do wrong? Because you must hate me to just ignore me when I am hurting so badly.

JOE: I don't hate you, and I'm sorry, Marn, you didn't deserve that as a kid. We have established I'm not the best at feelings, but I would not abandon you like your mother, I just can't always be stressed out like you are about the fertility stuff and I need a break.

THERAPIST: I get the sense, Joe, that this is a new way of talking to Marni and that you are taking a risk right now. What is this like to hear, Marni? How do you feel toward Joe right now? *[Therapist begins to make explicit how this current attachment experience differs from past attachment experiences for both Marni and Joe, while accepting whatever "crumbs" of vulnerability Joe offers.]*

MARNI: I don't know. I'm kind of overwhelmed.

THERAPIST: That's understandable. Just try to slow down and focus on Joe and how you feel around him right now?

MARNI: I feel less alone *[sniffling]*. I haven't felt this way in a long time.

THERAPIST: I wonder, Joe, if you know the impact you have on Marni? I think feeling disconnected from you, Joe, is very painful for Marni, and I wonder if you know that? *[Therapist helps Joe depict Marni's thoughts and feelings and the impact that his withdrawal has on her.]*

JOE: No, how would I know that? She is always angry and yelling at me! I thought the last person she would want to see after we got home from the clinic that day was me, the guy with the "bad" sperm.

THERAPIST: For you, the fact that Marni wants to be close to you gets drowned out by the intensity of her anger and disappointment. *[Joe nods in agreement.]* It would even make sense to me if there was a part of you that feels unwanted and retreats in response. *[Therapist tries to be validating without intrusive, while beginning to identify underlying attachment injuries.]*

JOE: I'm always disappointing her, and sometimes I honestly don't know what she wants from me. I knew she was upset when we got home from the clinic, but there was nothing I could do to make it better. Whether I try to help or not, I always end up disappointing her.

THERAPIST: What is it like for you to disappoint Marni? *[Therapist expresses curiosity into Joe's thoughts and feelings, sending the message that others care about his internal experience.]*

JOE: It doesn't affect me because I know that's just how Marni is, you know, very emotional, but I was hoping she would learn some strategies in here to calm down. *[Joe finds the therapist's curiosity threatening and stops internal exploration by focusing on Marni.]*

MARNI: You tell people I'm too emotional, but maybe you aren't emotional enough.

JOE: It's not going to help us get pregnant if I get emotional too. There is no point in that. You are worried and depressed enough for the both of us right now. I learned a long time ago that you can't let life get you down. No matter what life throws you, you just keep on going.

THERAPIST: You know, I think Marni would maybe agree that, despite anything else going on right now, she can always count on you to be a pillar of strength in times of crisis, and, at times, that is probably a great comfort and source of strength for you, Marni *[Marni nods her head in agreement]*. But, for some reason, which maybe is confusing to you, Joe, I think it feels like she doesn't appreciate the strength you are offering her, and like nothing you do is good enough.

JOE: Yes, exactly.

THERAPIST: On the other hand, to you, Marni, I think, and correct me if I'm off here, the strength Joe is offering you right now feels unempathic because you aren't looking for strength, you are looking for his emotional vulnerability *[Marni nods]*. *[The therapist validates Joe, pointing out the benefits of Joe's "strength," while exploring the possible costs.]*

JOE: I'm just not an emotional person like Marni is. I don't always know how to give her what she wants when it comes to that. I seemed to have said something before that you both liked, but I honestly don't quite understand what I did or why it helped.

THERAPIST: Marni, what if you take Joe at face value and believe him that he honestly doesn't always know how to give you the emotional response you are seeking from him. Can you help him out and be more specific about what you want from him?

MARNI: Well, to start, maybe you could share with me what you were thinking and feeling when you disappeared to your woodshed that day after the semen analysis came back?

JOE: Why don't you tell me what I should say so we can skip the fight?

THERAPIST: Let's put a pause on this for a moment. Do you believe her, Joe, that she really wants to know how you're feeling, that she cares enough to want to know?

JOE: No, I guess I don't. I think she's angry at me and wants to put me in my place as the inadequate husband who can't get her pregnant.

THERAPIST: It feels like Marni asked you to talk about your feelings not because she genuinely wants to understand or comfort you, but because she wants to humiliate you? *[Joe nods his head in agreement.]* No wonder you withdraw to your woodshed if you feel that way; I would too! *[Therapist is validating and accepting.]*

JOE: Sometimes maybe I do hide out back because no matter what I do, I can never actually seem to give Marni what she wants.

THERAPIST: Like a baby?

JOE: *[nods, and a spark of emotion seems to come across his face]*

THERAPIST: I want to give you your space, but I also want to acknowledge that you seem to have some feelings right now. So, this is me asking from outside your shed, knowing that I won't come in unless you invite me: What's going through your mind right now? *[Therapist works to strike a balance between emotionally joining with Joe and overwhelming him.]*

JOE: *[Looking at Marni]* I thought about coming out, Marni and finding you, but I couldn't; maybe that makes me weak. I didn't want to see that look of disgust on your face.

THERAPIST: What does that look of disgust bring up for you?

JOE: I think of it like kryptonite. Like I get anywhere near that look and all my superpowers melt away, and I become nothing more than a fragile mortal.

THERAPIST: That's very powerful. In a sense, withdrawing to your woodshed is a way of protecting yourself from feeling hurt and weakened to the point of feeling destroyed.

JOE: Marni's look of disgust could put bullets through a man, and I'm no softy. I guess I go to the woodshed to avoid saying the wrong thing, disappointing her, and getting that look.

THERAPIST: So, you would rather not say anything at all than risk saying the wrong thing and disappointing Marni and seeing that look of disgust on her face.

JOE: I want her to see me as a man. I feel like all she sees when she looks at me now is an empty sperm bank with nothing to offer her.

THERAPIST: What would it be like to turn to Marni right now and tell her how you feel? *[Therapist builds Joe's affective and relational capacities by facilitating a secure attachment experience in which Joe can safely share his feelings with Marni and feel validated by her.]*

JOE: Marni doesn't want to hear me cry and moan with everything she's dealing with.

THERAPIST: Is that true, Marni?

MARNI: I've never heard you talk like this before, Joe. I had no idea you felt this way. I thought you were rejecting me. It never occurred to me that you hide out back because you are afraid of me rejecting you. I want to hear you cry and moan! I do it all the time!

THERAPIST: Joe, is it hard to imagine a scenario where you feel comforted by sharing your feelings with Marni? Is that something that doesn't feel possible or familiar to you? *[Therapist explores the connection between past and present attachment experiences.]*

JOE: I can't imagine that. I think she would just tell me more about how we need to go to some other guy for sperm and then get mad at me for not being more excited about it. Either way, I'm out in the cold, in the doghouse or the woodshed.

MARNI: Joe, I don't want you to think I'm disgusted with you. I get angry when I feel abandoned, but you are the only person I want right now. I'm just scared.

JOE: I wish I knew how to give you what you wanted, Marni. You know me, I'm not good at the touchy-feely stuff. You want help with injections, a ride to the clinic, financial support, 'cause having a baby isn't cheap, I'm your guy.

THERAPIST: You said earlier, Joe, that you can't imagine sharing feelings with one another and something good coming from that. Marni talked about her experiences growing up; I wonder what it was like for you when you were younger? Who did you go to when upset or hurt? I know you are very self-reliant now, but as a kid, I imagine you sometimes needed an adult.

JOE: Not really, I've been self-reliant since I was 8. I learned not to rely on others for anything. I did it all myself.

THERAPIST: You sound like a very resourceful and resilient kid. What happened at 8? *[Therapist validates Joe's self-reliance.]*

JOE: I guess that's when I was diagnosed with dyslexia and a host of other learning disabilities you probably don't want to know about. I learned life throws you curveballs and you just gotta deal with tough situations on your own, no one is going to give you a handout.

THERAPIST: How did you learn that at such a young age?

JOE: From my parents. When I was diagnosed, the school started in with "Oh, he needs such-and-such accommodations," and my parents said, "No, you have to man up and work harder and do this on your own, or you will always be at the mercy of other people to help you in life." They were like,

"You can be lazy and labeled 'slow' all your life or work harder and prove them wrong." I learned to do it on my own. I owe my parents a lot, they made me strong. That's why I don't feel the same way about the fertility stuff as Marni. To me, anyone offering you help has an agenda. The doctor is going to suggest sperm donation, IVF, expensive drugs, because there is a financial incentive in that for him. We gotta keep trying, and we can do this on our own.

MARNI: Joe hates when I say bad things about his parents, but that story is awful. How could they not have helped you as a child? Children with learning disabilities need support, not a lecture on "manning up." Your mother is one of the coldest people I have ever met, and she just can't tolerate anyone being vulnerable about anything. She was over at our house once when I got my period. She saw me crying and I guess Joe told her why, and she actually came up to me and told me that me being so emotional was the reason we can't get pregnant.

JOE: She doesn't mean any harm. She just doesn't want people to waste time being upset about things they can't change. She helped me become strong and independent and today I have a very successful business despite not finishing school.

THERAPIST: Now you are strong and successful, and I see how you have done that on your own with hard work and perseverance, and that's commendable, but what about then? Do you have any memories of what it was like for that 8-year-old at the time? *[Therapist strikes a balance between validating Joe's self-reliance and exploring possible costs.]*

JOE: I do remember going to my parents after some stupid kids at school were picking on me for not being able to read. I asked my parents to put me in the special class that the school kept pushing for. They told me to stand up to those bullies or they would see I was an easy target. I remember my dad telling me, "Son, you can't whine and complain all the time. Don't ask for help because no one is going to give it out for free in life."

THERAPIST: So, it wasn't really OK for that 8-year-old to need help or to be vulnerable?

JOE: You could put it that way, but another way to put it is that they were teaching me to be independent and strong.

MARNI: Your parents think anyone who needs help is lazy and weak and a fool for asking.

JOE: That's the way the world works; people will take advantage of you if you let them.

THERAPIST: For you, in your world, all you have ever known is that asking for help, *needing* help or support, is like kryptonite that other people can use against you.

JOE: Yup, that's what I tell Marni, you can't let them see you cry.

THERAPIST: And do you happen to remember the look on your mother's face when you asked her for help in school?

JOE: *[Becomes emotional, seems to be fighting back tears]* She looked disgusted.

THERAPIST: How does that 8-year-old little boy feel in response, looking at the disgust on his mother's face, but needing her help and support? Can you visualize it in your mind?

JOE: He's a wuss and a coward and he is scared and humiliated, he, I, didn't understand why she hated me so much. I just wanted to please her but never could—everything I did was wrong. I remember once she asked, "Why can't you just read like the other kids your age," and I felt like she punched me. I barricaded myself in my room for days trying to teach myself how to read, but I couldn't, the letters would get all mixed up, and I hated myself. I was a stupid kid.

THERAPIST: Marni, you seem to be really in there with Joe right now. Is there something you want to say to that 8-year-old boy who is barricaded in his room, afraid to see the look of contempt on his mother's face? [Therapist tries to establish Marni as a secure attachment figure who will validate and accept Joe's need for comfort and support, not humiliate or criticize it.]

MARNI: Yes, I'd want to give him a hug and tell him there is nothing wrong with him.

JOE: How can you say that? You have that same look of disgust every month when you get your period, like I let you down again, and when the semen analysis came back it was like confirmation that you have every right to despise me for being inadequate.

MARNI: I am so sorry I ever made you feel that way. And I'm sorry if I made you feel like you couldn't come and tell me this earlier. Look, you married me knowing that I had fertility issues. If you are inadequate or defective, then so am I. I don't care about any of that, Joe. Like I said, I just want to feel like we are in this together. I don't look down on you because of the fertility issues, but I know what that's like because for a long time I looked down on myself for not being able to have a healthy pregnancy, and I still do.

THERAPIST: Do you believe her, Joe? What's your reaction to what Marni is saying?

JOE: I don't know. I don't know what to think.

THERAPIST: Does that 8-year-old boy believe her?

JOE: He's needy and desperate to believe anyone who throws him a bone?

THERAPIST: Marni, do you see him as needy and desperate?

MARNI: No, not at all. He's such a strong little boy for going through all of that alone, but he shouldn't have had to. Needing help is not a crime and it wasn't his, your, fault, Joe.

JOE: [almost in a whisper] . . . and if I do have bad swimmers, Marni, what then?

MARNI: Then we deal with that like we have always done.

THERAPIST: What is your fear, Joe?

JOE: I don't know, I just picture that look of disgust permanently implanted on her face.

THERAPIST: Can you look at Marni now? What do you see on her face?

JOE: I don't know, but she doesn't seem angry. Maybe pity, which is worse.

MARNI: It's not pity, it's concern!

THERAPIST: Look again, Joe, really look at her and try to take her in. What do you see or feel from her right now? *[Therapist tries to separate past from present attachment experiences and build Joe's relational capacities by making explicit what feels different in this relationship.]*

JOE: It's like the opposite of the disgusted/angry look she usually gives me; it's almost like she likes me *[the two smile]*.

THERAPIST: What we are talking about now feels so important. You both have been under such intense stress so need each other right now, which has maybe brought up past experiences for the both of you, in different ways, of not feeling like you could turn to someone for support and comfort. But, in this relationship, I think the question is, Marni, what can you do to help Joe feel less afraid that if he comes out of his woodshed, you will humiliate or scold him, and Joe, what can you do to reassure Marni that she doesn't need to get angry or work so hard to pursue you for you to be emotionally present when she needs you?

CLINICAL CHALLENGES TO THERAPIST RESPONSIVENESS TO CLIENT ATTACHMENT

Therapists who are more insecurely attached may get pulled into the client's insecure attachment dynamics, reacting in an extreme complementary or noncomplementary manner to the client's attachment style. Clients with an insecure attachment often engage in interpersonal and nonverbal behaviors that elicit strong reactions from others, and therapists are no exception to this. Therapist self-awareness and personal therapy or supervision are all key to managing this situation. Therapists, beginning in graduate training programs, need training on how to identify attachment dynamics in the therapy relationship and on how to manage their countertransference reactions. In therapy for RPL and infertility in particular, clients and therapists alike can often be pulled into focusing on the latest fertility setback or crisis, rather than on the attachment needs and fears that these experiences activate.

CLINICAL IMPLICATIONS

- Therapists should assess client attachment style from the beginning of treatment and adjust their relational style and approach to meet the attachment needs of the client.
- Pregnancy loss and infertility, and the experience of not feeling supported and understood during these stressful life events, open the door to past feelings and experiences related to not feeling supported

and understood during earlier instances of separation distress or traumatic loss. Psychotherapy for pregnancy loss and infertility can help clients grieve current and past losses by giving them a different and more secure attachment relationship in which feelings of distress related to separation and loss are validated, understood, and co-regulated.

10

Where Do We Go From Here?

Future Research Directions, Training Recommendations, and Practice Implications

The field of reproductive trauma is a relatively new and understudied area that psychotherapy researchers, clinicians, and trainers should all work together to better understand and treat. Pregnancy loss represents one form of reproductive trauma that commonly occurs within the context of other reproductive traumas, such as invasive medical procedures and fertility struggles. As reviewed in Chapter 2, although past studies lend insight into the symptoms commonly associated with pregnancy loss, particularly anxiety, depression, and PTSD, very little research has been conducted on how to treat individuals, couples, and families suffering from the effects of pregnancy loss, particularly the underlying psychological wounds inflicted by such losses (Diamond & Diamond, 2016). Current research typically focuses on treating symptoms associated with pregnancy loss in the short term; however, some clients, particularly those experiencing RPL, stillbirth, termination due to fetal anomaly, pregnancy after loss, and/or infertility (Herbert et al., 2022), may need psychotherapy treatments that address the effects of pregnancy loss in the long term and/or that go beyond observable symptoms to underlying feelings of trauma and loss that impact a person's sense of self and identity. Essentially, as others have similarly argued (Jaffe & Diamond, 2011; Leon, 2010, 2015), in this book, pregnancy loss has been conceptualized as a traumatic loss that can damage a bereaved parent's healthy self-esteem and sense of self. Furthermore, the psychotherapy relationship has been put forth as a vehicle for processing feelings of trauma and loss and restoring the client's sense of self and identity. From this theoretical framework, below, future directions and recommendations for research, training, and practice are suggested.

Psychotherapy for Pregnancy Loss. Rayna D. Markin, Oxford University Press. © Oxford University Press 2024.
DOI: 10.1093/oso/9780197693353.003.0010

FUTURE RESEARCH DIRECTIONS

- More research is needed to identify women at risk for chronic and severe grief and/or post-traumatic stress reactions after pregnancy loss and in most need of psychotherapy. The author suggests avoiding labels such as "pathological" or "complicated" grief and instead qualitatively describing various grief reactions, which have been known to vary after pregnancy loss (e.g., Lin & Lasker, 1996). Future research can explore the psychotherapy needs associated with different grief reactions following pregnancy loss.
- Pregnancy loss does not happen in a vacuum. Research shows that such losses impact mothers, fathers/partners, and siblings (see Diamond & Diamond, 2016, for a review). More research is needed on couples and family therapies for such losses.
- More research is needed on what treatments are effective for whom. Different treatments may be more or less effective for different bereaved parents/clients, depending on a number of client factors including attachment style, therapy preferences, cultural factors, stage of grief, stage of readiness for change, type and timing of loss, and trauma history. This is consistent with Norcross and Wampold's (2019) idea of *psychotherapy responsiveness*, or the need to adapt or fit psychotherapy to the individual client.
- Future research should explore which clients are likely to benefit from short-term supportive therapy after pregnancy loss and which clients are likely in need of relatively longer-term treatments after loss. Relatedly, future research should examine whether certain evidence-based relationship components have a larger effect on outcome in short-term versus long-term treatments for pregnancy loss. For instance, in short-term therapy for uncomplicated grief, empathy and validation may have the strongest effect on outcome, whereas in long-term treatment for complicated grief, attachment may have a stronger association with outcome.
- We need research on *why* treatments are found to be effective. In particular, future studies should examine the relation between various evidence-based relationship components (e.g., countertransference management, alliance, empathy) and the process and outcome of psychotherapy for pregnancy loss. Exploring how a relational element or component is expressed and utilized to promote positive outcomes in psychotherapy for pregnancy loss across different theoretical orientations is an interesting future area of research.
- Future research needs to go beyond whether or not more of some relationship element predicts less of some set of symptoms, to explore how a relational element is built, maintained, and utilized to the benefit of the treatment over time.
- Psychotherapy outcome should be assessed from a multifaceted perspective and include not only measures of depression and anxiety but

also measures of traumatic stress, unresolved trauma, perinatal grief, and self-esteem. Studies should examine not only the reduction of something that feels "bad" (i.e., grief, anxiety, and depression) but also the increase in something that feels "good" (i.e., constructing a sense of personal meaning from the tragedy of loss and/or gaining greater attachment security) (Markin, 2017).

- Relationship elements occur in context of one another and should not be treated as unrelated and distinct elements in research. Studies should assess multiple process/relationship variables (e.g., emotional expression, countertransference management, attachment) that predict multiple outcomes (e.g., post-traumatic growth, depression and anxiety, post-traumatic stress, quality of marital/partner relationship), and use standardized measures and control groups whenever possible (Markin, 2017).

- More research is needed on how psychotherapy relationships and techniques should be adjusted based on client culture in psychotherapy for pregnancy loss. In general, we need more research on culturally sensitive psychotherapy treatments for perinatal loss that focus on building trust and safety in the therapy relationship and empowering the client. For example, future research on culturally sensitive interventions for Black women suffering from pregnancy loss is needed, given that these women, as a cohort, are at increased risk of experiencing such losses (Mukherjee et al., 2013).

- Future research should investigate culturally sensitive psychotherapy treatments and relationships with LGBTQ+ clients experiencing pregnancy loss and/or fertility issues. Because these clients often experience double disenfranchisement in the context of pregnancy loss, empathy and validation may be particularly important to outcome and therapists may need to express empathy and validation in specific ways. Future research should also pay attention to the therapy needs of patients who identify as transgender and experience pregnancy loss, and to specific considerations to building an alliance.

- Future research should investigate the role of clients' diverse religious beliefs in their adjustment following perinatal loss. Pregnancy and pregnancy loss often carry religious meaning for clients and therapists alike. Understanding the religious context and significance around a pregnancy loss may be important for therapists to establish good alliances and empathy with clients. Further, special countertransference management considerations may be needed when the therapist is of a different religious background than the client. Differing religious attitudes between the therapist and client, and the impact that these divergent attitudes or beliefs have on the relationship, may be particularly important to pay attention to in cases of fetal terminations due to a genetic anomaly.

TRAINING RECOMMENDATIONS

- Graduate programs should teach students evidence-based relationship principles in conjunction with evidence-based treatments (Norcross & Lambert, 2019), and, furthermore, should train students on how to cultivate, maintain, and utilize various evidence-based relationship principles in psychotherapy with specific client populations, such as parents and families grieving a pregnancy loss. In particular, helping trainees identify and manage countertransference reactions to pregnancy loss seems critical to facilitating other important relational components like empathy and the repair of ruptures.
- Given the sheer number of women impacted by pregnancy loss and other reproductive traumas that often occur in conjunction with pregnancy loss, and who experience complicated grief reactions (Saraiya et al., 1999), graduate programs should offer trainees specific training in the psychological experience and consequences of pregnancy loss and how to treat the effects of such losses. Research, theory, and clinical practice suggest that we cannot adequately prepare psychotherapists to treat pregnancy loss clients without sufficient training in the kind of relationship that these clients need in order to mourn, process feelings of trauma and loss, and restore healthy self-esteem.

PRACTICE IMPLICATIONS

- Clinicians should regularly assess for client history of pregnancy loss and other reproductive traumas. From the start of therapy with affected clients, clinicians should focus more on empathy and building a safe and trusting alliance than a formal intake (Diamond & Diamond, 2016).
- Clinicians should apply empirically based relationship principles to therapy for pregnancy loss and continually assess the client's perspective of the relationship.
- With clients affected by pregnancy loss, clinical practice should move beyond exclusively focusing on symptom reduction to building a safe and trusting therapy relationship in which clients can mourn and process the trauma and grief associated with pregnancy loss and in which therapist empathy and validation helps to rebuild client self-esteem. Further, for clients with an insecure attachment, treatment should work toward rewiring insecure internal working models to more secure through giving the client an experience in which feelings of sadness and loss are understood, emotionally contained, and co-regulated.

Table A.1. Easy-to-Administer and Easy-to-Score Measures of Important Relationship Components That Can Be Used in Clinical Practice

Relationship Construct	Measure	Rater	Description
Working alliance	Working Alliance Inventory (WAI; Horvath & Greenberg, 1989)	Client and/or therapist	Based on Bordin's (1975) pan-theoretical tripartite model of the alliance; assesses agreement on goals, tasks, and the bond dimension of the alliance
Couple's working alliance	Working Alliance Inventory—Couples (WAI-CO; Symonds, 1999)	Each partner/client and/or therapist	Adapted from the WAI, based on Bordin's (1975) tripartite model of the alliance; includes separate scales for client, partner, and couple. Client form asks for perceptions of alliance between therapist and (a) respondent, (b) respondent's partner, and (c) couple as a unit. Therapist form asks for perceptions of the alliance with each partner and with the couple as a unit. Can be used to assess for a split alliance (see Friedlander et al., 2019, for full description)
Empathy	Barrett-Lennard Relationship Inventory; Other to Self version (Barrett-Lennard, 1981)	Client	Consists of four subscales: level of regard (R), empathic understanding (E), congruence (C), and unconditionality of regard (U)
Emotional awareness	The Toronto Alexithymia Scale (Bagby et al., 1994)	Client	Self-report measure of emotional awareness that assesses clients' inability to accurately label and identify their emotions
Perinatal grief	Perinatal Grief Scale (Toedter et al., 2001)	Client	Multidimensional measure of grief after perinatal loss, with subscales for Active Grief (PGS-AG; crying, sadness, and missing the baby); Difficulty Coping (PGS-DC; difficulty performing usual activities and relating to others); Despair (PGS-D; feelings of hopelessness and worthlessness)

(continued)

Relationship Construct	Measure	Rater	Description
Alliance rupture-repair events	*Post-Session Questionnaire* (Muran et al., 1992)	Client and/or therapist	Popular self-report measure that asks participants to rate the occurrence and intensity of rupture and resolution moments across several single-items on a 5-point scale, ranging from *not at all* to *very much* (see Eubanks et al., 2018, for the specific items)
Countertransference management	*Countertransference Factor Inventory* (CFI; Van Wagoner et al., 1991)	Supervisor	This measure consists of five factors of therapist qualities theorized to facilitate countertransference management, as described by Hayes et al. (2019): (1) *self-insight*, or the extent to which therapists are aware of their own feelings, including countertransference feelings, and understand their basis, (2) *conceptualizing ability*, or the therapist's ability to draw on theory in the work and grasp the client's dynamics in terms of the therapeutic relationship, (3) *empathy*, or the ability to partially identify with and put oneself in the other's shoes, (4) *self-integration*, or the therapist's possession of an intact basically healthy character structure, including a recognition of interpersonal boundaries and ability to differentiate self from other, and (5) *anxiety management*, or therapists allowing themselves to experience anxiety and possessing the internal skills needed to control and understand this anxiety.
Attachment style in close relationships	*Experiences in Close Relationship Scale—Revised* (ECR-R; Fraley et al., 2000; also see Brennan et al., 1998)	Client	A 36-item measure of adult attachment style. The ECR-R measures individuals on two subscales of attachment: Avoidance and Anxiety. Avoidant individuals find discomfort with intimacy and seek independence, whereas Anxious individuals tend to fear rejection and abandonment.

| Client attachment to therapist | *Client Attachment to Therapist Scale* (CATS; Mallinckrodt et al., 1995) | Client | A 36-item self-report measure developed to assess clients' perceptions of the client–therapist relationship from the perspective of attachment theory. The scale consisted of three dimensions: (1) *secure attachment* (clients feel encouraged to explore frightening or troubling material in therapy and experience the therapist as responsive, sensitive, emotionally available, and a comforting presence), (2) *avoidant-fearful attachment* (clients suspect that the therapist is disapproving and likely to be rejecting if displeased, are reluctant to make personal disclosures, and feel threatened or humiliated in the sessions), and (3) *preoccupied-merger attachment* (clients long for more contact and to be "at one" with the therapist, wish to expand the relationship beyond the bounds of therapy, and are preoccupied with the therapist and the therapist's other clients). |

For more information on scoring of these measures, please see the citations included in the table.

REFERENCES

Ackerman, S. J., & Hilsenroth, M. J. (2001). A review of therapist characteristics and techniques negatively impacting the therapeutic alliance. *Psychotherapy: Theory, Research, Practice, Training, 38*(2), 171–185. https://doi.org/10.1037/0033-3204.38.2.171

Ackerman, S. J., & Hilsenroth, M. J. (2003). A review of therapist characteristics and techniques positively impacting the therapeutic alliance. *Clinical Psychology Review, 23*(1), 1–33. https://doi.org/10.1016/S0272-7358(02)00146-0

Adolfsson, A. (2011). Meta-analysis to obtain a scale of psychological reaction after perinatal loss: Focus on miscarriage. *Psychology Research and Behavior Management, 2011*(4), 29–39. https://doi.org/10.2147/prbm.s17330

Ainsworth, M. D. S., Blehar, M. C., Waters, E., & Wall, S. (1978). *Patterns of attachment: A psychological study of the strange situation.* Lawrence Erlbaum.

Ainsworth, M. D. S., & Eichberg, C. (1991). Effects on infant–mother attachment of mother's unresolved loss of an attachment figure, or other traumatic experience. In C. M. Parkes, J. Stevenson-Hinde, & P. Marris (Eds.), *Attachment across the life cycle* (pp. 160–183). London: Routledge.

American College of Obstetricians and Gynecologists. (2022). Abortion care: Resources and glossary. https://www.acog.org/womens-health/faqs/induced-abortion

American Society for Reproductive Medicine. (2012). Evaluation and treatment of recurrent pregnancy loss: A committee opinion. *Fertility and Sterility, 98*(5), 1103–1111.

Amir, N., Stafford, J., Freshman, M. S., & Foa, E. B. (1998). Relationship between trauma narratives and trauma pathology. *Journal of Traumatic Stress, 11*(2), 358–392. https://doi.org/10.1023/A:1024415523495

Ammaniti, M. (1991). Maternal representations during pregnancy and early infant-mother interactions. *Infant Mental Health Journal, 12*(3), 246–255. https://doi.org/10.1002/1097-0355(199123)12:3<246::AID IMHJ2280120310>3.0.CO;2-8

Ammon Avalos, L., Galindo, C., & Li, D.-K. (2012). A systematic review to calculate background miscarriage rates using life table analysis. *Birth Defects Research Part A: Clinical and Molecular Teratology, 94*(6), 417–423. https://doi.org/10.1002/bdra.23014

Anchin, J. C., & Kiesler, D. J. (Eds.). (1982). *Handbook of interpersonal psychotherapy.* Pergamon Press.

Anker, M. G., Owen, J., Duncan, B. L., & Sparks, J. A. (2010). The alliance in couple therapy: Partner influence, early change, and alliance patterns in a naturalistic sample. *Journal of Consulting and Clinical Psychology, 78*(5), 635–645. https://doi.org/10.1037/a0020051

Armstrong, D. S., Hutti, M. H., & Myers, J. (2009). The influence of prior perinatal loss on parents' psychological distress after the birth of a subsequent healthy infant. *Journal of Obstetric, Gynecologic & Neonatal Nursing, 38*(6), 654–666. https://doi.org/10.1111/j.1552-6909.2009.01069.x

Atkinson, L., & Zucker, K. J. (Eds.). (1997). Attachment and psychopathology: From laboratory to clinic. In L. Atkinson & K. Zucker (Eds.), *Attachment and psychopathology* (pp. 3–16). Guilford Press.

Bagby, R. M., Taylor, G. J., & Parker, J. D. A. (1994). The twenty-item Toronto Alexithymia Scale: II. Convergent, discriminant, and concurrent validity. *Journal of Psychosomatic Research, 38*(1), 33–40. https://doi.org/10.1016/0022-3999(94)90006-X

Bandura, A., Lipsher, D. H., & Miller, P. E. (1960). Psychotherapists' approach-avoidance reactions to patients' expressions of hostility. *Journal of Consulting Psychology, 24*(1), 1–8. https://doi.org/10.1037/h0043403

Barrett-Lennard, G. T. (1981). The empathy cycle: Refinement of a nuclear concept. *Journal of Counseling Psychology, 28*(2), 91–100. https://doi.org/10.1037/0022-0167.28.2.91

Bartholomew, K., & Horowitz, L. M. (1991). Attachment styles among young adults: A test of a four-category model. *Journal of Personality and Social Psychology, 61*(2), 226–244. https://doi.org/10.1037//0022-3514.61.2.226

Bayley, T. M., Slade, P., & Lashen, H. (2009). Relationships between attachment, appraisal, coping and adjustment in men and women experiencing infertility concerns. *Human Reproduction, 24*(11), 2827–2837. https://doi.org/10.1093/humrep/dep235

Bayrampour, H., Ali, E., McNeil, D. A., Benzies, K., MacQueen, G., & Tough, S. (2016). Pregnancy-related anxiety: A concept analysis. *International Journal of Nursing Studies, 55*, 115–130. https://doi.org/10.1016/j.ijnurstu.2015.10.023

Beaudreau, S. A. (2007). Are trauma narratives unique and do they predict psychological adjustment? *Journal of Traumatic Stress, 20*(3), 353–357. https://doi.org/10.1002/jts.20206

Beck, J. S. (2011). *Cognitive behavior therapy: Basics and beyond* (2nd ed.). Guilford Press.

Beebe, B., & Lachmann, F. M. (1988). The contribution of mother-infant mutual influence to the origins of self- and object representations. *Psychoanalytic Psychology, 5*(4), 305–337. https://doi.org/10.1037/0736-9735.5.4.305

Beebe, B., & Lachmann, F. (2002). *Infant research and adult treatment: Co-constructing interactions.* Analytic Press.

Beebe, B., & Lachmann, F. (2013). *Infant research and adult treatment: Co-constructing interactions.* Routledge. https://doi.org/10.4324/9780203767498

Bennett, S. M., Litz, B. T., Maguen, S., & Ehrenreich, J. T. (2008). An exploratory study of the psychological impact and clinical care of perinatal loss. *Journal of Loss and Trauma, 13*(6), 485–510. https://doi.org/10.1080/15325020802171268

Benoit, D., Parker, K. C. H., & Zeanah, C. H. (1997). Mothers' representations of their infants assessed prenatally: Stability and association with infants' attachment classifications. *Child Psychology & Psychiatry & Allied Disciplines, 38*(3), 307–313. https://doi.org/10.1111/j.1469-7610.1997.tb01515.x

Berant, E., & Obegi, J. H. (2009). Attachment-informed psychotherapy research with adults. In J. H. Obegi & E. Berant (Eds.), *Attachment theory and research in clinical work with adults* (pp. 461–469). Guilford Press.

Bernecker, S. L., Levy, K. N., & Ellison, W. D. (2014). A meta-analysis of the relation between patient adult attachment style and the working alliance. *Psychotherapy Research, 24*, 12–24. https://doi.org/10.1080/10503307.2013.809561

Betchen, S. (2005). *Intrusive partners, elusive mates: The pursuer-distancer dynamic in couples.* Routledge.

Beutel, M., Deckardt, R., von Rad, M., & Weiner, H. (1995). Grief and depression after miscarriage: Their separation, antecedents, and course. *Psychosomatic Medicine, 57*(6), 517–526.

Beutler, L. E., Clarkin, J. F., & Bongar, B. (2000). *Guidelines for the systematic treatment of the depressed patient.* Oxford University Press. https://doi.org/10.1093/acprof:oso/9780195105308.001.0001

Black, S., Hardy, G., Turpin, G., & Parry, G. (2005). Self-reported attachment styles and therapeutic orientation of therapists and their relationship with reported general alliance quality and problems in therapy. *Psychology and Psychotherapy: Theory, Research and Practice, 78*, 363–377. https://doi.org/10.1348/147608305X43784

Blackmore, E., Côté-Arsenault, D., Tang, W., Glover, V., Evans, J., Golding, J., & O'Connor, T. (2011). Previous prenatal loss as a predictor of perinatal depression and anxiety. *British Journal of Psychiatry, 198*(5), 373–378. https://doi.org/10.1192/bjp.bp.110.083105

Bohart, A. C., Elliott, R., Greenberg, L. S., & Watson, J. C. (2002). Empathy. In J. C. Norcross (Ed.), *Psychotherapy relationships that work* (pp. 89–108). Oxford University Press.

Boivin, J., Bunting, L., Collins, J. A., & Nygren, K. G. (2007). International estimates of infertility prevalence and treatment-seeking: Potential need and demand for infertility medical care. *Human Reproduction, 22*(6), 1506–1512. https://doi.org/10.1093/humrep/dem046

Bonanno, G. (2009). *The other side of sadness: What the new science of bereavement tells us about life after loss.* New York: Basic Books.

Bonanno, G. A., Keltner, D., Holen, A., & Horowitz, M. J. (1995). When avoiding unpleasant emotions might not be such a bad thing: Verbal-autonomic response dissociation and midlife conjugal bereavement. *Journal of Personality and Social Psychology, 69*(5), 975–989. https://doi.org/10.1037/0022-3514.69.5.975

Booth, A., Trimble, T., & Egan, J. (2010). Body-centred countertransference in a sample of Irish clinical psychologists. *The Irish Psychologist, 36*, 284–289.

Bordin, E. S. (1975, September). *The working alliance: Basis for a general theory of psychotherapy.* [Paper presentation]. Society for Psychotherapy Research, Washington, DC.

Bordin, E. S. (1979). The generalizability of the psychoanalytic concept of the working alliance. *Psychotherapy: Theory, Research & Practice, 16*(3), 252–260. https://doi.org/10.1037/h0085885

Bordin, E. S. (1994). Theory and research on the therapeutic working alliance: New directions. In A. O. Horvath & L. S. Greenberg (Eds.), *The working alliance: Theory, research, and practice* (pp. 13–37). John Wiley & Sons.

Bowlby, J. (1969). *Attachment and loss, vol. 1: Loss, attachment.* Basic Books.

Bowlby, J. (1973). *Attachment and loss, vol. 2: Separation: Anxiety and anger.* Basic Books.

Bowlby, J. (1975). Attachment theory, separation anxiety, and mourning. *American Handbook of Psychiatry, 6,* 292–309.

Bowlby, J. (1977). The making and breaking of affectional bonds. *British Journal of Psychiatry, 130*(3), 201–210. https://doi.org/10.1192/bjp.130.3.201

Bowlby, J. (1980). *Attachment and loss, vol. 3: Loss, sadness and depression.* Basic Books.

Bowlby, J. (1982). *Attachment and loss, vol. 1. Attachment* (2nd ed.). Basic Books.

Bowlby, J. (1988). *A secure base: Clinical applications of attachment theory.* Routledge.

Bowles, S. V., Bernard, R. S., Epperly, T., Woodward, S., Ginzburg, K., Folen, R., Perez, T., & Koopman, C. (2006). Traumatic stress disorders following first-trimester spontaneous abortion: A pilot study of patient characteristics associated with these disorders. *Journal of Family Practice, 55*(11), 969–973.

Bowman, E. A., & Safran, J. D. (2007). An integrated developmental perspective on insight. In L. G. Castonguay & C. Hill (Eds.), *Insight in psychotherapy* (pp. 401–421). American Psychological Association. https://doi.org/10.1037/11532-019

Brandon, A. R., Pitts, S., Denton, W. H., Stringer, C. A., & Evans, H. M. (2009). A history of the theory of prenatal attachment. *Journal of Prenatal & Perinatal Psychology & Health, 23*(4), 201–222.

Brattland, H., Koksvik, J. M., Burkeland, O., Klöckner, C. A., Lara-Cabrera, M. L., Miller, S. D., Wampold, B., Ryum, T., & Iversen, V. C. (2019). Does the working alliance mediate the effect of routine outcome monitoring (ROM) and alliance feedback on psychotherapy outcomes? A secondary analysis from a randomized clinical trial. *Journal of Counseling Psychology, 66*(2), 234–246. https://doi.org/10.1037/cou 0000320

Brennan, K. A., Clark, C. L., & Shaver, P. R. (1998). Self-report measurement of adult attachment: An integrative overview. In J. A. Simpson & W. S. Rholes (Eds.), *Attachment theory and close relationships* (pp. 46–76). Guilford Press.

Brier, N. (2004). Anxiety after miscarriage: A review of the empirical literature and implications for clinical practice. *Birth, 31*(2), 138–142.

Brier, N. (2008). Grief following miscarriage: A comprehensive review of the literature. *Journal of Women's Health, 17*(3), 451–464. https://doi.org/10.1089/jwh.2007.0505

Bromberg, P. M. (1998). *Standing in the spaces: Essays on clinical process, trauma, and dissociation.* Analytic Press.

Brouquet, K. (1999). Psychological reactions to pregnancy loss. *Primary Care Update for OB/GYNS, 6*(1), 12–16.

Brown, E. J., & Heimberg, R. G. (2001). Effects of writing about rape: Evaluating Pennebaker's paradigm with a severe trauma. *Journal of Traumatic Stress, 14*(4), 781–790. https://doi.org/10.1023/A:1013098307063

Büchi, S., Mörgeli, H., Schnyder, U., Jenewein, J., Hepp, U., Jina, E., Neuhaus, R., Fauchère, J.-C., Bucher, H. U., & Sensky, T. (2007). Grief and post-traumatic growth in parents 2–6 years after the death of their extremely premature baby. *Psychotherapy and Psychosomatics, 76*(2), 106–114. https://doi.org/10.1159/000097969

Buckley, T., Sunari, D., Marshall, A., Bartrop, R., McKinley, S., & Tofler, G. (2012). Physiological correlates of bereavement and the impact of bereavement interventions. *Dialogues in Clinical Neuroscience, 14*(2), 129–139.

Butler, S. F., Flasher, L. V., & Strupp, H. H. (1993). Countertransference and qualities of the psychotherapist. In N. E. Miller, L. Luborsky, J. P. Barber, & J. P. Docherty (Eds.), *Psychodynamic treatment research: A handbook for clinical practice* (pp. 342–360). Basic Books.

Calhoun, L. G., & Tedeschi, R. G. (Eds.). (2006). *Handbook of posttraumatic growth: Research & practice*. Lawrence Erlbaum Associates Publishers.

Cain, A. C., & Cain, B. S. (1964). On replacing a child. *Journal of the American Academy of Child psychiatry, 3*, 443–456. doi:10.1016/s0002-7138(09)60158-8. PMID: 14179092.

Cassidy, J., & Kobak, R. R. (1988). Avoidance and its relationship with other defensive processes. In J. Belsky & T. Nezworski (Eds.), *Clinical implications of attachment* (pp. 300–323). Erlbaum.

Chen, S. L., Chang, S. M., Kuo, P. L., & Chen, C. H. (2020). Stress, anxiety and depression perceived by couples with recurrent miscarriage. *International Journal of Nursing Practice, 26*(2), e12796. https://doi.org/10.1111/ijn.12796

Christiansen, D. M. (2017). Posttraumatic stress disorder in parents following infant death: A systematic review. *Clinical Psychology Review, 51*, 60–74. https://doi.org/10.1016/j.cpr.2016.10.007

Christiansen, D. M., Olff, M., & Elklit, A. (2014). Parents bereaved by infant death: Sex differences and moderation in PTSD, attachment, coping and social support. *General Hospital Psychiatry, 36*(6), 655–661. https://doi.org/10.1016/j.genhosppsych.2014.07.012

Chung, M. C., & Reed, J. (2017). Posttraumatic stress disorder following stillbirth: Trauma characteristics, locus of control, posttraumatic cognitions. *Psychiatric Quarterly, 88*(2), 307–321. https://doi.org/10.1007/s11126-016-9446-y

Clarke, M., & Williams, A. J. (1979). Depression in women after perinatal death. *Lancet, 1*(8122), 916–917.

Cohen, J. (1988). *Statistical power analysis for the behavioral sciences* (2nd ed.). Erlbaum.

Condon, J. (2000). Pregnancy loss. In M. Steiner, P. Yonkers, & P. Eriksson (Eds.), *Mood disorders in women* (pp. 353–369). Martin Dunitz.

Côté-Arsenault, D., & Brody, D. (2009). Pregnancy as a rite of passage: Liminality, rituals & communitas. *Journal of Prenatal & Perinatal Psychology & Health, 24*, 69–87. https://birthpsychology.com/journal/article/pregnancy-rite-passage-liminality-rituals- communitas

Côte-Arsenault, D., & Mahlangu, N. (1999). Impact of perinatal loss on the subsequent pregnancy and self: Women's experiences. *Journal of Obstetric, Gynecologic, and Neonatal Nursing, 28*(3), 274–282. http://dx.doi.org/10.1111/j.1552-6909.1999.tb01992.x

Courtois, C. (2020). *It's not you, it's what happened to you: complex trauma and treatment*. Telemachus press.

Courtois, C. A., & Brown, L. S. (2019). Guideline orthodoxy and resulting limitations of the American Psychological Association's clinical practice guideline for the treatment of PTSD in adults. *Psychotherapy, 56*(3), 329–339. http://dx.doi.org/10.1037/pst0000239

Courtois, C. A., & Sack, D. A. (2014). *It's not you, it's what happened to you: Complex trauma and treatment*. Telemachus Press.

Cousineau, T. M., & Domar, A. D. (2007). Psychological impact of infertility. *Best Practice & Research in Clinical Obstetrics & Gynaecology, 21*(2), 293–308. https://doi.org/10.1016/j.bpobgyn.2006.12.003

Covington, S. N. (2005). Miscarriage and stillbirth. In A. Rosen & J. Rosen (Eds.), *Frozen dreams: Psychodynamic dimensions of infertility and assisted reproduction* (1st ed., pp. 197–218). Taylor & Francis.

Covington, S. N. (2006). Pregnancy loss. In S. N. Covington & L. H. Burns (Eds.), *Infertility counseling: A comprehensive handbook for clinicians* (2nd ed., pp. 290–304). Cambridge University Press. https://doi.org/10.1017/CBO9780511547263.018

Covington, S. N. (2015). *Fertility counseling: Clinical guide and case studies.* Cambridge University Press. doi:10.1017/CBO9781107449398

Covington, S. N., & Marosek, K. (1999, September). *Personal infertility experience among nurses and mental health professionals working in reproductive medicine* [Paper presentation]. Meeting of American Society for Reproductive Medicine, Toronto, Canada.

Daniel, S. I. (2006). Adult attachment patterns and individual psychotherapy: A review. *Clinical Psychology Review, 26*(8), 968–984. https://doi.org/10.1016/j.cpr.2006.02.001

Daniel, S. I. F. (2015). *Adult attachment patterns in a treatment context: Relationship and narrative.* Routledge/Taylor & Francis Group.

Dayal, M. B., et al. (2022). *Preimplantation Genetic Diagnosis.* Medscape. https://emedicine.medscape.com/article/273415-overview?form=fpf

Decety, J., & Lamm, C. (2009). Empathy versus personal distress: Recent evidence from social neuroscience. In J. Decety & W. Ickes (Eds.), *The social neuroscience of empathy* (pp. 199–213). MIT Press.

DeFrain, J., Millspaugh, E., & Xie, X. (1996). The psychosocial effects of miscarriage: Implications for health professionals. *Families, Systems, & Health, 14*(3), 331–347. https://doi.org/10.1037/h0089794

Del Re, A. C., Flückiger, C., Horvath, A. O., Symonds, D., & Wampold, B. E. (2012). Therapist effects in the therapeutic alliance–outcome relationship: A restricted-maximum likelihood meta-analysis. *Clinical Psychology Review, 32*(7), 642–649. https://doi.org/10.1016/j.cpr.2012.07.002

Diamond, D. J., & Diamond, M. O. (2016). Understanding and treating the psychosocial consequences of pregnancy loss. In A. Wenzel (Ed.), *The Oxford handbook of perinatal psychology* (pp. 487–523). Oxford University Press. https://doi.org/10.1093/oxfordhb/9780199778072.013.30

Diamond, D. J., & Diamond, M. O. (2017). Parenthood after reproductive loss: How psychotherapy can help with postpartum adjustment and parent–infant attachment. *Psychotherapy, 54*(4), 373–379. https://doi.org/10.1037/pst0000127

Diamond, M. O. (2011). Pregnancy and parenthood after infertility or reproductive loss. In J. Jaffe & M. O. Diamond (Eds.), *Reproductive trauma: Psychotherapy with infertility and pregnancy loss clients* (pp. 215–229). American Psychological Association. http://dx.doi.org/10.1037/12347-005

Diener, M. J., Hilsenroth, M. J., & Weinberger, J. (2007). Therapist affect focus and patient outcomes in psychodynamic psychotherapy: A meta-analysis. *American Journal of Psychiatry, 164*(6), 936–941. https://doi.org/10.1176/appi.ajp.164.6.936

Diener, M. J., & Monroe, J. M. (2011). The relationship between adult attachment style and therapeutic alliance in individual psychotherapy: A meta-analytic review. *Psychotherapy, 48*, 237–248. doi:10.1037/a0022425

Dingle, K., Alati, R., Clavarino, A., Najman, J. M., & Williams, G. M. (2008). Pregnancy loss and psychiatric disorders in young women: An Australian birth cohort study. *British Journal of Psychiatry*, *193*(6), 455–460. doi:10.1192/bjp.bp.108.055079. PMID: 19043146.

Doka, K. J. (Ed.). (1989). *Disenfranchised grief: Recognizing hidden sorrow*. Lexington Books.

Donarelli, Z., Lo Coco, G., Gullo, S., Marino, A., Volpes, A., & Allegra, A. (2012). Are attachment dimensions associated with infertility-related stress in couples undergoing their first IVF treatment? A study on the individual and cross-partner effect. *Human Reproduction*, *27*(11), 3215–3225. https://doi.org/10.1093/humrep/des307

Donarelli, Z., Lo Coco, G., Gullo, S., Marino, A., Volpes, A., Salerno, L., & Allegra, A. (2016). Infertility-related stress, anxiety and ovarian stimulation: Can couples be reassured about the effects of psychological factors on biological responses to assisted reproductive technology? *Reproductive Biomedicine & Society Online*, *3*, 16–23. https://doi.org/10.1016/j.rbms.2016.10.001

Dozier, M., Cue, K. L., & Barnett, L. (1994). Clinicians as caregivers: Role of attachment organization in treatment. *Journal of Consulting and Clinical Psychology*, *62*, 793–800. doi:10.1037/0022-006X.62.4.793

Dozier, M., Stovall, K., & Albus, K. (1999). Attachment and psychopathology in adulthood. In J. Cassidy & P. Shaver (Eds.), *Handbook of attachment: Theory, research and clinical applications* (pp. 718–744). Guilford.

Duan, C., & Kivlighan, D. M., Jr. (2002). Relationships among therapist presession mood, therapist empathy, and session evaluation. *Psychotherapy Research*, *12*(1), 23–37. https://doi.org/10.1093/ptr/12.1.23

Dyregrov, A. (1990). Parental reactions to the loss of an infant child: A review. *Scandinavian Journal of Psychology*, *31*(4), 266–280. https://doi.org/10.1111/j.1467-9450.1990.tb00839.x

Dyregrov, K., Nordanger, D., & Dyregrov, A. (2003). Predictors of psychosocial distress after suicide, SIDS and accidents. *Death Studies*, *27*(2), 143–165. https://doi.org/10.1080/07481180302892

Dyson, L., & While, A. (1998). The lifelong shadow of perinatal bereavement. *British Journal of Community Nursing*, *3*, 432–439.

Eames, V., & Roth, A. (2000). Patient attachment orientation and the early working alliance: Study of patient and therapist reports of alliance quality and ruptures. *Psychotherapy Research*, *10*, 421– 434. doi:10.1093/ptr/10.4.421

Earle, S., Foley, P., Komaromy, C., & Lloyd, C. (2008). Conceptualizing reproductive loss: A social sciences perspective. *Human Fertility*, *11*(4), 259–262.

Ekman, P. (2007). *Emotions revealed* (2nd ed.). Holt Paperbacks.

Elliott, R., Bohart, A. C., Watson, J. C., & Greenberg, L. S. (2011). Empathy. *Psychotherapy*, *48*(1), 43–49. https://doi.org/10.1037/a0022187

Elliott, R., Bohart, A. C., Watson, J. C., & Murphy, D. (2018). Therapist empathy and client outcome: An updated meta-analysis. *Psychotherapy*, *55*(4), 399–410. https://doi.org/10.1037/pst0000175

Elliott, R., Bohart, A. C., Watson, J. C., & Murphy, D. (2019). Empathy. In J. C. Norcross & M. J. Lambert (Eds.), *Psychotherapy relationships that work: Volume 1: Evidence-based therapist contributions* (3rd ed., pp. 245–287). Oxford University Press.

Elliott, R., Watson, J. C., Goldman, R. N., & Greenberg, L. S. (2004). *Learning emotion-focused therapy: The process-experiential approach to change*. American Psychological Association. https://doi.org/10.1037/10725-000

Ellis, A. E., Simiola, V., Brown, L., Courtois, C., & Cook, J. M. (2018). The role of evidence-based therapy relationships on treatment outcome for adults with trauma: A systematic review. *Journal of Trauma & Dissociation, 19*, 185–213. https://doi.org/10.1080/15299732.2017.1329771

Engelhard, I. M. (2004). Miscarriage as a traumatic event. *Clinical Obstetrics and Gynecology, 47*(3), 547–551. https://doi.org/10.1097/01.grf.0000129920.38874.0d

Engelhard, I. M., van den Hout, M. A., & Arntz, A. (2001). Posttraumatic stress disorder after pregnancy loss. *General Hospital Psychiatry, 23*(2), 62–66.

Engelhard, I. M., van den Hout, M. A., Kindt, M., Arntz, A., & Schouten, E. (2003a). Peritraumatic dissociation and posttraumatic stress after pregnancy loss: A prospective study. *Behaviour Research and Therapy, 41*(1), 67–78. https://doi.org/10.1016/s0005-7967(01)00130-9

Engelhard, I. M., van den Hout, M. A., & Vlaeyen, J. W. (2003b). The sense of coherence in early pregnancy and crisis support and posttraumatic stress after pregnancy loss: A prospective study. *Behavioral Medicine, 29*(2), 80–84. https://doi.org/10.1080/08964280309596060

Engelkemeyer, S. M., & Marwitt, S. J. (2008). Posttraumatic growth in bereaved parents. *Journal of Traumatic Stress, 21*(3), 344–346.

Escudero, V., Boogmans, E., Loots, G., & Friedlander, M. L. (2012). Alliance rupture and repair in conjoint family therapy: An exploratory study. *Psychotherapy, 49*(1), 26–37. https://doi.org/10.1037/a0026747

Escudero, V., & Friedlander, M. L. (2017). *Therapeutic alliances with families: Empowering clients in challenging cases*. Springer International. https://doi.org/10.1007/978-3-319-59369-2

Essig, T. (2005). Riding the elephant in the room: How I use countertransference in couples therapy. In A. Rosen & J. Rosen (Eds.), *Frozen dreams: Psychodynamic dimensions of infertility and assisted reproduction* (pp. 103–127). The Analytic Press/Taylor & Francis Group.

Eubanks, C. F., Burckell, L. A., & Goldfried, M. R. (2018). Clinical consensus strategies to repair ruptures in the therapeutic alliance. *Journal of Psychotherapy Integration, 28*(1), 60–76. https://doi.org/10.1037/int0000097

Eubanks, C. F., Lubitz, J., Muran, J. C., & Safran, J. D. (2018). Rupture resolution rating system (3RS): Development and validation. *Psychotherapy Research, 29*(3), 306–319. https://doi.org/10.1080/10503307.2018.1552034

Eubanks, C. F., Muran, J. C., & Safran, J. D. (2018). Alliance rupture repair: A meta-analysis. *Psychotherapy, 55*, 508–519. http://dx.doi.org/10.1037/pst0000185

Eubanks-Carter, C. F., Muran, J. C., & Safran, J. D. (2010). Alliance ruptures and resolution. In J. C. Muran & J. P. Barber (Eds.), *The therapeutic alliance: An evidence-based approach to practice and training* (pp. 74–94). Guilford Press.

Eubanks-Carter, C., Muran, J. C., & Safran, J. D. (2015). Alliance-focused training. *Psychotherapy, 52*(2), 169–173. https://doi.org/10.1037/a0037596

Eugene Declercq et al., The U.S. Maternal Health Divide: The Limited Maternal Health Services and Worse Outcomes of States Proposing New Abortion Restrictions (Commonwealth Fund, 2022). https://doi.org/10.26099/z7dz-8211

Farber, B. A., Suzuki, J. Y., & Lynch, D. A. (2018). Positive regard and psychotherapy outcome: A meta-analytic review. *Psychotherapy, 55*(4), 411–423. https://doi.org/10.1037/pst0000171

Feeney, J. A., & Noller, P. (1990). Attachment style as a predictor of adult romantic relationships. *Journal of Personality and Social Psychology, 58*(2), 281–291. https://doi.org/10.1037/0022-3514.58.2.281

Fenstermacher, K., & Hupcey, J. E., (2013). Perinatal bereavement: A principle-based analysis. *Journal of Advanced Nursing, 69*(11), 2389–2400. http://doi.org/10.1111/jan.12119

Fernández Ordóñez, E., Rengel Díaz, C., Morales Gil, I. M., & Labajos Manzanares, M. T. (2018). Post-traumatic stress and related symptoms in a gestation after a gestational loss: Narrative review. *Salud Mental, 41*(5), 237–243. https://doi.org/10.17711/sm.0185-3325.2018.035

Flemons, J. (2018). *Infertility and PTSD: The uncharted storm*. CreateSpace Independent Publishing Platform.

Flückiger, C., Del Re, A. C., Wampold, B. E., & Horvath, A. O. (2018). The alliance in adult psychotherapy: A meta-analytic synthesis. *Psychotherapy, 55*(4), 316–340. http://dx.doi.org/10.1037/pst0000172

Flückiger, C., Del Re, A. C., Wampold, B. E., Symonds, D., & Horvath, A. O. (2012). How central is the alliance in psychotherapy? A multilevel longitudinal meta-analysis. *Journal of Counseling Psychology, 59*(1), 10–17. https://doi.org/10.1037/a0025749

Flückiger, C., Hilpert, P., Goldberg, S. B., Caspar, F., Wolfer, C., Held, J., & Vîslă, A. (2019). Investigating the impact of early alliance on predicting subjective change at posttreatment: An evidence-based souvenir of overlooked clinical perspectives. *Journal of Counseling Psychology, 66*(5), 613–625. https://doi.org/10.1037/cou0000336

Fonagy, P., Leigh, T., Steele, M., Steele, H., Kennedy, R., Mattoon, G., Target, M., & Gerber, A. (1996). The relation of attachment status, psychiatric classification, and response to psychotherapy. *Journal of Consulting and Clinical Psychology, 64*(1), 22–31. https://doi.org/10.1037//0022-006x.64.1.22

Fonagy, P., Target, M., Steele, H., & Steele, M. (1998). *Reflective functioning manual. Version 5 for application to adult attachment interviews*. University College London.

Fosha, D. (2000). *The transforming power of affect: A model for accelerated change*. Basic Books.

Fraley, R. C. (2002). Attachment stability from infancy to adulthood: Meta-analysis and dynamic modeling of developmental mechanisms. *Personality and Social Psychology Review, 6*(2), 123–151. https://doi.org/10.1207/S15327957PSPR0602_03

Fraley, R. C., Niedenthal, P. M., Marks, M., Brumbaugh, C., & Vicary, A. (2006). Adult attachment and the perception of emotional expressions: Probing the hyperactivating strategies underlying anxious attachment. *Journal of Personality, 74*(4), 1163–1190. https://doi.org/10.1111/j.1467-6494.2006.00406.x

Fraley, R. C., & Shaver, P. R. (2016). Attachment, loss, and grief: Bowlby's views, new developments, and current controversies. In J. Cassidy & P. R. Shaver (Eds.), *Handbook of attachment: Theory, research, and clinical applications* (3rd Edition, pp. 40–62). New York: Guilford Press.

Frank, J. D. (1971). Therapeutic factors in psychotherapy. *American Journal of Psychotherapy, 25*(3), 350–361. https://doi.org/10.1176/appi.psychotherapy.1971.25.3.350

Freeman, N. (2005). When the therapist is infertile. In A. Rosen & J. Rosen (Eds.), *Frozen dreams: Psychodynamic dimensions of infertility and assisted reproduction* (pp. 50–68). Taylor & Francis.

Freud, S. (1910/1957). Future prospects of psychoanalytic therapy. In J. Strachey (Ed.), *The standard edition of the complete works of Sigmund Freud* (Vol. 11, pp. 139–151). Hogarth Press.

Freud, S. (1913). On the beginning of treatment: Further recommendations on the technique of psychoanalysis. In J. Strachey (Ed.), *The standard edition of the complete psychological works of Sigmund Freud* (Vol. 13, pp. 122–144). Hogarth Press.

Freud, S. (1927/1961). The future of an illusion, civilization and its discontents, and other works. In J. Strachey (Ed.), *The standard edition of the complete psychological works of Sigmund Freud* (Vol. 21, pp. 5–58). Hogarth Press.

Friedlander, M. L., Bernardi, S., & Lee, H.-H. (2010). Better versus worse family therapy sessions as reflected in clients' alliance-related behavior. *Journal of Counseling Psychology, 57*(2), 198–204. https://doi.org/10.1037/a0019088

Friedlander, M. L., Escudero, V., Heatherington, L., & Diamond, G. M. (2011). Alliance in couple and family therapy. *Psychotherapy (Chicago), 48*(1), 25–33. doi:10.1037/a0022060. PMID: 21401271

Friedlander, M. L., Escudero, V., & Heatherington, L. (2006). Repairing split alliances. In M. L. Friedlander, V. Escudero, & L. Heatherington, *Therapeutic alliances in couple and family therapy: An empirically informed guide to practice* (pp. 161–177). American Psychological Association. https://doi.org/10.1037/11410-008

Friedlander, M. L., Escudero, V., Welmers-van de Poll, M. J., & Heatherington, L. (2019). Alliances in couple and family therapy. In J. C. Norcross & M. J. Lambert (Eds.), *Psychotherapy relationships that work: Volume 1: Evidence-based therapist contributions* (3rd ed., pp. 117–166). Oxford University Press. https://doi.org/10.1093/med-psych/9780190843953.003.0004

Friedman, T., & Garth, D. (1989). The psychiatric consequences of spontaneous abortion. *British Journal of Psychiatry, 155*, 810–813.

Frost, M., & Condon, J. T. (1996). The psychological sequelae of miscarriage: A critical review of the literature. *Australian and New Zealand Journal of Psychiatry, 30*(1), 54–62. https://doi.org/10.3109/00048679609076072

Gaudet, C., Séjourné, N., Camborieux, L., Rogers, R., & Chabrol, H. (2010). Pregnancy after perinatal loss: Association of grief, anxiety and attachment. *Journal of Reproductive and Infant Psychology, 28*, 240–251. http://dx.doi.org/10.1080/02646830903487342

Gausia, K., Moran, A. C., Ali, M., Ryder, D., Fisher, C., & Koblinsky, M. (2011). Psychological and social consequences among mothers suffering from perinatal loss: Perspective from a low-income country. *BMC Public Health, 11*(1), Article number 451. https://doi.org/10.1186/1471-2458-11-451

Geerinck-Vercammen, C. R., & Kanhai, H. H. H. (2003). Coping with termination of pregnancy for fetal abnormality in a supportive environment. *Prenatal Diagnosis, 23*(7), 543–548. https://doi.org/10.1002/pd.636

Geller, J. D., Norcross, J. C., & Orlinsky, D. E. (Eds.). (2005). *The psychotherapist's own psychotherapy.* Oxford University Press.

Geller, P. A., Kerns, D., & Klier, C. M. (2004). Anxiety following miscarriage and the subsequent pregnancy: A review of the literature and future directions. *Journal of Psychosomatic Research, 56*(1), 34–45. https://doi.org/10.1016/S0022-3999(03)00042-4

Geller, P. A., Klier, C. M., & Neugebauer, R. (2001). Anxiety disorders following miscarriage. *Journal of Clinical Psychiatry, 62*(6), 432–438.

Geller, P. A., Psaros, C., & Kornfield, S. L. (2010). Satisfaction with pregnancy loss after-care: Are women getting what they want? *Archives of Women's Mental Health*, *13*(2), 111–124. https://doi.org/10.1007/s00737-010-0147-5

Gelso, C. J., & Carter, J. A. (1985). The relationship in counseling and psycho-therapy: Components, consequences, and theoretical antecedents. *The Counseling Psychologist*, *13*(2), 155–243. https://doi.org/10.1177%2F0011000085132001

Gelso, C. J., & Hayes, J. A. (1998). *The psychotherapy relationship: Theory, research, and practice*. John Wiley & Sons Inc.

Gelso, C. J., & Hayes, J. A. (2001). Countertransference management. *Psychotherapy: Theory, Research, Practice, Training,38*(4),418–422. https://doi.org/10.1037/0033-3204.38.4.418

Gelso, C. J., & Hayes, J. A. (2007). *Countertransference and the therapist's inner experi-ence: Perils and possibilities*. Lawrence Erlbaum Associates Publishers.

Gillies, J., & Neimeyer, R. A. (2006). Loss, grief, and the search for significance: Toward a model of meaning reconstruction in bereavement. *Journal of Constructivist Psychology*, *19*(1), 31–65. https://doi.org/10.1080/10720530500311182

Gilligan, C. (2002). *The birth of pleasure: A new map of love*. Vintage.

Ginzburg, K., Ein-Dor, T., & Solomon, Z. (2010). Comorbidity of posttraumatic stress disorder, anxiety and depression: A 20-year longitudinal study of war vet-erans. *Journal of Affective Disorders*, *123*(1–3), 249–257. https://doi.org/10.1016/j.jad.2009.08.006

Glebova, T., Bartle-Haring, S., Gangamma, R., Knerr, M., Delaney, R. O., Meyer, K., McDowell, T., Adkins, K., & Grafsky, E. (2011). Therapeutic alliance and progress in couple therapy: Multiple perspectives. *Journal of Family Therapy*, *33*(1), 42–65. https://doi.org/10.1111/j.1467-6427.2010.00503.x

Gold, K. (2007). Navigating care after a baby dies: A systematic review of parent experiences with health providers. *Journal of Perinatology*, *27*, 230–237. https://doi.org/10.1038/sj.jp.7211676

Gold, K. J., Leon, I., Boggs, M. E., & Sen, A. (2015). Depression and posttraumatic stress symptoms after perinatal loss in a population-based sample. *Journal of Women's Health*, *25*(3), 263–269. https://doi.org/10.1089/jwh.2015.5284

Gosai, S., & Markin, R. D. (2019). Alliance formation, rupture and repair themes in psychotherapy for reproductive trauma patients: The therapist perspective. Unpublished dissertation.

Goubert, L., Craig, K. D., & Buysee, A. (2009). Perceiving others in pain: Experimental and clinical evidence of the role of empathy. In J. Decety & W. Ickes (Eds.), *The social neuroscience of empathy* (pp. 153–165). MIT Press.

Grauerholz, K. R., Berry, S. N., Capuano, R. M., & Early, J. M. (2021). Uncovering pro-longed grief reactions subsequent to a reproductive loss: Implications for the primary care provider. *Frontiers in Psychology*, *12*, 673050. doi:10.3389/fpsyg.2021.673050. PMID: 34054675; PMCID: PMC8149623.

Greenberg, L. (2014). The therapeutic relationship in emotion-focused therapy. *Psychotherapy*, *51*(3), 350–357. https://doi.org/10.1037/a0037336

Greenberg, L. S. (2015). *Emotion-focused therapy: Coaching clients to work through their feelings* (2nd ed.). American Psychological Association. https://doi.org/10.1037/14692-000

Greenberg, L. S. (2016). The clinical application of emotion in psychotherapy. In L. F. Barrett, M. Lewis, & J. M. Haviland-Jones (Eds.), *Handbook of emotions* (4th ed., pp. 670–684). Guilford Press.

Greenberg, L. S., & Pascual-Leone, A. (2006). Emotion in psychotherapy: A 'practice-friendly research review. *Journal of Clinical Psychology*, *62*(5), 611–630. https://doi.org/10.1002/jclp.20252

Greenberg, L. S., & Safran, J. D. (1989). Emotion in psychotherapy. *American Psychologist*, *44*(1), 19–29. https://doi.org/10.1037/0003-066X.44.1.19

Greenfield, D., & Walther, V. (1991). Psychological aspects of recurrent pregnancy loss. *Infertility and Reproductive Clinics of North America*, *2*, 235–247.

Gupta, S., & Bonanno, G. A. (2011). Complicated grief and deficits in emotional expressive flexibility. *Journal of Abnormal Psychology*, *120*(3), 635–643. https://doi.org/10.1037/a0023541

Haidich, A. B. (2010). Meta-analysis in medical research. *Hippokratia*, *14*(1), 29–37.

Hakim, R. B., Gray, R. H., & Zacur, H. (1995). Infertility and early pregnancy loss. *American Journal of Obstetrics and Gynecology*, *172*(5), 1510–1517. https://doi.org/10.1016/0002-9378(95)90489-1

Halford, T. C., Owen, J., Duncan, B. L., Anker, M. G., & Sparks, J. A. (2016). Pre-therapy relationship adjustment, gender and the alliance in couple therapy. *Journal of Family Therapy*, *38*(1), 18–35. https://doi.org/10.1111/1467-6427.12035

Hamama, L., Rauch, S. A. M., Sperlich, M., Defever, E., & Seng, J. S. (2010). Previous experience of spontaneous or elective abortion and risk for posttraumatic stress and depression during subsequent pregnancy. *Depression and Anxiety*, *27*(8), 699–707. https://doi.org/10.1002/da.20714

Harb, H. M., Al-rshoud, F., Dhillon, R., Harb, M., & Coomarasamy, A. (2014). Ethnicity and miscarriage: A large prospective observational study and meta-analysis. *Fertility and Sterility*, *102*(3S), E81. https://doi.org/10.1016/j.fertnstert.2014.07.276

Harper, H. (1989a). *Coding guide I: Identification of confrontation challenges in exploratory therapy*. University of Sheffield.

Harper, H. (1989b). *Coding guide II: Identification of withdrawal challenges in exploratory therapy*. University of Sheffield.

Hart, V. A. (2002). Infertility and the role of psychotherapy. *Issues in Mental Health Nursing*, *23*(1), 31–41. doi:10.1080/01612840252825464

Hatcher, R. L. (2015). Interpersonal competencies: Responsiveness, technique, and training in psychotherapy. *American Psychologist*, *70*(8), 747–757. https://doi.org/10.1037/a0039803

Hatcher, R. L., & Barends, A. W. (2006). How a return to theory could help alliance research. *Psychotherapy: Theory, Research, Practice, Training*, *43*(3), 292–299. https://doi.org/10.1037/0033-3204.43.3.292

Hayes, J. A., & Gelso, C. J. (1991). Effects of therapist-trainees' anxiety and empathy on countertransference behavior. *Journal of Clinical Psychology*, *47*(2), 284–290. https://doi.org/10.1002/1097-4679(199103)47:2<284::AID-JCLP2270470216>3.0.CO;2- N

Hayes, J. A., & Gelso, C. J. (1993). Counselors' discomfort with gay and HIV-infected clients. *Journal of Counseling Psychology*, *40*(1), 86–93. http://dx.doi.org/10.1037/0022- 0167.40.1.86

Hayes, J. A., Gelso, C. J., Kivlighan, D. M., & Goldberg, S. B. (2019). Managing countertransference. In J. C. Norcross & M. J. Lambert (Eds.), *Psychotherapy relationships that work: Volume 1: Evidence-based therapist contributions* (3rd ed., pp. 522–548). Oxford University Press.

Hayes, J. A., Yeh, Y.-J., & Eisenberg, A. (2007). Good grief and not-so-good grief: Countertransference in bereavement therapy. *Journal of Clinical Psychology*, 63(4), 345–355. https://doi.org/10.1002/jclp.20353

Heazell, A. E., Siassakos, D., Blencowe, H., Burden, C., Bhutta, Z. A., Cacciatore, J., Dang, N., Das, J., Flenady, V., Gold, K. J., Mensah, O. K., Millum, J., Nuzum, D., O'Donoghue, K., Redshaw, M., Rizvi, A., Roberts, T., Toyin Saraki, H. E., Storey, C., . . . Downe, S. (2016). Stillbirths: Economic and psychosocial consequences. *Lancet*, 387(10018), 604–616. https://doi.org/10.1016/s0140-6736(15)00836-3

Heimann, P. (1950). Countertransference. *British Journal of Medical Psychology*, 33, 9–15.

Hein, G., & Singer, T. (2010). Neuroscience meets social psychology: An integrative approach to human empathy and prosocial behaviour. In M. Mikulincer & P. R. Shaver (Eds.), *Prosocial motives, emotions, and behavior: The better angels of our nature* (pp. 109–124). American Psychological Association.

Henschel, D. N., & Bohart, A. C. (1981). *The relationship between the effectiveness of a course in paraprofessional training and level of cognitive functioning.* [Paper presentation]. American Psychological Association, Los Angeles, CA.

Herbert, D., Young, K., Pietrusińska, M., & MacBeth, A. (2022). The mental health impact of perinatal loss: A systematic review and meta-analysis. *Journal of Affective Disorders*, 297, 118–129. https://doi.org/10.1016/j.jad.2021.10.026

Herman, J. L. (1992). *Trauma and recovery.* Basic Books.

Hersoug, A. G., Høglend, P., Havik, O., von der Lippe, A., & Monsen, J. (2009). Therapist characteristics influencing the quality of alliance in long-term psychotherapy. *Clinical Psychology & Psychotherapy*, 16(2), 100–110. https://doi.org/10.1002/cpp.605

Hill, C. E. (2014). *Helping skills: Facilitating exploration, insight, and action* (4th ed.). American Psychological Association.

Hill, C. E., Gelso, C. J., Chui, H., Spangler, P. T., Hummel, A., Huang, T., Jackson, J., Jones, R. A., Palma, B., Bhatia, A., Gupta, S., Ain, S. C., Klingaman, B., Lim, R. H., Liu, J., Hui, K., Jezzi, M. M., & Miles, J. R. (2014). To be or not to be immediate with clients: The use and perceived effects of immediacy in psychodynamic/interpersonal psychotherapy. *Psychotherapy Research*, 24(3), 299–315. https://doi.org/10.1080/10503307.2013.812262Hill, C. E., Helms, J. E., Spiegel, S. B., & Tichenor, V. (1988). Development of a system for categorizing client reactions to therapist interventions. *Journal of Counseling Psychology*, 35(1), 27–36. https://doi.org/10.1037//0022-0167.35.1.27

Hill, C. E., & Knox, S. (2002). Self-disclosure. In J. C. Norcross (Ed.), *Psychotherapy relationships that work: Therapist contributions and responsiveness to patients* (pp. 255–265). Oxford University Press.

Hill, C. E., Knox, S, & Pinto-Coelho, K. G. (2019). Self-disclosure and immediacy. In J. C. Norcross & M. J. Lambert (Eds.), *Psychotherapy relationships that work: Volume 1: Evidence-based therapist contributions* (3rd ed., pp. 379–420). Oxford University Press.

Hofer, M. A. (1984). Relationships as regulators: A psychobiologic perspective on bereavement. *Psychosomatic Medicine*, 46(3), 183–197. https://doi.org/10.1097/00006842-198405000-00001

Holley, S., & Pasch, L. (2015). Counseling lesbian, gay, bisexual and transgender patients. In S. Covington (Ed.), *Fertility counseling: Clinical guide and case studies* (pp. 180–196). Cambridge University Press. https://doi.org/10.1017/CBO9781107449398.014

Holmes, B. M., & Johnson, K. R. (2009). Adult attachment and romantic partner preference: A review. *Journal of Social and Personal Relationships*, 26(6–7), 833–852.
https://doi.org/10.1177/0265407509345653

Holmes, J. (2001). *The search for the secure base: Attachment theory and psychotherapy.*
Brunner-Routledge.

Horvath, A. Q., & Bedi, R. P. (2002). The alliance. In J. C. Norcross (Ed.), *Psychotherapy
relationships that work: Therapist contributions and responsiveness to patients* (pp.
37–69). Oxford University Press.

Horvath, A. O., Del Re, A. C., Fluckiger, C., & Symonds, D. (2011). Alliance in individual psychotherapy. In J. C. Norcross (Ed.), *Psychotherapy relationships that
work: Evidence-based responsiveness* (2nd ed., pp. 24–69). Oxford University Press.

Horvath, A. O., & Greenberg, L. S. (1989). Development and validation of the Working
Alliance Inventory. *Journal of Counseling Psychology*, 36(2), 223–233. https://doi.
org/10.1037/0022-0167.36.2.223

Horvath, A. O., & Symonds, B. D. (1991). Relation between working alliance and outcome in psychotherapy: A meta-analysis. *Journal of Counseling Psychology*, 38(2),
139–149. https://doi.org/10.1037/0022-0167.38.2.139

Hughes, P., Turton, P., & Hopper, E. (2001). Behaviour among infants born subsequent
to stillbirth. *Journal of Child Psychology and Psychiatry*, 42(6), 791–801.

Hughes, P., Turton, P., Hopper, E., & Evans, C. D. H. (2002). Assessment of guidelines for
good practice in psychosocial care of mothers after stillbirth: A cohort study. *Lancet*,
360, 114–118. http://dx.doi.org/10.1016/S0140-6736(02)09410-2.

Hughes, P., Turton, P., Hopper, E., McGauley, G. A., & Fonagy, P. (2004). Factors associated with the unresolved classification of the Adult Attachment Interview in women
who have suffered stillbirth. *Development and Psychopathology*, 16(1), 215–230.
http://doi.org/10.1017/S0954579404044487

Hunter, A., Tussis, L., & MacBeth, A. (2017). The presence of anxiety, depression and
stress in women and their partners during pregnancies following perinatal loss: A
meta-analysis. *Journal of Affective Disorders*, 223, 153–164. https://doi.org/10.1016/
j.jad.2017.07.004

Hutti, M. H. (1992). Parents' perceptions of the miscarriage experience. *Death Studies*,
16(5), 401–415. https://doi.org/10.1080/07481189208252588

Hutti, M. H., Armstrong, D. S., & Myers, J. (2013). Evaluation of the Perinatal Grief
Intensity Scale in the subsequent pregnancy after perinatal loss. *Journal of
Obstetric, Gynecologic & Neonatal Nursing*, 42(6), 697–706. https://doi.org/10.1111/
1552-6909.12249

Hutti, M. H., dePacheco, M., & Smith, M. (1998). A study of miscarriage: Development validation of the Perinatal Grief Intensity Scale. *Journal of Obstetric, Gynecologic &Neonatal
Nursing*, 27(5), 547–555. https://doi.org/10.1111/j.1552-6909.1998.tb02621.x

Hutti, M. H., Polivka, B., White, S., Hill, J., Clark, P., Cooke, C., Clemens, S., & Abell,
H. (2016). Experiences of nurses who care for women after fetal loss. *Journal of
Obstetric, Gynecologic & Neonatal Nursing*, 45(1), 17–27. https://doi.org/10.1016/
j.jogn.2015.10.010

Iwakabe, S., Rogan, K., & Stalikas, A. (2000). The relationship between client emotional
expressions, therapist interventions, and the working alliance: An exploration of
eight emotional expression events. *Journal of Psychotherapy Integration, 10*, 375–401.

Jaffe, J., & Diamond, M. O. (2011). Self-disclosure, transference, and countertransference.
In J. Jaffe & M. O. Diamond, Reproductive trauma: Psychotherapy with infertility

and pregnancy loss clients (pp. 159–177). American Psychological Association. https://doi.org/10.1037/12347-008

Jaffe, J. (2014). The reproductive story: Dealing with miscarriage, stillbirth, or other perinatal demise. In D. L. Barnes (Ed.), *Women's reproductive mental health across the lifespan* (pp. 159–176). Springer International Publishing. https://doi.org/10.1007/978-3-319-05116-1_9

Jaffe, J. (2015). The view from the fertility counselor's chair. In S. N. Covington (Ed.), Fertility counseling: Clinical guide and case studies (pp. 239–251). Cambridge University Press. https://doi.org/10.1017/CBO9781107449398.018

Jaffe, J., Diamond, M. O., & Diamond, D. J. (2005). *Unsung lullabies: Understanding and coping with infertility*. St. Martin's Griffin.

Janssen, H. J. E. M., Cuisinier, M. C. J., & Hoogduin, K. A. L. (1996). A critical review of the concept of pathological grief following pregnancy loss. *Omega: Journal of Death and Dying, 33*(1), 21–42.

Jerga, A. M., Shaver, P. R., & Wilkinson, R. B. (2011). Attachment insecurities and identification of at-risk individuals following the death of a loved one. *Journal of Social and Personal Relationships, 28*, 891–914.

Johnson, S. M. (2019). *Attachment theory in practice: Emotionally focused therapy (EFT) with individuals, couples, and families*. Guilford Publications.

Johnson, J. E., Burlingame, G. M., Olsen, J. A., Davies, R., & Gleave, R. L. (2005). Group climate, cohesion, alliance, and empathy in group psychotherapy: Multilevel structural equation models. *Journal of Counseling Psychology, 52*(3), 310–320. https://doi.org/10.1037/0022-0167.52.3.310

Johnson, O. P., & Langford, R. W. (2015). A randomized trial of a bereavement intervention for pregnancy loss. *Journal of Obstetric, Gynecologic & Neonatal Nursing, 44*(4), 492–499. https://doi.org/10.1111/1552-6909.12659

Johnson, S. M. (2004). *The practice of emotionally focused couple therapy: Creating connection* (2nd ed.). Routledge.

Johnson, S., & Sims, A. (2000). Attachment theory: A map for couples therapy. In T. M. Levy (Eds.), *Handbook of attachment interventions* (pp. 169–191). Academic Press.

Kaluzeviciute, G. (2020). The role of empathy in psychoanalytic psychotherapy: A historical exploration. *Cogent Psychology, 7*(1), Article 1748792. https://doi.org/10.1080/23311908.2020.1748792

Kanninen, K., Salo, J., & Punamaki, R. L. (2000). Attachment patterns and working alliance in trauma therapy for victims of political violence. *Psychotherapy Research, 10*, 435–449. doi:10.1093/ptr/10.4.435

Kenny, D. A., & Cook, W. L. (1999). Partner effects in relationship research: Conceptual issues, analytic difficulties, and illustrations. *Personal Relationships, 6*, 433–448. https://doi.org/10.1111/j.1475-6811.1999.tb00202.x

Keren, M. (2010). Perinatal loss: Its immediate and long-term impact on parenting. In S. Tyano, M. Keren, H. Herrman, & J. Cox (Eds.), *Parenthood and mental health: A bridge between infant and adult psychiatry* (pp. 161–170). Wiley-Blackwell. https://doi.org/10.1002/9780470660683.ch15

Kernberg, O. (1965). Notes on countertransferences. *Journal of the American Psychoanalytic Association, 13*(1), 38–56. https://doi.org/10.1177/000306516501300102

Kersting, A., Dölemeyer, R., Steinig, J., Walter, F., Kroker, K., Baust, K., & Wagner, B. (2013). Brief internet-based intervention reduces posttraumatic stress and prolonged grief in parents after the loss of a child during pregnancy: A randomized

controlled trial. *Psychotherapy and Psychosomatics, 82*, 372–381. https://doi.org/
10.1159/000348713

Kersting, A., Kroker, K., Schlicht, S., Baust, K., & Wagner, B. (2011). Efficacy of cognitive
behavioral internet-based therapy in parents after the loss of a child during pregnancy: Pilot data from a randomized controlled trial. *Archives of Women's Mental
Health, 14*, 465–477. https://doi.org/10.1007/s00737-011-0240-4

Kersting, A., & Wagner, B. (2012). Complicated grief after perinatal loss. *Bereavement
and Complicated Grief, 14*(2), 187–194. https://doi.org/10.31887/dcns.2012.14.2/
akersting

Kiesler, D. J. (2001). Therapist countertransference: In search of common themes and
empirical referents. *Journal of Clinical Psychology, 57*(8), 1053–1063. https://doi.org/
10.1002/jclp.1073

Kilpatrick, D. G., Resnick, H. S., Milanak, M. E., Miller, M. W., Keyes, K. M., & Friedman,
M. J. (2013). National estimates of exposure to traumatic events and PTSD prevalence using DSM-IV and DSM-5 criteria. *Journal of Traumatic Stress, 26*, 537–547.
https://doi.org/10.1002/jts.21848

Kivlighan, D. M., Jr., Patton, M. J., & Foote, D. (1998). Moderating effects of client attachment on the counselor experience-working alliance relationship. *Journal of
Counseling Psychology, 45*, 274–278. doi:10.1037/ 0022-0167.45.3.274

Klier, C. M., Geller, P. A., & Neugebauer, R. (2000). Minor depressive disorder in the
context of miscarriage. *Journal of Affective Disorders, 59*(1), 13–21. https://doi.org/
10.1016/S0165-0327(99)00126-3

Klier, C. M., Geller, P. A., & Ritsher, J. B. (2002). Affective disorders in the aftermath of
miscarriage: A comprehensive review. *Archives of Women's Mental Health, 5*, 129–
149. https://doi.org/10.1007/s00737-002-0146-2

Knobloch-Fedders, L., Pinsof, W. M., & Mann, B. J. (2007). Therapeutic alliance and
treatment progress in couple psychotherapy. *Journal of Marital and Family Therapy,
33*(2), 245–257. https://doi.org/10.1111/j.1752-0606.2007.00019.x

Knox, S., Hess, S. A., Petersen, D. A., & Hill, C. E. (1997). A qualitative analysis of
client perceptions of the effects of helpful therapist self-disclosure in long-term
therapy. *Journal of Counseling Psychology, 44*(3), 274–283. https://doi.org/10.1037/
0022-0167.44.3.274

Knox, S., & Hill, C. E. (2003). Therapist self-disclosure: Research-based suggestions
for practitioners. *Journal of Clinical Psychology, 59*(5), 529–539. https://doi.org/
10.1002/jclp.10157

Koopmans, L., Wilson, T., Cacciatore, J., & Flenady, V. (2013). Support for mothers, fathers and families after perinatal death. *Cochrane Database of Systematic Reviews, 6*,
Article CD000452. https://doi.org/10.1002/14651858.cd000452.pub3

Kotler, T., Buzwell, S., Romeo, Y., & Bowland, J. (1994). Avoidant attachment as a risk
factor for health. *British Journal of Medical Psychology, 67*(3), 237–245. https://doi.
org/10.1111/j.2044-8341.1994.tb01793.x

Kronen, J. (1995). Infertility and psychotherapy. *Issues in Psychoanalytic Psychology,
17*(1), 52–64.

Krosch, D. J., & Shakespeare-Finch, J. E. (2017). Grief, traumatic stress, and
posttraumatic growth in women who have experienced pregnancy loss. *Psychological
Trauma: Theory, Research, Practice, and Policy, 9*(4), 425–433. https://doi.org/
10.1037/tra0000183

Kübler-Ross, E. (1975). *Death: The final stage of growth.* Touchstone.

Kulathilaka, S., Hanwella, R., & de Silva, V. A. (2016). Depressive disorder and grief following spontaneous abortion. *BMC Psychiatry*, *16*(1), Article 100. https://doi.org/10.1186/s12888-016-0812-y

Lafarge, C., Mitchell, K., & Fox, P. (2014). Termination of pregnancy for fetal abnormality: A meta-ethnography of women's experiences. *Reproductive Health Matters*, *22*(44), 191–201. https://doi.org/10.1016/S0968-8080(14)44799-2

Lamb, E. H. (2002). The impact of previous perinatal loss on subsequent pregnancy and parenting. *Journal of Perinatal Education*, *11*(2), 33–40. https://doi.org/10.1891/1058-1243.11.2.33

Lambert, M. J., Whipple, J. L., & Kleinstäuber, M. (2019). Collecting and delivering client feedback. In J. C. Norcross & M. J. Lambert (Eds.), *Psychotherapy relationships that work: Volume 1: Evidence-based therapist contributions* (3rd ed., pp. 580–630). Oxford University Press. https://doi.org/10.1093/med-psych/9780190843953.003.0017

Lang, A., Fleiszer, A. R., Duhamel, F., Sword, W., Gilbert, K. R., & Corsini-Munt, S. (2011). Perinatal loss and parental grief: The challenge of ambiguity and disenfranchised grief. *Omega: Journal of Death and Dying*, *63*(2), 183–196. https://doi.org/10.2190/OM.63.2.e

Layne, L. L. (2003). *Motherhood lost: A feminist account of pregnancy loss in America.* Routledge.

Lee, C., & Slade, P. (1996). Miscarriage as a traumatic event: A review of the literature and new implications for intervention. *Journal of Psychosomatic Research*, *40*(3), 235–244.

Lee, C., Slade, P., & Lygo, V. (1996). The influence of psychological debriefing on emotional adaptation in women following early miscarriage: A preliminary study. *British Journal of Medical Psychology*, *69*, 47–58. https://doi.org/10.1111/j.2044-8341.1996.tb01849.x

Leon, I. G. (1990). *When a baby dies: Psychotherapy for pregnancy and newborn loss.* Yale University Press.

Leon, I. G. (1996). Revising psychoanalytic understandings of perinatal loss. *Psychoanalytic Psychology*, *13*(2), 161–176. https://doi.org/10.1037/h0079646

Leon, I. G. (2010). Understanding and treating infertility: Psychoanalytic considerations. *Journal of the American Academy of Psychoanalysis and Dynamic Psychiatry*, *38*(1), 47–75.

Leon, I. G. (2015). Pregnancy and loss counseling. In S. N. Covington (Ed.), *Fertility counseling: Clinical guide and case studies* (pp. 226–238). Cambridge University Press. https://doi.org/10.1017/CBO9781107449398.017

Leon, I. G. (2017). Empathic psychotherapy for pregnancy termination for fetal anomaly. *Psychotherapy*, *54*(4), 394–399. doi:10.1037/pst0000124. PMID: 29251959.

Levenson, H. (1995). *Time-limited dynamic psychotherapy.* Basic Books.

Levy, K., Ellison, W. D., Scott, L. N., & Bernecker, S. L. (2019). Attachment style. In J. C. Norcross (Eds.), *Psychotherapy relationships that work: Evidence-based responsiveness.* Oxford Scholarship Online. DOI:10.1093/acprof:oso/9780199737208.003.0019

Lin, S. X., & Lasker, J. N. (1996). Patterns of grief reaction after pregnancy loss. *American Journal of Orthopsychiatry*, *66*, 262–271. http://dx.doi.org/10.1037/h0080177

Little, M. (1951). Counter-transference and the patient's response to it. *International Journal of Psychoanalysis*, *32*, 32–40.

Littlewood, J. (1996). Stillbirth and neonatal death. In C. A. Niven & A. Walker (Eds.),*Conception, pregnancy and birth* (pp. 148–158). Butterworth and Heinemann.

Lobb, E. A., Kristjanson, L. J., Aoun, S. M., Monterosso, L., Halkett, G. K. B., & Davies, A. (2010). Predictors of complicated grief: A systematic review of empirical studies. *Death Studies, 34*(8), 673–698. https://doi.org/10.1080/07481187.2010.496686

Lok, I. H., & Neugebauer, R. (2007). Psychological morbidity following miscarriage. *Best Practice & Research Clinical Obstetrics & Gynaecology, 21*(2), 229–247.

Lowyck, B., Vermote, R., Luyten, P., Franssen, M., Verhaest, Y., Vertommen, H., & Peuskens, J. (2009). Comparison of reflective functioning as measured on the Adult Attachment Interview and the Object Relations Inventory in patients with a personality disorder: A preliminary study. *Journal of the American Psychoanalytic Association, 57*(6), 1469–1472. https://doi.org/10.1177/00030651090570060803

Luborsky, L. (1976). Helping alliances in psychotherapy. In J. L. Cleghhorn (Ed.), *Successful psychotherapy* (pp. 92–116). Brunner/Mazel.

Lui, P. P., & Rollock, D. (2013). Tiger mother: Popular and psychological scientific perspectives on Asian culture and parenting. *American Journal of Orthopsychiatry, 83*(4), 450–456. https://doi.org/10.1111/ajop.12043

Luyten, P., Mayes, L. C., Nijssens, L., & Fonagy, P. (2017). The Parental Reflective Functioning Questionnaire: Development and preliminary validation. *PLoS ONE, 12*(5), Article e0176218. https://doi.org/10.1371/journal.pone.0176218

MacDorman, M. F., & Gregory, E. (2015, July 23). *Fetal and perinatal mortality: United States, 2013*. Centers for Disease Control and Prevention. Retrieved March 6, 2022, from https://stacks.cdc.gov/view/cdc/61389

Magnus, M. C., Wilcox, A. J., Morken, N.-H., Weinberg, C. R., & Håberg, S. E. (2019). Role of maternal age and pregnancy history in risk of miscarriage: Prospective register-based study. *BMJ, 364*, l869. https://doi.org/10.1136/bmj.l869

Main, M. (1995). Recent studies in attachment: Overview, with selected implications for clinical work. In S. Goldberg, R. Muir, & J. Kerr (Eds.), *Attachment theory: Social, developmental, and clinical perspectives* (pp. 407–474). Analytic Press.

Main, M., & Hesse, E. (1990). Parents' unresolved traumatic experiencesare related to infant disorganized attachment status: Is frightened and/orfrightening parental behavior the linking mechanism? In M. T. Green-berg, D. Cicchetti, & E. M. Cummings (Eds.), *Attachment in the pre-school years: Theory, research, and intervention* (pp. 161–182). Chi-cago: University of Chicago Press.

Main, M., & Hesse, E. (1992). Disorganized disoriented behavior in the strange situation, lapses in the monitoring of reasoning and discourse during the parent's adult attachment interview, and disassociate stress. In M. S. Ammaniti, D. Rome, G. Laterza, & S. Figl (Eds.), *Attachment and psycho-analysis* (pp. 80–140). Chicago, IL: University of Chicago Press.

Main, M., & Weston, D. R. (1982). The quality of the toddler's relationship to mother and to father: Related to conflict behavior and the readiness to establish new relationships. *Child Development, 52*(3), 932–940. https://doi.org/10.2307/1129097

Malan, D. (1995). *Individual psychotherapy and the science of psychodynamics* (2nd ed.). Butterworth-Heinemann.

Mallinckrodt, B. (2010). The psychotherapy relationship as attachment: Evidence and implications. *Journal of Personal and Social Relationships, 27*, 262–270. doi:10.1177/0265407509360905

Mallinckrodt, B., Gantt, D. L., & Coble, H. M. (1995). Attachment patterns in the psychotherapy relationship: Development of the Client Attachment to Therapist

Scale. *Journal of Counseling Psychology, 42*(3), 307–317. https://doi.org/10.1037/0022-0167.42.3.307

Mallinckrodt, B., & Jeong, J. (2015). Meta-analysis of client attachment to therapist: Associations with working alliance and client pretherapy attachment. *Psychotherapy, 52*(1), 134–139. http://dx.doi.org/10.1037/a0036890

Marerro, S. J. (2013). *The role of the psychologist in reproductive medicine* [Doctoral dissertation, Rutgers University]. ProQuest Dissertations Publishing, Publication No. 3602900.

Markin, R. D. (2014). Toward a common identity for relationally oriented clinicians: A place to hang one's hat. *Psychotherapy, 51*(3), 327–333. https://doi.org/10.1037/a0037093

Markin, R. D. (2016). What clinicians miss about miscarriages: Clinical errors in the treatment of early term perinatal loss. *Psychotherapy, 53*(3), 347–353. https://doi.org/10.1037/pst0000062

Markin, R. D. (2017). An introduction to the special section on psychotherapy for pregnancy loss: Review of issues, clinical applications, and future research direction. *Psychotherapy, 54*(4), 367–372. http://doi.org/10.1037/pst0000134

Markin, R. D. (2018). "Ghosts" in the womb: A mentalizing approach to understanding and treating prenatal attachment disturbances during pregnancies after loss. *Psychotherapy, 55*(3), 275–288. https://doi.org/10.1037/pst0000186

Markin, R. D. (2022). "A little bit pregnant": Counseling for recurrent pregnancy loss. In S. Covington (Ed.), *Fertility counseling: A clinical guide* (2nd ed., pp. 195–254). Cambridge University Press.

Markin, R. D., & McCarthy, K. S. (2020). The process and outcome of psychodynamic psychotherapy for pregnancy after loss: A case study analysis. *Psychotherapy, 57*(2), 273–288. https://doi.org/10.1037/pst0000249

Markin, R. D., & Zilcha-Mano, S. (2018). Cultural processes in psychotherapy for perinatal loss: Breaking the cultural taboo against perinatal grief. *Psychotherapy, 55*(1), 20–26. https://doi.org/10.1037/pst0000122

Marmarosh, C. L., Kivlighan, D. M., Bieri, K., LaFauci Schutt, J. M., Barone, C., & Choi, J. (2014). The insecure psychotherapy base: Using client and therapist attachment styles to understand the early alliance. *Psychotherapy, 51*(3), 404–412. https://doi.org/10.1037/a0031989

Marmarosh, C. L., Markin, R. D., & Spiegel, E. B. (2013). *Attachment in group psychotherapy*. American Psychological Association. https://doi.org/10.1037/14186-000

Marmarosh, C. L., & Tasca, G. A. (2013). Adult attachment anxiety: Using group therapy to promote change. *Journal of Clinical Psychology, 69*(11), 1172–1182. https://doi.org/10.1002/jclp.22044

Martin, D. J., Garske, J. P., & Davis, M. K. (2000). Relation of the therapeutic alliance with outcome and other variables: A meta-analytic review. *Journal of Consulting and Clinical Psychology, 68*(3), 438–450. https://doi.org/10.1037/0022-006X.68.3.438

Matthiesen, S. M., Frederiksen, Y., Ingerslev, H. J., & Zachariae, R. (2011). Stress, distress and outcome of assisted reproductive technology (ART): A meta-analysis. *Human Reproduction, 26*(10), 2763–2776. https://doi.org/10.1093/humrep/der246

McClintock, A. S., Anderson, T., Patterson, C. L., & Wing, E. H. (2018). Early psychotherapeutic empathy, alliance, and client outcome: Preliminary evidence of indirect effects. *Journal of Clinical Psychology, 74*(6), 839–848. https://doi.org/10.1002/jclp.22568

McCoyd, J. (2009). What do women want? Experiences and reflections of women after prenatal diagnosis and termination for anomaly. *Health Care for Women International*, 30(6), 507–535.

McCullough, L., Kuhn, N., Andrews, S., Kaplan, A., Wolf, J., & Hurley, C. L. (2003). *Treating affect phobia: A manual for short-term dynamic psychotherapy*. Guilford Press.

Mcleod, S. (2019, July 10). *Effect size*. Simply Psychology. https://www.simplypsychol ogy.org/effect-size.html

McWilliams, N. (1994). *Psychoanalytic diagnosis: Understanding personality structure in the clinical process*. Guilford Press.

McWilliams, N. (2011). *Psychoanalytic diagnosis: Understanding personality structure in the clinical process* (2nd ed.). Guilford Press.

Meier, A. M., Carr, D. R., Currier, J. M., & Neimeyer, R. A. (2013). Attachment anxiety and avoidance in coping with bereavement: Two studies. *Journal of Social and Clinical Psychology*, 32(3), 315–334. https://doi.org/10.1521/jscp.2013.32.3.315

Mikulincer, M. (1998). Adult attachment style and affect regulation: Strategic variations in self-appraisals. *Journal of Personality and Social Psychology*, 75(2), 420–435. https://doi.org/10.1037/0022-3514.75.2.420

Mikulincer, M., & Florian, V. (1999). Maternal-fetal bonding, coping strategies, and mental health during pregnancy–the contribution of attachment style. *Journal of Social and Clinical Psychology*, 18(3), 255–276.

Mikulincer, M., Horesh, N., Levy-Shiff, R., Manovich, R., & Shalev, J. (1998). The contribution of adult attachment style to the adjustment to infertility. *British Journal of Medical Psychology*, 71(3), 265–280. https://doi.org/10.1111/j.2044-8341.1998. tb00991.x

Mikulincer, M., & Nachshon, O. (1991). Attachment styles and patterns of self-disclosure. *Journal of Personality and Social Psychology*, 61(2), 321– 331. https://doi. org/10.1037/0022-3514.61.2.321

Mikulincer, M., & Shaver, P. R. (2003). The attachment behavioral system in adulthood: Activation, psychodynamics, and interpersonal processes. In M. P. Zanna (Ed.), *Advances in experimental social psychology* (Vol. 35, pp. 53–152). Elsevier Academic Press. https://doi.org/10.1016/S0065-2601(03)01002-5

Mikulincer, M., & Shaver, P. R. (2005). Attachment theory and emotions in close relationships: Exploring the attachment-related dynamics of emotional reactions to relational events. *Personal Relationships*, 12, 149–168. doi:10.1111/ j.1350-4126.2005.00108.x

Mikulincer, M., & Shaver, P. R. (2007). *Attachment in adulthood: Structure, dynamics, and change*. Guilford Press.

Mikulincer, M., & Shaver, P. R. (2008). An attachment perspective on bereavement. In M. Stroebe, R. O. Hansson, H. A. W. Schut, & W. Stroebe (Eds.), *Handbook of bereavement research and practice: 21st century perspectives* (pp. 87–112). Washington, DC: American Psychological Association.

Mikulincer, M., & Shaver, P. R. (2013). Attachment insecurities and disordered patterns of grief. In M. Stroebe, H. Schut, & J. van den Bout (Eds.), *Complicated grief: Scientific foundations for health care professionals* (pp. 190–203). Routledge/ Taylor & Francis Group.

Mikulincer, M., Shaver, P. R., Sapir-Lavid, Y., & Avihou-Kanza, N. (2009). What's inside the minds of securely and insecurely attached people? The secure-base script and its associations with attachment-style dimensions. *Journal of Personality and Social Psychology, 97*(4), 615–633. https://doi.org/10.1037/a0015649

Miller-Bottome, M., Talia, A., Eubanks, C. F., Safran, J. D., & Muran, J. C. (2019). Secure in-session attachment predicts rupture resolution: Negotiating a secure base. *Psychoanalytic Psychology, 36*(2), 132–138. https://doi.org/10.1037/pap0000232

Miller-Bottome, M., Talia, A., Safran, J. D., & Muran, J. C. (2018). Resolving alliance ruptures from an attachment-informed perspective. *Psychoanalytic Psychology, 35*(2), 175–183. https://doi.org/10.1037/pap0000152

Mohr, J. J., Gelso, C. J., & Hill, C. E. (2005). Client and counselor trainee attachment as predictors of session evaluation and countertransference behavior in first counseling sessions. *Journal of Counseling Psychology, 52*, 298–309. doi:10.1037/0022-0167.52.3.298

Molo, M. W., Kelly, M., Balos, R., Mullaney, K., & Radwanska, E. (1993). Incidence of fetal loss in infertility patients after detection of fetal heart activity with early transvaginal ultrasound. *Journal of Reproductive Medicine, 38*(10), 804–806.

Mukherjee, S., Velez Edwards, D. R., Baird, D. D., Savitz, D. A., & Hartmann, K. E. (2013). Risk of miscarriage among black women and white women in a US prospective cohort study. *American Journal of Epidemiology, 177*(11), 1271–1278. https://doi.org/10.1093/aje/kws393

Muran, J. C. (2017). Confessions of a New York rupture researcher: An insider's guide and critique. *Psychotherapy Research, 29*(1), 1–14. https://doi.org/10.1080/10503307.2017.1413261

Muran, J. C., & Eubanks, C. F. (2020). *Therapist performance under pressure: Negotiating emotion, difference, and rupture.* American Psychological Association. https://doi.org/10.1037/0000182-000

Muran, J. C., Safran, J. D., Samstag, L. W., & Winston, A. (1992). *Patient and therapist postsession questionnaires, Version 1992.* Beth Israel Medical Center, NY.

Muran, J. C., Safran, J. D., Samstag, L. W., & Winston, A. (2005). Evaluating an alliance-focused treatment for personality disorders. *Psychotherapy: Theory, Research, Practice, Training, 42*(4), 532–545. https://doi.org/10.1037/0033-3204.42.4.532

Nakano, Y., Akechi, T., Furukawa, T. A., & Sugiura-Ogasawara, M. (2013). Cognitive behavior therapy for psychological distress in patients with recurrent miscarriage. *Psychology Research and Behavior Management, 6*, 37–43. http://dx.doi.org/10.2147/PRBM.S44327

Navidian, A., Saravani, Z., & Shakiba, M. (2017). Impact of psychological grief counseling on the severity of post-traumatic stress symptoms in mothers after stillbirths. *Issues in Mental Health Nursing, 38*(8), 650–654. https://doi.org/10.1080/01612840.2017.1315623

Neria, Y., & Litz, B. T. (2004). Bereavement by traumatic means: The complex synergy of trauma and grief. *Journal of Loss and Trauma, 9*(1), 73–87.

Neugebauer, R., Kline, J., Bleiberg, K., Baxi, L., Markowitz, J. C., Rosing, M., Levin, B., & Keith, J. (2007). Preliminary open trial of interpersonal counseling for subsyndromal depression following miscarriage. *Depression and Anxiety, 24*(3), 219–222. https://doi.org/10.1002/da.20150

Neugebauer, R., Kline, J., O'Connor, P., Shrout, P., Johnson, J., & Skodol, A. (1992). Determinants of depressive symptoms in the early weeks after miscarriage. *American Journal of Public Health, 82*(10), 1332–1339.

Nienhuis, J. B., Owen, J., Valentine, J. C., Winkeljohn Black, S., Halford, T. C., Parazak, S. E., Budge, S., & Hilsenroth, M. (2018). Therapeutic alliance, empathy, and genuineness in individual adult psychotherapy: A meta-analytic review. *Psychotherapy Research, 28*(4), 593–605. https://doi.org/10.1080/10503307.2016.1204023

Nødtvedt, Ø. O., Binder, P.-E., Stige, S. H., Schanche, E., Stiegler, J. R., & Hjeltnes, A. (2019)."You feel they have a heart and are not afraid to show it" : Exploring how clients experience the therapeutic relationship in emotion-focused therapy. *Frontiers in Psychology, 10*, Article 1996. https://doi.org/10.3389/fpsyg.2019.01996

Norcross, J. C. (Ed.). (2002). *Psychotherapy relationships that work.* Oxford University Press.

Norcross, J. C. (Ed.). (2011). *Psychotherapy relationships that work* (2nd ed.). Oxford University Press.

Norcross, J. C., & Lambert, M. J. (2019). (Eds.). *Psychotherapy relationships that work. Vol. 1: Evidence-based therapist contributions* (3rd ed.). Oxford University Press.

Norcross, J. C., Lambert, M. J., & Wampold, B. E. (2018). Report of the third interdivisional APA task force on evidence-based relationships and responsiveness. Society for the Advancement of Psychotherapy (APA Division 29) and the Society of Counseling Psychology (APA Division 17).

Norcross, J. C., & Wampold, B. E. (2019). (Eds.). *Psychotherapy relationships that work. Vol. 2: Evidence-based responsiveness* (3rd ed.). Oxford University Press.Nybo Andersen, A.-M., Wohlfahrt, J., Christens, P., Olsen, J., & Melbye, M. (2000). Maternal age and fetal loss: Population-based register linkage study. *BMJ, 320*(7251), 1708–1712. https://doi.org/10.1136/bmj.320.7251.1708Obst, K. L., Due, C., Oxlad, M., & Middleton, P. (2020). Men's grief following pregnancy loss and neonatal loss: A systematic review and emerging theoretical model. *BMC Pregnancy and Childbirth, 20*(1), Article 11. https://doi.org/10.1186/s12884-019-2677-9

O'Leary, J. (2004). Grief and its impact on prenatal attachment in the subsequent pregnancy. *Archives of Women's Mental Health, 7*, 7–18. http://dx.doi.org/10.1007/s00 737-003-0037-1

Owen, J., & Hilsenroth, M. J. (2014). Treatment adherence: The importance of therapist flexibility in relation to therapy outcomes. *Journal of Counseling Psychology, 61*(2), 280–288.

Pando-Mars, K. (2016). Tailoring AEDP interventions to attachment style. *Transformance Journal, 6*(2).

Pascual-Leone, A., & Yeryomenko, N. (2017). The client "experiencing" scale as a predictor of treatment outcomes: A meta-analysis on psychotherapy process. *Psychotherapy Research, 27*(6), 653–665. https://doi.org/10.1080/10503307.2016.1152409

Peabody, S. A., & Gelso, C. J. (1982). Countertransference and empathy: The complex relationship between two divergent concepts in counseling. *Journal of Counseling Psychology, 29*, 240–245.

Peluso, P. R., & Freund, R. R. (2019). Emotional expression. In J. C. Norcross & M. J. Lambert (Eds.), *Psychotherapy relationships that work: Volume 1: Evidence-based therapist contributions* (3rd ed., pp. 421–460). Oxford University Press. https://doi. org/10.1093/med-psych/9780190843953.003.0012

Peterson, B. (2015). Fertility counseling for couples. In S. N. Covington (Ed.), *Fertility counseling: Clinical guide to case studies* (pp. 60–73). Cambridge University Press.

Peterson, B., Newton, C., Rosen, K., Schulman, R. (2006). Coping processes of couples experiencing infertility. *Family Relations, 55*(2), 227–239. https://doi.org/10.1111/ j.1741-3729.2006.00372.x

Pinsof, W. M., & Catherall, D. R. (1986). The integrative psychotherapy alliance: Family, couple and individual therapy scales. *Journal of Marital and Family Therapy, 12*(2), 137–151. https://doi.org/10.1111/j.1752-0606.1986.tb01631.x

Practice Committee of the American Society for Reproductive Medicine. (2020). Definitions of infertility and recurrent pregnancy loss: A committee opinion. *Fertility & Sterility, 113,* 533–535. doi:10.1016/j.fertnstert.2019.11.025

Prigerson, H. G., Bierhals, A. J., Kasl, S. V., & Reynolds, C. F., III. (1997). Traumatic grief as a risk factor for mental and physical morbidity. *American Journal of Psychiatry, 154*(5), 616–623.

Raphael-Leff, J. (2012). The baby makers: Conscious and unconscious psychological reactions to infertility and "baby-making"—An in-depth single case study. In P. Mariotti (Ed.), *The maternal lineage: Identification, desire and transgenerational issues* (pp. 212–230). Routledge/Taylor and Francis Group.

Reich, A. (1951). On countertransference. *International Journal of Psychoanalysis, 32,* 25–31.

Robbins, S. B., & Jolkovski, M. P. (1987). Managing countertransference feelings: An interactional model using awareness of feeling and theoretical framework. *Journal of Counseling Psychology, 34*(3), 276–282. https://doi.org/10.1037/0022-0167.34.3.276

Robinson, G. E., Stirtzinger, R., Stewart, D. E., & Ralevski, E. (1994). Psychological reactions in women followed for 1 year after miscarriage. *Journal of Reproductive and Infant Psychology, 12*(1), 31–36. https://doi.org/10.1080/02646839408408865

Robinson, M., Baker, L., & Nackerud, L. (1999). The relationship of attachment theory and perinatal loss. *Death Studies, 23*(3), 257–270. http://dx.doi.org/10.1080/074811899201073

Rogers, C. R. (1957). The necessary and sufficient conditions of therapeutic personality change. *Journal of Consulting Psychology, 21*(2), 95–103. https://doi.org/10.1037/h0045357

Rogers, C. R. (1980). *A way of being.* Houghton Mifflin.

Romano, V., Fitzpatrick, M., & Janzen, J. (2008). The secure-base hypothesis: Global attachment, attachment to counselor, and session exploration in psychotherapy. *Journal of Counseling Psychology, 55*(4), 495–504. https://doi.org/10.1037/a0013721

Rosenberger, E. W., & Hayes, J. A. (2002). Origins, consequences, and management of countertransference: A case study. *Journal of Counseling Psychology, 49*(2), 221–232. https://doi.org/10.1037/0022-0167.49.2.221

Rothaupt, J., & Becker, K. (2007). A literature review of Western bereavement theory: From decathecting to continuing bonds. *Family Journal, 15,* 6–15. https://doi.org/10.1177/1066480706294031

Rottenberg, J., & Gross, J. J. (2007). Emotion and emotion regulation: A map for psychotherapy researchers. *Clinical Psychology: Science and Practice, 14*(4), 323–328. https://doi.org/10.1111/j.1468-2850.2007.00093.x

Rowlands, I., & Lee, C. (2010). Adjustment after miscarriage: Predicting positive mental health trajectories among young Australian women. *Psychology, Health & Medicine, 15*(1), 34–49. https://doi.org/10.1080/13548500903440239

Rubino, G., Barker, C., Roth, T., & Fearon, P. (2000). Therapist empathy and depth of interpretation in response to potential alliance ruptures: The role of therapist and patient attachment styles. *Psychotherapy Research, 10,* 408–420. doi:10.1093/ptr/10.4.408

Safran, J. D. (1993). Breaches in the therapeutic alliance: An arena for negotiating authentic relatedness. *Psychotherapy: Theory, Research, Practice, Training, 30*(1), 11–24. https://doi.org/10.1037/0033-3204.30.1.11

Safran, J. D., Crocker, P., McMain, S., & Murray, P. (1990). Therapeutic alliance rupture as a therapy event for empirical investigation. *Psychotherapy: Theory, Research, Practice, Training, 27*(2), 154–165. https://doi.org/10.1037/0033-3204.27.2.154

Safran, J. D., & Kraus, J. (2014). Alliance ruptures, impasses, and enactments: A relational perspective. *Psychotherapy, 51*(3), 381–387. https://doi.org/10.1037/a0036815

Safran, J. D., & Muran, J. C. (2000). *Negotiating the therapeutic alliance: A relational treatment guide*. Guilford Press.

Safran, J. D., Muran, J. C., & Eubanks-Carter, C. (2011). Repairing alliance ruptures. *Psychotherapy, 48*(1), 80–87. https://doi.org/10.1037/a0022140

Safran, J. D., & Segal, Z. V. (1990). *Interpersonal process in cognitive therapy*. Basic Books.

Samadaee-Gelehkolaee, K., McCarthy, B. W., Khalilian, A., Hamzehgardeshi, Z., Peyvandi, S., Elyasi, F., & Shahidi, M. (2016). Factors associated with marital satisfaction in infertile couples: A comprehensive literature review. *Global Journal of Health Science, 8*(5), 96–109. https://doi.org/10.5539/gjhs.v8n5p96

Sandelowski, M., & Barroso, J. (2005). The travesty of choosing after positive prenatal diagnosis. *Journal of Obstetric, Gynecologic, & Neonatal Nursing, 34*(3), 307–318. doi:10.1177/0884217505276291. PMID: 15890829.

Sapra, K. J., Buck Louis, G. M., Sundaram, R., Joseph, K. S., Bates, L. M., Galea, S., & Ananth, C. V. (2016). Signs and symptoms associated with early pregnancy loss: Findings from a population-based preconception cohort. *Human Reproduction, 31*(4), 887–896. https://doi.org/10.1093/humrep/dew010

Saraiya, M., Berg, C. J., Shulman, H., Green, C. A., & Atrash, H. K. (1999). Estimates of the annual number of clinically recognized pregnancies in the United States, 1981–1991. *American Journal of Epidemiology, 149*(11), 1025–1029.

Sauer, E. M., Lopez, F. G., & Gormley, B. (2003). Respective contributions of therapist and client adult attachment orientations to the development of the early working alliance: A preliminary growth modeling study. *Psychotherapy Research, 13*, 371–382. doi:10.1093/ptr/kpg027

Scheidt, C. E., Hasenburg, A., Kunze, M., Waller, E., Pfeifer, R., Zimmermann, P., Hartmann, A., & Waller, N. (2012). Are individual differences of attachment predicting bereavement outcome after perinatal loss? A prospective cohort study. *Journal of Psychosomatic Research, 73*(5), 375–382. https://doi.org/10.1016/j.jpsychores.2012.08.017

Schenck, L. K., Eberle, K. M., & Rings, J. A. (2015). Insecure attachment styles and complicated grief severity: Applying what we know to inform future directions. *Omega: Journal of Death and Dying, 73*(3), 231–249. https://doi.org/10.1177/00302 22815576124

Schore, A. N. (1994). *Affect regulation and the origin of the self: The neurobiology of emotional development*. Erlbaum.

Schore, A. N. (2002). Advances in neuropsychoanalysis, attachment theory, and trauma research: Implications for self psychology. *Psychoanalytic Inquiry, 22*(3), 433–484. https://doi.org/10.1080/07351692209348996

Schore, A. N. (2003). *Affect regulation and the repair of the self*. W.W. Norton.

Schore, A. N. (2012). *The science and art of psychotherapy*. Norton.

Schore, A. N. (2014). The right brain is dominant in psychotherapy. *Psychotherapy, 51*(3), 388–397. https://doi.org/10.1037/a0037083

Schore, J. R., & Schore, A. N. (2008). Modern attachment theory: The central role of affect regulation in development and treatment. *Clinical Social Work Journal, 36*(1), 9–20. https://doi.org/10.1007/s10615-007-0111-7

Schwerdtfeger, K. L., & Shreffler, K. M. (2009). Trauma of pregnancy loss and infertility among mothers and involuntarily childless women in the United States. *Journal of Loss and Trauma, 14*(3), 211–227. https://doi.org/10.1080/1532502080 2537468

Séjourné, N., Callahan, S., & Chabrol, H. (2010). The utility of a psychological intervention for coping with spontaneous abortion. *Journal of Reproductive and Infant Psychology, 28*(3), 287–296. https://doi.org/10.1080/02646830903487334

Sereshti, M., Nahidi, F., Simbar, M., Ahmadi, F., Bakhtiari, M., & Zayeri, F. (2016). Mothers' perception of quality of services from health centers after perinatal loss. *Electronic Physician, 8*(2), 2006–2017. https://doi.org/10.19082/2006

Serrano, E., & Warnock, J. J. K. (2007). Depressive disorders related to female reproductive transitions. *Journal of Pharmacy Practice, 20*(5), 385–391. https://doi.org/ 10.1177/0897190007304984

Serrano, F., & Lima, M. L. (2006). Recurrent miscarriage: Psychological and relational consequences for couples. *Psychology and Psychotherapy: Theory, Research and Practice, 79*(4), 585–594. https://doi.org/10.1348/147608306X96992

Sham, A. K. H., Yiu, M. G. C., & Ho, W. Y. B. (2010). Psychiatric morbidity following miscarriage in Hong Kong. *General Hospital Psychiatry, 32*, 284–293. https://doi. org/10.1016/j.genhosppsych.2009.12.002

Shamay-Tsoory, S. G. (2009). Empathic processing: Its cognitive and affective dimensions and neuroanatomical basis. In J. Decety & W. Ickes (Eds.), *The social neuroscience of empathy* (pp. 215–232). MIT Press. https://doi.org/10.7551/mitpress/9780262012 973.003.0017

Shaohua, L., & Shorey, S. (2021). Psychosocial interventions on psychological outcomes of parents with perinatal loss: A systematic review and meta-analysis. *International Journal of Nursing Studies, 117*, 103871. https://doi.org/10.1016/j.ijnur stu.2021.103871

Shechtman, Z., & Dvir, V. (2006). Attachment style as a predictor of children's behavior ingroup psychotherapy. *Group Dynamics: Theory, Research, and Practice, 10*(1), 29–42.

Siddiqui, A., & Hägglöf, B. (2000). Does maternal prenatal attachment predict postnatal mother-infant interaction? *Early Human Development, 59*(1), 13–25. https://doi. org/10.1016/s0378-3782(00)00076-1

Siegel, D. J. (1999). *The developing mind: Toward a neurobiology of interpersonal experience*. Guilford Press.

Siegel, D. J. (2001). Toward an interpersonal neurobiology of the developing mind: Attachment relationships, "mindsight," and neural integration. *Infant Mental Health Journal, 22*(1–2), 67–94. https://doi.org/10.1002/1097-0355(200101/ 04)22:1<67::AID-IMHJ3>3.0.CO;2-G

Siegel, R. S., Hoeppner, B., Yen, S., Stout, R. L., Weinstock, L. M., Hower, H. M., Birmaher, B., Goldstein, T. R., Goldstein, B. I., Hunt, J. I., Strober, M., Axelson, D. A., Gill, M. K., & Keller, M. B. (2015). Longitudinal associations between interpersonal relationship functioning and mood episode severity in youth with bipolar disorder. *Journal of Nervous and Mental Disease, 203*(3), 194–204.https://doi.org/10.1097/ NMD.0000000000000261

Silverman, G. K., Johnson, J. G., & Prigerson, H. G. (2001). Preliminary explorations of the effects of prior trauma and loss on risk for psychiatric disorders in recently widowed people. *Israel Journal of Psychiatry and Related Sciences, 38,* 202–215.

Simpson, J. A., & Rholes, W. S. (2017). Adult attachment, stress, and romantic relationships. *Current Opinion in Psychology, 13,* 19–24. https://doi.org/10.1016/j.copsyc.2016.04.006

Slade, P. (1994). Predicting the psychological impact of miscarriage. *Journal of Reproductive and Infant Psychology, 12*(1), 5–16. https://doi.org/10.1080/026468 39408408862

Sroufe, L. A., Egeland, B., Carlson, E., & Collins, W. A. (2005). Placing early attachment experiences in developmental context: The Minnesota longitudinal study. In K. E. Grossmann, K. Grossmann, & E. Waters (Eds.), *Attachment from infancy to adulthood: The major longitudinal studies* (pp. 48–70). Guilford Publications.

Sroufe, L. A., Fox, N. E., & Pancake, V. R. (1983). Attachment and dependency in developmental perspective. *Child Development, 54*(6), 1615–1627. https://doi.org/10.2307/1129825

Stalikas, A., & Fitzpatrick, M. (1995). Client good moments: An intensive analysis of a single session. *Canadian Journal of Counseling, 29*(2), 160–175.

Stirtzinger, R., & Robinson, G. E. (1989). The psychologic effects of spontaneous abortion. *Canadian Medical Association Journal, 140*(7), 799.

Strauss, B. M., & Petrowski, K. (2017). The role of the therapist's attachment in the process and outcome of psychotherapy. In L. G. Castonguay & C. E. Hill (Eds.), *How and why are some therapists better than others?: Understanding therapist effects* (pp. 117–138). American Psychological Association. https://doi.org/10.1037/0000034-008

Suedfeld, P., Fell, C., & Krell, R. (1998). Structural aspects of survivors' thinking about the Holocaust. *Journal of Traumatic Stress, 11,* 323–336. https://doi.org/10.1023/A:1024455204839

Sullins, D. P. (2019). Affective and substance abuse disorders following abortion by pregnancy intention in the United States: A longitudinal Cohort Study. *Medicina (Kaunas), 55*(11), 741. doi:10.3390/medicina55110741. PMID: 31731786; PMCID: PMC6915619.

Sutan, R., Amin, R. M., Ariffin, K. B., Teng, T. Z., Kamal, M. F., & Rusli, R. Z. (2010). Psychosocial impact of mothers with perinatal loss and its contributing factors: An insight. *Journal of Zhejiang University SCIENCE B, 11*(3), 209–217. https://doi.org/10.1631/jzus.b0900245

Swanson, K. M. (2000). Predicting depressive symptoms after miscarriage: A path analysis based on the Lazarus paradigm. *Journal of Women's Health & Gender-Based Medicine, 9*(2), 191–206. https://doi.org/10.1089/152460900318696

Swanson, K. M., Chen, H.-T., Graham, J. C., Wojnar, D. M., & Petras, A. (2009). Resolution of depression and grief during the first year after miscarriage: A randomized controlled clinical trial of couples-focused interventions. *Journal of Women's Health, 18*(8), 1245–1257. https://doi.org/10.1089/jwh.2008.1202

Swanson-Kauffman, K. M. (1986). Caring in the instance of unexpected early pregnancy loss. *Topics in Clinical Nursing, 8,* 37–46.

Symonds, B. D. (1999). *The measurement of alliance in short-term couples therapy* [Unpublished doctoral dissertation]. Simon Fraser University.

Tasca, G. A., Balfour, L., Ritchie, K., & Bissada, H. (2007). The relationship between attachment scales and group therapy alliance growth differs by treatment type for women with binge-eating disorder. *Group Dynamics: Theory, Research, and Practice*, *11*(1), 1–14. https://doi.org/10.1037/1089-2699.11.1.1

Tavoli, Z., Mohammadi, M., Tavoli, A., Moini, A., Effatpanah, M., Khedmat, L., & Montazeri, A. (2018). Quality of life and psychological distress in women with recurrent miscarriage: A comparative study. *Health and Quality of Life Outcomes*, *16*(1), Article 150. https://doi.org/10.1186/s12955-018-0982-z

Tedeschi, R. G., & Calhoun, L. G. (1996). The Posttraumatic Growth Inventory: Measuring the positive legacy of trauma. *Journal of Traumatic Stress*, *9*(3), 455–472. https://doi.org/10.1002/jts.2490090305

Thapar, A. K., & Thapar, A. (1992). Psychological sequelae of miscarriage: A controlled study using the General Health Questionnaire and the Hospital Anxiety and Depression Scale. *British Journal of General Practice*, *42*(356), 94–96.

Tian, X., & Solomon, D. H. (2020). Grief and post-traumatic growth following miscarriage: The role of meaning reconstruction and partner supportive communication. *Death Studies*, *44*(4), 237–247. https://doi.org/10.1080/07481187.2018.1539051

Timulak, L., McElvaney, J., Keogh, D., Martin, E., Clare, P., Chepukova, E., & Greenberg, L. S. (2017). Emotion-focused therapy for generalized anxiety disorder: An exploratory study. *Psychotherapy*, *54*(4), 361–366. https://doi.org/10.1037/pst0000128

Toedter, L. J., Lasker, J. N., & Alhadeff, J. M. (1988). The Perinatal Grief Scale: Development and initial validation. *American Journal of Orthopsychiatry*, *58*(3), 435–449.

Toedter, L. J., Lasker, J. N., & Janssen, H. J. (2001). International comparison of studies using the Perinatal Grief Scale: A decade of research on pregnancy loss. *Death Studies*, *25*(3), 205–228. https://doi.org/10.1080/074811801750073251

Town, J. M., Salvadori, A., Falkenström, F., Bradley, S., & Hardy, G. (2017). Is affect experiencing therapeutic in major depressive disorder? Examining associations between affect experiencing and changes to the alliance and outcome in intensive short-term dynamic psychotherapy. *Psychotherapy*, *54*(2), 148–158. https://doi.org/10.1037/pst0000108

Tronick, E. Z. (1989). Emotions and emotional communication in infants. *American Psychologist*, *44*(2), 112–119. https://doi.org/10.1037/0003-066X.44.2.112

Turton, P., Hughes, P., Evans, C., & Fainman, D. (2001). Incidence, correlates and predictors of post-traumatic stress disorder in the pregnancy after stillbirth. *British Journal of Psychiatry*, *178*(6), 556–560. https://doi.org/10.1192/bjp.178.6.556

Tyrrell, C. L., Dozier, M., Teague, G. B., & Fallot, R. D. (1999). Effective treatment relationships for persons with serious psychiatric disorders: The importance of attachment states of mind. *Journal of Consulting and Clinical Psychology*, *67*, 725–733. doi:10.1037/0022-006X.67.5.725

Vanderwerker, L. C., Jacobs, S. C., Parkes, C. M., & Prigerson, H. G. (2006). An exploration of associations between separation anxiety in childhood and complicated grief in later-life. *Journal of Nervous and Mental Diseases*, *194*, 121–123.

van Minnen, A., Wessel, I., Dijkstra, T., & Roelofs, K. (2002). Changes in PTSD patients' narratives during prolonged exposure therapy: A replication and extension. *Journal of Traumatic Stress*, *15*(3), 255–258. https://doi.org/10.1023/A:1015263513654

Van Wagoner, S. L., Gelso, C. J., Hayes, J. A., & Diemer, R. A. (1991). Countertransference and the reputedly excellent therapist. *Psychotherapy: Theory, Research, Practice, Training, 28*(3), 411–421. https://doi.org/10.1037/0033-3204.28.3.411

Verkuijlen, J., Verhaak, C., Nelen, W. L., Wilkinson, J., & Farquhar, C. (2016). Psychological and educational interventions for subfertile men and women. *Cochrane Database of Systematic Reviews, 3,* CD011034. https://doi.org/10.1002/14651858.CD011034

Voss, P., Schick, M., Langer, L., Ainsworth, A., Ditzen, B., Strowitzki, T., Wischmann, T., & Kuon, R. J. (2020). Recurrent pregnancy loss: A shared stressor. Couple-orientated psychological research findings. *Fertility and Sterility, 114*(6), 1288–1296. https://doi.org/10.1016/j.fertnstert.2020.08.1421

Walker, T. M., & Davidson, K. M. (2001). A preliminary investigation of psychological distress following surgical management of early pregnancy loss detected at initial ultrasound scanning: A trauma perspective. *Journal of Reproductive and Infant Psychology, 19,* 7–16. https://doi.org/10.1080/02646830020032365

Wallin, D. J. (2007). *Attachment in psychotherapy.* Guilford Press.

Waskowic, T. D., & Chartier, B. M. (2003). Attachment and the experience of grief following the loss of a spouse. *Omega: Journal of Death and Dying, 47*(1), 77–91. https://doi.org/10.2190/0CMC-GYP5-N3QH-WEH4

Watson, R. I., Jr. (2005). When the patient has experienced severe trauma. In A. Rosen & J. Rosen (Eds.), *Frozen dreams: Psychodynamic dimensions of infertility and assisted reproduction* (pp. 219–235). Analytic Press/Taylor & Francis Group.

Westmaas, J. L., & Silver, R. C. (2001). The role of attachment in responses to victims of life crises. *Journal of Personality and Social Psychology, 80,* 425–438. doi:10.1037/0022-3514.80.3.425

Whelton, W. J. (2004). Emotional processes in psychotherapy: Evidence across therapeutic modalities. *Clinical Psychology & Psychotherapy, 11*(1), 58–71. https://doi.org/10.1002/cpp.392

Woods-Giscombé, C. L., Lobel, M., & Crandell, J. L. (2010). The impact of miscarriage and parity on patterns of maternal distress in pregnancy. *Research in Nursing & Health, 33*(4), 316–328. https://doi.org/10.1002/nur.20389

Wright, P. M. (2011). Barriers to a comprehensive understanding of pregnancy loss. *Journal of Loss and Trauma, 16*(1), 1–12. https://doi.org/10.1080/15325024.2010.519298

Youngblut, J. M., Brooten, D., Cantwell, G. P., del Moral, T., & Totapally, B. (2013). Parent health and functioning 13 months after infant or child NICU/PICU death. *Pediatrics, 132,* 1295–1301. https://doi.org/10.1542/peds.2013-1194

Yulis, S., & Kieser, D. J. (1968). Countertransference response as a function of therapist anxiety and content of patient talk. *Journal of Consulting and Clinical Psychology, 32*(4), 413–419. https://doi.org/10.1037/h0026107

Zeanah, C. H., Danis, B., Hirshberg, L., & Dietz, L. (1995). Initial adaptation in mothers and fathers following perinatal loss. *Infant Mental Health Journal, 16*(2), 80–93. https://doi.org/10.1002/1097-0355(199522)16:2<80::AID-IMHJ2280160203>3.0.CO;2-J

Zegers-Hochschild, F., Adamson, G. D., & Dyer, S., Racowsky, C., De Mouzon, J., Sokol, R., . . . Van Der Poel, S. (2017). The international glossary of infertility and fertility care: Led by ICMART in partnership with ASRM, ESHRE, IFFS, March of

Dimes, AFS, GIERAF, ASPIRE, MEFS, REDLARA, FIGO. *Fertility Sterility*, *108*(3), 393–406.

Zetzel, E. R. (1956). An approach to the relation between concept and content in psychoanalytic theory. *Psychoanalytic Study of the Child*, *11*, 99–124.

Zisook, S., & DeVaul, R. (1985). Unresolved grief. *The American Journal of Psychoanalysis*, *45*(4), 370–379. https://doi.org/10.1007/BF01252871

Zuroff, D. C., & Blatt, S. J. (2006). The therapeutic relationship in the brief treatment of depression: Contributions to clinical improvement and enhanced adaptive capacities. *Journal of Consulting and Clinical Psychology*, *74*(1), 199–206.https://doi.org/10.1037/0022-006X.74.1.130

For the benefit of digital users, indexed terms that span two pages (e.g., 52–53) may, on occasion, appear on only one of those pages.

Tables and boxes are indicated by *t* and *b* following the page number